Wearable Medical Device Security and Network Protection for Reliable Healthcare

Pandimurugan V.
https://orcid.org/0000-0003-4766-996X
Acharya University, Uzbekistan

Rajaram V.
https://orcid.org/0000-0002-7023-8327
SRM Institute of Science and Technology, India

Chinnasamy A.
SRM Institute of Science and Technology, India

Sountharrajan S.
Amrita Vishwa Vidyapeetham, India

Amudhavel Jayavel
De Montfort University, UK

IGI Global
Scientific Publishing
Publishing Tomorrow's Research Today

Vice President of Editorial Melissa Wagner
Director of Acquisitions Mikaela Felty
Director of Book Development Jocelynn Hessler
Production Manager Mike Brehm
Cover Design Jose Rosado

Published in the United States of America by
IGI Global Scientific Publishing
701 East Chocolate Avenue
Hershey, PA, 17033, USA
Tel: 717-533-8845 | Fax: 717-533-7115
Website: https://www.igi-global.com E-mail: cust@igi-global.com

Library of Congress Cataloging-in-Publication Data

LCCN: 2025036226 (CIP Data Pending)
ISBN13: 9798337344126
Isbn13Softcover: 9798337344133
EISBN13: 9798337344140
British Cataloguing in Publication Data
A Cataloguing in Publication record for this book is available from the British Library.

Table of Contents

Detailed Table of Contents

Wearable medical devices (WMDs) are one of the most interesting ways that technology and healthcare are coming together. Digital health care has come a long way since fitness trackers were just basic tools. They are now complicated tools for diagnosis and treatment. Today, WMDs include a wide range of devices, such as smartwatches that can do an ECG, patches that can check glucose levels, wearable defibrillators, biosensors, and smart textiles that can always keep track of important physiological data. These devices not only enable people keep an eye on their own health, but they also send doctors real-time, nonstop, and very personalized data streams that can help them make better diagnoses, treatment plans, and disease management. One of the most crucial ways that WMDs can improve things is by making healthcare more proactive and predictive. Patients and healthcare providers can now access health information all the time instead of only when they go to the hospital.

This chapter examines the convergence of healthcare IoT, artificial intelligence, and data privacy within modern connected care systems. It explores how the Internet of Medical Things (IoMT) enables continuous monitoring through wearable devices and cloud platforms while introducing complex cybersecurity and regulatory challenges. The discussion highlights AI-driven threat detection, explainable and privacy-preserving models, and the use of federated learning and blockchain for secure data sharing. It also reviews global frameworks such as HIPAA, GDPR, and emerging AI regulations, emphasizing transparency, accountability, and patient trust.

Finally, it outlines best practices and future policy directions aimed at achieving resilient, ethical, and compliant healthcare innovation in an increasingly digital and data-driven environment.

M. Sindhuja, SRM Institute of Science and Technology, Kattankulathur, India
Eugene Berna I., Bannari Amman Institute of Technology, Erode, India
K. Vijay, Rajalakshmi Engineering College, India
Vigneshwaran Pandi, Acharya University, Karakul, Uzbekistan

As healthcare institutions incorporate digital innovations, connected gadgets and data-driven services have complicated and networked patient care. Communication between WMDs, hospital systems, cloud platforms, and remote monitoring technologies that send sensitive patient data requires healthcare network security. Connectivity boosts creativity but adds risk. This chapter covers hospital network and WMD integration defenses against ransomware, MITM, illegal access, DoS, and APT. Zero-trust architectures, IDS/IPS, segmentation, and E2E encryption are essential because breaches jeopardize lives and compliance. Anomaly detection using SDN, NFV, and AI/ML is also examined. HIPAA and ISO/IEC 27001 demonstrate network security. Policy, governance, and personnel training are resilient system priorities. The chapter discusses dangers, remedies, and industry benchmarks to improve hospital network security.

S. P. Maniraj, SRM Institute of Science and Technology, India
K. Priyadarsini, SRM Institute of Science and Technology, India
J. Jeba Sonia, SRM Institute of Science and Technology, India
R. Thamizhamuthu, SRM Institute of Science and Technology, India
P. Selvakumari, Rajalakshmi Institute of Technology, India

The health industry is being overwhelmed by cybersecurity threats with digitization increasing the attack surface and exposing vulnerable patient information and essential medical infrastructure at risk of becoming targets of enhanced attacks. Network security within healthcare settings is of paramount interest with the industry depending on interconnected devices, cloud-based health information. Alignment with stringent regulations such as HIPAA, GDPR, and NIST compliance also adds to the complexity in security strategies is required between availability and strong defense mechanisms. This chapter looks at the special vulnerabilities of healthcare networks, such as legacy system threats, human-factor risks, and suggests the use of mitigation techniques such as zero-trust security models, and AI-based threat

and privacy risks. Unauthorized access, data breaches, and device malfunctions are critical concerns, as these vulnerabilities can jeopardize patient safety. This chapter delves into the security challenges associated with wearable and implantable devices, focusing on threats like remote attacks, signal interference, and potential device compromise. The chapter concludes by exploring future directions for secure, reliable, and user-friendly medical devices to ensure patient safety in an increasingly interconnected healthcare landscape.

Implantable Medical Devices (IMDs) play vital role in modern healthcare by enabling treatments, health monitoring, and improved patient capabilities. However, integrating electronics into IMDs raises serious security concerns. Unauthorized access can compromise patient privacy, manipulate data, and even threaten lives. Biometric authentication, including iris scans and patient-specific biometrics, is suggested to enhance security. Lightweight protocols are proposed to ensure authentication and confidentiality while conserving energy and extending battery life. The paper addresses risks associated with unauthorized access to radio channels used by IMDs, highlighting the importance of encryption and secure communication. Advanced cryptographic techniques, such as block ciphers and lightweight encryption schemes, are explored to reinforce IMD security. These cryptographic methods help maintain data integrity and confidentiality, safeguarding sensitive patient information from malicious threats.

The chapter highlights a novel approach towards predicting blood pressure without the necessity of using invasive methods like cuff-based measurements. This chapter proposes the use of vibration sensors based on the Doppler principle to capture movements within the blood vessels, primarily the movement of arterial walls. The signals acquired from vibration sensor technology are analysed with the various characteristics of cardiovascular dynamics and deployed advanced Spectro-temporal deep learning approaches, thereby predicting blood pressure in real-time and with great precision. In recent years, there has been a sudden proliferation of cuffless blood pressure devices, faring away from the standard method of inflating a cuff around the limb. These devices could hold immeasurable promise in providing continuous, beat-to-beat blood pressure monitoring, creating a more informative record of cardiovascular health trends. Beyond traditional clinical settings, there is application potential for telemedicine, wearables, and integrated healthcare systems.

Tuberculosis (TB) remains a major global health challenge, particularly in low-resource settings where traditional diagnostic methods are slow, often leading to disease progression and increased transmission. To overcome these limitations, this study introduces an IoT-based patient monitoring system for early TB diagnosis, employing an Optimized Hyperbolic NasNet Attention Sea-horse Graph Network (OpHyp-NASH-Gra-Net). The system uses a wearable IoT sensor to collect patient data, which is transmitted via mobile device to cloud storage. Data is then clustered using an Adaptively Regularized Kernel-Based Fuzzy C-Means algorithm, filtered via a Fast Guided Median Filter (FGMF) for enhanced quality, and processed with a Scale-Aware Modulation Meet Transformer (SA2MT) for feature extraction. The OpHyp-NASH-Gra-Net model classifies the data to distinguish between TB and non-TB cases, achieving 99% accuracy in simulations conducted with Python. This approach enables real-time, high-accuracy diagnosis, reducing delays and improving outcomes in resource-constrained environments.

As wearable medical devices become integral to modern healthcare, ensuring their safety, security, and regulatory compliance is paramount. This chapter explores the key pillars of testing, auditing, and compliance, focusing on the distinct challenges posed by dynamic, software-intensive, and network-connected environments in which these devices operate. Beyond surveying existing standards such as ISO 14971, IEC 62304, and FDA guidance, this chapter proposes a comprehensive,

Preface

OVERVIEW OF THE SUBJECT MATTER

The fast development of wearable medical devices has revolutionized the healthcare industry through being able to constantly, personalized, and remotely monitor a patient. Smartwatches, biosensors, implantables, and AI-based diagnostic wearables have become a significant part of preventing diseases, early detection, and real-time health control. Nevertheless, with the vast amounts of sensitive data produced and delivered by these devices via Internet of Medical Things (IoMT), the problem of security, privacy, and network reliability has taken top priority.

The book Wearable Medical Device Security and Network Protection to Reliable Healthcare offers a thorough discussion of the intersectional blind spot of wearable devices technology, cybersecurity, and healthcare informatics. It touches upon contemporary risks, privacy-saving systems, data integrity applications, and blockchain-enhanced systems that guarantee credibility and confidence in computerized healthcare systems.

This edited book is a collection of multidisciplinary views of the academic and industry, with academics and experts in computer science, biomedical engineering, healthcare IT, and artificial intelligence. Together, the chapters attempt to establish a plan on how to safeguard next-generation medical devices and data-driven health networks.

With the shift to the digitization and smart connectivity of the healthcare sector, the credibility of wearable data has become a priority in clinical decisions and individualized treatment. The integration of AI analytics, edge computing, and cloud services opens up additional opportunities in the context of innovation, but at the same time increases the chance of data breaches and unauthorized access. The given book attempts to fill this gap by providing detailed discourses on security architectures, encryption standards, and intrusion detection mechanisms specific to medical IoT settings.

Besides, the volume highlights the moral, legal, and cultural consequences of the wearable medical data processing, which are in accordance with the global regulations in the sphere of privacy, including HIPAA and GDPR. It offers useful information on how a collaborative system between the engineering, health care practitioners and policy makers can improve resilience to new cyber threats. This book is useful as both a technical resource and a strategic roadmap that can be used by every individual that is determined to craft safe and sustainable digital healthcare systems by combining theory and practical case studies.

Finally, it motivates researchers, developers, and clinicians to dream of a world where technology and trust can co-exist so that healthcare ecosystems can be safer, smarter, and more patient-centered.

Where the Topic Fits in the World Today

In the context of the digital revolution and the global shift to smart healthcare systems, wearable devices have become an indispensable point of contact between the patients and healthcare professionals. The safety of these interconnected systems has become a social concern with the development of AI-assisted diagnostics, telemedicine, and cloud-based medical services.

Malicious interference of medical equipment, ransomware attacks, as well as data breach are not only a threat to the financial and operational aspect but also to human life. Achieving the confidentiality, integrity and access of medical data are therefore, a moral and ethical responsibility of the researchers and developers and also of the healthcare organizations.

The book is a mirror of all the current advances in cybersecurity, digital health, and data governance, in a manner that is amenable to the objectives of such frameworks as GDPR, HIPAA, and WHO digital health strategies. It is also a contribution to the research ecosystem surrounding the Internet of Things (IoT), Blockchain, and Artificial Intelligence in a medical setting, which can give pertinent ideas about the medical systems of the future.

Target Audience

This volume has been carefully curated to serve a diverse audience, including:

- **Researchers and Academicians** exploring IoT, network security, blockchain, and AI in healthcare.

- **Healthcare Professionals and Policy Makers** seeking to understand the technological safeguards behind digital health infrastructures.
- **Industry Practitioners and Developers** designing secure wearable systems, sensors, and medical IoT solutions.
- **Graduate and Doctoral Students** engaged in interdisciplinary studies spanning computer science, health informatics, and biomedical systems.
- **Cybersecurity Analysts and Data Protection Officers** aiming to strengthen the resilience of healthcare networks.

By addressing the technical, ethical, and regulatory dimensions of wearable medical devices, this book ensures broad applicability across multiple professional domains.

Importance of Each Chapter Submission

1. Introduction to Wearable Medical Devices in Healthcare

Wearable medical devices are transforming modern healthcare by enabling continuous monitoring and personalized treatment. This chapter explains their evolution, applications, and growing importance in patient care. It sets the foundation for understanding all advanced technologies discussed in later chapters.

2. Securing Healthcare IoT – AI Threat Detection, Data Privacy, and Regulatory Frameworks

As healthcare becomes more connected, securing IoT ecosystems is essential to protect sensitive patient data. This chapter highlights how AI-driven threat detection, privacy-preserving methods, and global regulations work together to ensure safety. It establishes the security principles necessary for managing intelligent healthcare systems.

3. Network Protection in Healthcare Environments

Healthcare networks must be safeguarded from cyberattacks to ensure uninterrupted medical services. This chapter explains cybersecurity frameworks, defensive strategies, and secure network architectures. It strengthens the reader's understanding of how network-level protection supports safe device operation.

4. AI-Driven Threat Detection in Healthcare Networks

Artificial intelligence enhances the ability to detect anomalies and cyber threats in real time. This chapter explores intrusion detection techniques, machine learning models, and intelligent monitoring systems. It demonstrates how AI significantly improves the security of healthcare networks.

5. Integrating Blockchain and IoT for Wearable Device Security

Blockchain brings transparency and trust to IoT-based wearable environments by securing shared data. This chapter explains how decentralized structures protect communication between connected devices. It introduces the powerful combination of blockchain and IoT for strengthening wearable ecosystems.

6. Blockchain-Empowered Data Security and Privacy-Preserving Framework for Wearable Medical Devices

Protecting sensitive medical data requires strong privacy-preserving methods and secure architectures. This chapter provides an in-depth look at blockchain frameworks designed for wearable healthcare systems. It highlights how blockchain ensures safe, private, and trustworthy communication channels.

7. Strengthening Data Integrity in Healthcare Through Blockchain Technology for Enhanced Patient Privacy in the Digital Age

Healthcare systems must maintain accurate, untampered data to support patient safety and reliable diagnosis. This chapter shows how blockchain's immutability enhances data integrity and transparency. It reinforces the importance of trustworthy records in digital healthcare environments.

8. Hardware Security and Challenges in Wearable and Implantable Medical Devices

Wearable and implantable devices face several hardware-level vulnerabilities that threaten patient safety. This chapter discusses tamper resistance, secure design, and encryption at the device level. It emphasizes why robust hardware security is essential for dependable medical technologies.

9. Implantable Medical Devices: Types, Risks, and Securing Solutions

Implantable medical devices are life-saving technologies but come with unique security risks. This chapter explores device types, vulnerabilities, and methods to safeguard them. It highlights the need for strong, device-specific security solutions to protect patients.

10. Futuristic Approach for Wearable Blood Pressure Prediction Using Doppler Radar

Advanced sensing using Doppler radar enables non-contact, accurate blood pressure prediction. This chapter explains how radar principles and machine learning improve monitoring efficiency. It showcases a futuristic approach to patient-friendly health assessments.

11. Smart IoT Health Monitor for Early TB Diagnosis Using Optimized Hyperbolic NasNet Attention Sea-Horse

Early diagnosis of tuberculosis can save lives, and intelligent IoT devices make this possible. This chapter explores a deep learning–powered system designed for accurate TB detection. It demonstrates how AI and IoT revolutionize infectious disease screening.

12. Testing, Auditing & Compliance for Medical Devices

Medical devices undergo strict testing, auditing, and certification to ensure global safety standards. This chapter explains compliance requirements and governance processes essential for device approval. It stresses the importance of regulatory adherence in healthcare technology.

CONCLUSION: CONTRIBUTION TO THE FIELD

This book marks an important step forward in the study and practice of wearable medical device security. It consolidates the latest advances in cybersecurity, AI, and blockchain as applied to healthcare, offering a unified perspective that bridges theory and practice. By connecting global expertise from multiple continents, the volume serves as both a research reference and a practical guide for the secure design, deployment, and management of medical wearables. It reinforces the commitment of the scientific community toward building trustworthy, patient-centered, and technologically robust healthcare ecosystems. The insights shared within these pages not only address current security challenges but also lay the groundwork for future innovations that will define the next decade of digital health.

Chapter 1
Introduction to Wearable Medical Devices in Healthcare

Biswajit Saha
https://orcid.org/0000-0001-8000-6733
JIS University, Kolkata, India & Dr. B.C. Roy Engineering College, Durgapur, India

Dharmpal Singh
JIS University, Kolkata, India

Gour Sundar Mitra Thakur
https://orcid.org/0000-0001-8907-9058
Dr. B.C. Roy Engineering College, Durgapur, India

ABSTRACT

Wearable medical devices (WMDs) are one of the most interesting ways that technology and healthcare are coming together. Digital health care has come a long way since fitness trackers were just basic tools. They are now complicated tools for diagnosis and treatment. Today, WMDs include a wide range of devices, such as smartwatches that can do an ECG, patches that can check glucose levels, wearable defibrillators, biosensors, and smart textiles that can always keep track of important physiological data. These devices not only enable people keep an eye on their own health, but they also send doctors real-time, nonstop, and very personalized data streams that can help them make better diagnoses, treatment plans, and disease management. One of the most crucial ways that WMDs can improve things is by

DOI: 10.4018/979-8-3373-4412-6.ch001

making healthcare more proactive and predictive. Patients and healthcare providers can now access health information all the time instead of only when they go to the hospital.

1 INTRODUCTION

Wearable Medical Devices (WMDs) are one of the most transformative technologies we have seen in the healthcare arena this century. These devices can be as simple as a fitness tracking device or as complex as a biosensor capable of monitoring in real time a patient's vital signs, cardiac activity, or glucose levels. They can also be something in between. What is certain is that these devices and the accompanying technologies are starting to reshape the ways healthcare is delivered. It is widely known that healthcare systems currently face rising costs, aging populations, and the growing burden of chronic diseases. Wearable technologies present an opportunity to enhance patient outcomes, improve care efficiency, and enable remote and preventive health monitoring. However, their integration into healthcare infrastructures also raises various concerns. These concerns are particularly related to data security, device interoperability, user privacy, and regulatory compliance.

WMDs are high-tech, sensor-equipped gadgets that are made to be worn on the body so that they may continuously or intermittently collect, monitor, and send physiological and biometric data. These devices can be used for real-time or retrospective clinical assessments, and they are becoming more common in preventative care, chronic illness management, rehabilitation, and telemedicine. WMDs help make personalized, data-driven, and remote healthcare delivery models possible by making it easy for them to work with health information systems and decision-support platforms.

Wearable medical gadgets have become more popular in recent years thanks to improvements in miniaturized sensors, wireless communication, and artificial intelligence. Wearables may now not only passively gather data, but also actively give users information about their health thanks to these technologies. Smartwatches, for instance, may now let users know when their heart rhythms are out of rhythm, and wearable glucose monitors give those with diabetes constant feedback on ways to manage their condition. The fact that these gadgets are easy to find and use has led to more patients taking charge of their own health and being more involved in their care. This has led to a more proactive healthcare culture.

Figure 1. Information Flow Saad et al. (2024)

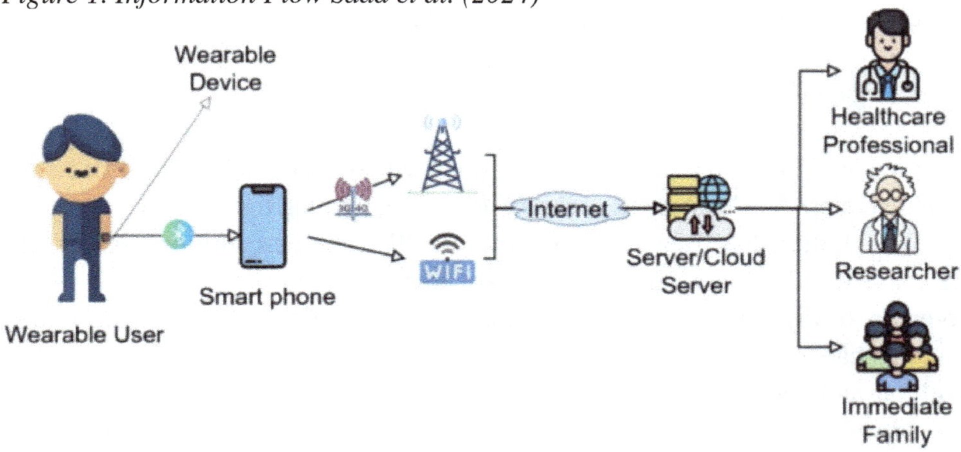

Figure 1 shows the flow of information of WMDs that occur when they are in use. WMDs are also very important for connecting patients and clinicians, especially in communities that do not have enough healthcare services or are hard to reach. Healthcare experts may keep an eye on patients' development from afar, change therapies in real time, and step in quickly when something goes wrong. This ability not only makes clinical infrastructure less of a burden, but it also makes healthcare delivery more fair and continuous. Wearable technology is becoming more common, along with data analytics platforms and cloud-based health records. WMDs are going to be an important part of next-generation healthcare systems.

We can consider an introductory framework or a central model to explain how a wearable turns raw signals into real health value. At first data needs to be captured followed by aggregation of data which in turn is followed by reason.

The last one is engage. So the model can be called the CARE Loop (Capture; Aggregate; Reason; Engage) through which IoT devices transform raw sensor data into meaningful clinical actions through the four stage CARE process. Each stage is briefly described below:

- **Capture:**

  Sensors on the body collect signals (heart rate, SpO_2, activity).

- **Aggregate:** • Data moves via phone/gateway to secure storage. Constraints: connectivity costs, offline use, interoperability, encryption.
- **Reason:**

Edge/cloud analytics turn data into risk scores and alerts. Constraints: compute cost, model transparency, bias, regulatory validation.

- **Engage:**

Insights fit into lives and workflows—patient nudges, clinician dashboards, automated referrals. Constraints: usability, language, training time, re- imbursement.

Though there has been a fast growth in WMDs, the literature remains largely descriptive and siloed by device or disease area. Few sources synthesize the end-to-end pathway—from sensing and communication to data integration, analytics, and clinical action—or explicitly connect environmental exposure measurements with physiological responses captured by wearables. On looking at the comparative analyses of security/privacy risks, interoperability/standards, and regulatory expectations across regions it is found them to be fragmented. Also due to limited longitudinal or diverse-population studies, the evidence on equity, cost, usability, reliability, calibration/validation, and real-world adoption (workflow fit, EHR integration, reimbursement) is inconsistent.

The purpose of this chapter is to provide the readers with an overview of WMDs - starting from definitions and taxonomy and moving to clinical use, cross-cutting challenges, regulation, ethics/equity, and future directions. This chapter discusses about the various categories of WMDs ranging from individual measurement devices to advanced devices designed for using under the super- vision of doctors'. Any discussion of technology is incomplete without a foun- dational understanding of its historical evolution. This chapter also attempts to provide the readers with an understanding on the historical evolution and market growth of WMDs. The chapter also provides the readers with a com- prehensive overview of clinical applications, challenges, regulatory landscape, ethical and societal considerations, future trends and innovations of WMDs.

The next section categorizes WMDs into two major divisions: the ones that monitor our health and the ones that are used under a physician's watchful eye.

2 CATEGORIES OF WMDS

There are various types of WMDs spanning from consumer-grade to clinician-supervised wearables. In this section the reader will be guided through various categories of WMDs. The figure below 3 shows the various categories of WMDs. According to C¸ elik et al. (2024) WMDs can be categorized into two groups:

(a) those that are used for individual measurement and (b) those that have advanced patient tracking systems that can only be used under the supervision of a healthcare expert. Individual measurement is a new trend that lets us keep an eye on the health of users in real time by measuring data about how their bodies work. Individual measuring apps keep track of a number of different metrics. Stress level, amount of steps taken each day, meal pattern, sleep pattern, and medical parameters like blood oxygen level, heart function, body weight, blood sugar level, and blood pressure are all examples of recorded individual mea- suring parameters that might affect health. These categories show how flexible WMDs may be, from simple health tracking tools to complex clinical monitoring systems. Figure 2 shows some of the various categories of WMDs in use.

Figure 2. Categories of WMDs Saad et al. (2024)

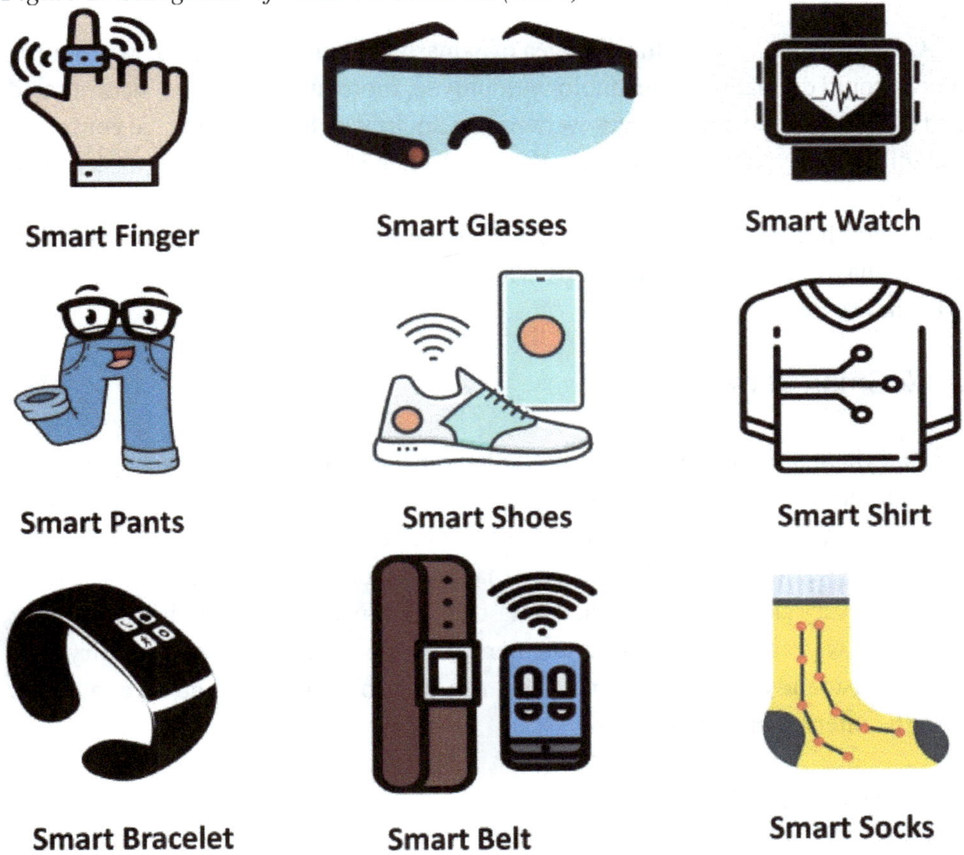

2.1 Individual Measurement Devices

C¸ elik et al. (2024) emphasizes that getting knowledge and using it well is really important these days. As technology has advanced quickly, clothes, smart- phones, and watches have become one of the best ways to get and evaluate personal data. Wearable technology gives users individual measurements that let them make changes to improve their quality of life and understand and con- trol their lifestyles to make health management more user-friendly. Wearable technology can help us get things done faster and better every day.

2.1.1 Smart Watches

Cottle (2017) explains that the idea of "smartness" initially came up when time-pieces could do maths. As technology improved, more functions were incorporated and timepieces of different sizes were made. Smart watches offer a voice command capability that makes it easy to do things like keep track of our daily tasks, send messages, and make calls. Smartwatches can connect to phones over the internet or Bluetooth. People use these watches for more than just regular chores. They can also manage programs, count steps while working out, save data, measure heart rate, and more.

2.1.2 Smart Jewelry

Kaewkannate and Kim (2016) states that the technology is also starting to show itself in the world of jewelry. Smart jewelry is a great example of how technology and design can work together in this way. Smart gadgets make rings, bracelets, necklaces, earrings, and other jewelry that can record what the people who wear them do every day. They can track data over long periods of time by connecting wirelessly to smart devices like computers and mobile phones. Smart jewelry, like rings, wristbands, spectacles, and belts, can talk to each other and to computers over the internet or Bluetooth.

2.1.3 Smart Clothes

Smart clothes are clothes that have sensors, wires, or chips integrated into them that can track things like body motions, temperature, heart rate, and other health information. It looks like normal clothes, but it can gather and transfer information to a computer or smartphone. People wear smart clothes in sports, healthcare, or everyday life to monitor their health or do better. Ju and Lee (2021) states that the expectations for smart clothing improvements have been demonstrated to make people less resistant to smart clothing. However, in order to get more people to buy smart clothing, the risks that people think they face need to be lowered, and the performance, durability, and availability of smart clothing need to be improved.

2.2 Advanced Wearable Devices Designed for Using Under Supervision of Doctors

Teng et al. (2008) discusses that the main reason for which smart gadgets are used in healthcare is that they can collect data to check on a person's health and find out what disorders they have. So, other health data, including loss of balance and an abnormal heart rhythm, that smart devices can collect could be very important. These systems can let the user know when there is a problem with the data, and some of them can even take action.

While taxonomy clarifies 'what' WMDs are, understanding 'how' we arrived here requires historical and market context. Before we investigate the therapeutic implications further, it is helpful to understand how WMDs have evolved historically. This perspective not only demonstrates their advancements in technology but also underscores their rapidly expanding market presence. After having discussed about the different types of WMDs in this the next section we shall bring forward the historical evolution and market growth of WMDs in the following section.

3 HISTORICAL EVOLUTION AND MARKET GROWTH

In this section evolution of WMDs, their commercialization and market growth are discussed. We trace the evolution and commercialization of WMDs to ex- plain adoption patterns and the technical inflection points that enabled current capabilities.

Many fields, such as healthcare and biomedical monitoring systems, are seeing more and more use of wearable technologies. These devices make it possible to constantly check vital indicators for medical diagnostics, monitoring and evaluating physiological health, and more. As the number of older individuals around the world grows, more and more chronic and acute diseases become important. The need for point-of-care (POC) diagnostics and real-time monitoring of long-term health problems is making a big difference in the medical industry. Wearable tech has changed over time from accessories to garments with built-in tech to attachments and inserts that go on the body. Over the past few decades, electronics, biocompatible materials, and nanotechnology have made a lot of progress. As a result, implanted devices that use small sensors and biomedical equipment to find and anticipate health problems have been made. The quality and effectiveness of medical services have substantially increased thanks to these gadgets.

Zhu et al. (2020) emphasizes in their research that the traditional system of hospitals is changing into a system that focuses on individuals since chronic diseases are common, treatments are expensive, and the population is getting older. Early diagnosis to stop diseases is better and cheaper than treating them after an outbreak. The most essential thing that has changed is the rise of wearable technology. Wearable medical technologies can keep an eye on physiological parameters for long periods of time. So, it will be easier to get health care, and diseases can be found and treated early, and possible health hazards can be dealt with.

Figure 3. Wearable Medical Devices Market by Device Type, 2021-2034 (USD Billion) Global Market Insights (2024)

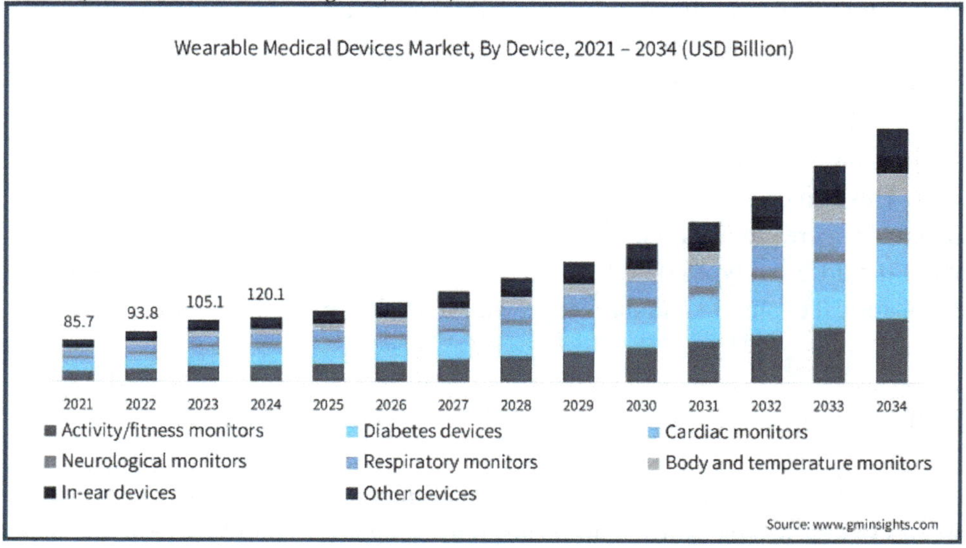

The market segmentation shown in Figure 3 illustrates the diverse categories of wearable medical devices driving this growth (Global Market Insights, 2024). Activity/fitness monitors represent the largest segment, followed by diabetes devices, cardiac monitors, neurological monitors, respiratory monitors, body and temperature monitors, in-ear devices, and other specialized devices. This diversification demonstrates the broad applicability and market penetration of wearable technologies across various healthcare domains.

The market data presented in Table 1 demonstrates the substantial growth trajectory of the wearable medical devices industry. The market size has grown from USD 120.1 billion in 2024 and is projected to reach USD 543.9 billion by 2034, representing a compound annual growth rate (CAGR) of 16.5% during the forecast period 2025-2034.

In recent years, the global market for medical wearables has grown tremendously. Thanks to technology, connections have gone wireless, sensors have become tiny, and Artificial Intelligence (AI) now plays a part in everything. With no pain or harm involved, the 'new' devices can take constant readings of all kinds of health indicators—blood pressure, heart rate, the level of glucose in the blood of any person, the amount of oxygen in blood of any person, and so on. These are not 'new' programs in the sense of new processes or technologies. They are new in the sense that they are now being used to anything like the promised level. And they have become particularly ubiquitous and useful in the diagnosis and treatment of the kinds of health problems that many face as they age and that many more are likely to have thanks to the COVID-19 pandemic. WMDs are designed to be used within the home by patients with a variety of

Table 1. Wearable Medical Devices Market Report Attributes (Global Market Insights, 2024)

Key Takeaway	Details
Market Size & Growth	
Base Year	2024
Market Size in 2024	USD 120.1 Billion
Forecast Period 2025–2034 CAGR	16.5%
Market Size in 2034	USD 543.9 Billion
Key Market Trends	
Growth Drivers	• Increasing awareness about physical fitness and wearable devices among the population in developing countries • Growing prevalence of chronic diseases globally • Technological advancements in wearable devices • Rising disposable income and healthcare expenditure in emerging countries
Pitfalls & Challenges	• Issues related to data security • Cost-intensive nature of wearable devices

health conditions, and they allow for continuous monitoring and recording of vital signs and other significant health data. The devices utilize wireless technology to communicate with a central hub that aggregates data from multiple devices. The home hub is fundamentally an edge computing device, and home health monitors can be viewed as Internet of Things (IoT) devices that allow for remote patient monitoring (RPM) and virtual health visits.

In short, the history of WMDs and their quick rise in the market show their growing importance and the wide spread use in healthcare. Now after having discussed about how the industry has evolved and how it has changed over time, it is time to look at the ways WMDs are influencing the way doctors work. The next section guides the reader about various clinical application of WMDs.

4 CLINICAL APPLICATIONS OF WMDS

Using the device categorization as a guide, this section discusses about various applications and outcomes of WMDs across specialties. WMDs are being used more and more in clinical practice to help with diagnosis, monitoring, treatment, and rehabilitation in a wide range of medical professions. One of the key purposes is to keep an eye on patients all the time. For example, smartwatches and biosensors can keep track of key indications including blood pressure, heart rate, glucose levels, and oxygen saturation. These devices help people with long- term illnesses like diabetes, heart disease, and lung disease discover problems early and do something about them before they grow worse. Guk et al. (2019) discusses about the various wearable gadgets that have been produced thus far and how they are used in the medical field.

In cardiology, wearable electrocardiogram (ECG) monitors provide real-time data on cardiac rhythms, assisting in the diagnosis and management of arrhythmia and other heart-related issues. Similarly, glucose monitoring wearables, such as Continuous Glucose Monitoring (CGM) systems, are helpful in the diabetes field because they allow clinicians to monitor glucose levels in continuously. Immediate data concerning glucose levels allows for more precise and timely adjustments to be made regarding a treatment regimen of a patient.

Neurology also benefits from wearable devices. Seizure-prone individuals can use an Electroencephalogram or Electroencephalography (EEG) headband to help detect when a seizure is happening or about to happen. In the field of rehabilitation medicine, sensors can be used to spatially track an individual's movements with a high degree of fidelity. Such devices can also measure the electrical activity in muscles—information that is crucial when determining the best course of physical therapy for an individual recovering from some type of neurological event. Remote Patient Monitoring (RPM), especially for post- surgical or rural patients, is another big area. Wearables let healthcare providers keep an eye on how well patients are doing after an operation. The technology cuts down on the number of hospital trips patients have to make and allows for quicker action if something goes wrong.

Also, sleep-monitoring gadgets can assist doctors figure out what is wrong with people who have sleep disorders like sleep apnea and help them decide what to do about it. Wearables that detect stress signals, heart rate variability, help mental health professionals figure out how stressed their patients are and ways to best help them. WMDs are becoming more popular in a number of other significant clinical fields, in addition to their principal uses.

Some of them are:

- **Respiratory Monitoring**

Wearable equipment like spirometers and respiratory rate monitors help people with chronic obstructive pulmonary disease (COPD), asthma, and other lung problems. These let us not only keep an eye on how our patients breathe, but they also assist us find early indicators of respiratory distress.

- **Orthopedics and Musculoskeletal Care**

Wearable motion sensors and smart braces watch how patients move their joints and how they sit and stand after an injury or orthopaedic surgery. They help with recovery in real time by letting us know how well a person moves, which makes it less likely that for the person to get hurt again.

- **Pregnancy and Neonatal Monitoring**

Wearable foetal monitors help with obstetric care by keeping track of the contractions of the mother and the heart rate of the baby in real time. Sensors that may be worn can keep a check on newborns' vital signs without having to touch them. This is especially helpful for preterm babies who need constant care.

- **Oncology**

Wearable devices are used to track cancer patients' activity levels, fatigue levels, and how their bodies respond to chemotherapy or radiation. This information helps doctors make treatment plans that are right for each person and keep an eye on their overall health.

- **Pain Management**

More and more individuals are utilizing wearable devices like Transcuta- neous Electrical Nerve Stimulation (TENS) units, which send electrical signals via the skin to stimulate nerves. One does not need drugs to get rid of arthritis, chronic back pain, or to heal after surgery.

- **Wound Care**

Smart bandages have sensors built in that check on how wounds are healing by measuring things like temperature, moisture levels, and pH balance. This helps doctors find diseases early and change how they treat them.

- **Geriatric Care**

Wearable devices can help older people who live alone by sending out emergency alerts, keeping track of what they're doing, and letting them know when they fall. This makes their lives better and keeps them safe.

- **Medication Adherence Monitoring**

Some wearables have sensors or built-in reminders that help individuals remember to take their medicine and follow their treatment plans.

These different clinical uses all show how wearable medical technologies may make healthcare more personalized, efficient, and successful. Overall, WMDs are transforming clinical practice by enabling personalized, real-time healthcare delivery, improving patient outcomes, and reducing healthcare costs through early detection and timely interventions.

In this review by Farabolini et al. (2025), the use of wearable sensors for at-home continuous monitoring of motor behavior is considered. It centered on the objective, type, feasibility and potential use of these sensors in neurolog- ical, musculoskeletal or rheumatologic diseases. The articles included in this review were obtained from PubMed, Scopus, and Web of Science according to the PRISMA guidelines. Seventy-two studies that involved 7949 patients met the inclusion criteria. Most of the research focused on neurological diseases, in particular Parkinson's. Sensors such as inertial measurement units (IMUs), accelerometers, and gyroscopes are widely used and frequently integrated in trackers, smart phones and medical devices. Duration of monitoring varied from 24 hours to 2 years. Feasibility studies showed high patient compliance, greater than equal to 70% and good acceptance, with strong agreement with clinical assessments. However, only half of the studies were controlled trials, and just 5.6% were randomized. They concluded that though wearable sensors offer strong potential for real-world motor function monitoring some challenges including ethical issues, data privacy, standardization, and healthcare access persist. Artificial intelligence integration may help in boosting predictive accu- racy and personalized care.

Table 2. WMDs vs. Clinical Applications

Device Type	Use Case		Key Parameters Monitored	Healthcare Specialty
Smart watch	Daily tracking; mia	activity arrhyth- screening;	Heart rate (HR), heart rhythm/ ECG, step count/activity	Cardiology; Preven- tive care

Table 2 shows comparison of WMDs with clinical applications.

WMDs possess a lot of therapeutic benefit, but they also have a lot of ractical and technical drawbacks. The following section talks about the primary challenges that need to be solved in order to make the greatest possible use of WMDs in healthcare.

5 CHALLENGES IN THE USE OF WEARABLE DEVICES

In this section we discuss about the challenges, distinguishing mature capabilities from unresolved gaps that recur across applications. The review by Lu et al. (2020) reveals that the WMDs that have been made so far can be used on all regions of the body, including the head, arms, and torso. There are four main uses for these devices: (1) keeping an eye on health and safety, (2) managing chronic diseases, (3) diagnosing and treating diseases, and (4) rehabilitation. However, the wearable medical device industry is currently facing a number of major issues that make it hard to use wearable technology in medical practice. These include problems with making solutions that are easy to use, concerns about security and privacy, the lack of industry standards, and various technical problems. They states that as science and technology improve and personalized health ideas grow more popular, wearable gadgets will become more important in health care and be more incorporated into people's daily lives. But further research is needed to find other ways that wearable devices can be used in medicine.

When making technical solutions for real-world use, it is crucial to know what kinds of gadgets work best. For example, low-cost commercial gadgets are considerably easier to use in real life than high-cost research-grade ones. Even said, using low-cost commercial gadgets to better mirror real-world settings comes with its own set of problems.

The work by K¨onig et al. (2023) performs three studies with participants to find out what problems come up while utilizing cheap commercial wearable devices. Specifically, data accessibility, the variety of wearable devices (inter- operability), and if they are right for the intended use (fit-for-purpose). They discusses about three investigations in the study that used cheap, commercially available wearable equipment. Then they highlights the problems that they faced during these experiments, and how they are applicable to other studies. Finally, they discusses ways to solve these problems, while still using low-cost, commercially available wearables.

Wearable electronics are getting better, which opens the door to a new type of device that can sense, process, and communicate all at the same time. These devices can be used for many things, including as keeping an eye on the health of a person, tracking his or her activities, and interacting with computers. But three big problems keep wearable devices from being used by a lot of people. To start, people cease using these devices fast since they need to be charged often. Second, the materials used to make current wearable gadgets are stiff, which makes them heavy and uncomfortable. Third, high-impact applications have not yet shown the usefulness of wearable devices. The Table 3 gives an overview of the areas of WMDs which have matured and areas which are challenging to this day.

Bhat et al. (2019) gives a list of possible ways to solve these three problems. More specifically, they begin with a method for optimizing runtime that can make it possible to run without recharging. Next, they specifies ways to make gadgets that are physically flexible and stretchable so that they are comfortable to wear. Finally, they focuses on wearable apps that have a big influence, such as health monitoring and interacting with computers.

5.1 IoT/Wearable Data Security Challenges and Technical Solutions

A major concern with IoT communications is security and privacy. No one would like to compromise with the security and privacy of users. For example, if we have smart locker which can communicate with smart band to operate then security is crucial. Same way the smart band contains health record and other IoT devices can communicate, so we never want our health record to be shared only eith doctors and not with others. All this control and security poses a challenge for designing solutions keeping in mind the way IoT development grow with wearable devices. IoT communication protocols and selection of devices with security parameters are the key factor for the IoT solution design and implementations. Bhushan and Agrawal (2019) discussed about various design and security challenges for Wearable Devices and IoT.

In their research Cook et al. (2023) five key areas impacting IoT security are identified. By doing an extensive analysis of each area, the article discusses about future research opportunities for IoT privacy and security for the next generation of network technologies. The challenges identified in the research are as follows:

- **Device Constraints**
- **Human-centric Weaknesses**

- **Lack of security standards/secure-by-design**
- **Data misuse and surveillance risk**
- **Known device exploits**
- **Physical-layer exposure and next-gen networks**
- **Over-reliance on "contemporary tech"**

The research also discusses or recommends some technical solutions as below:

- **Embed cryptography on the device**
- **Hardening the update/patch pipeline**
- **Use AI/ML and blockchain judiciously**
- **Explore alternative physical-layer defenses**
- **Push standards and secure-by-design**
- **Prioritize device-level encryption as hardware improves**

5.2 Common Cyber Security Vulnerabilities and Potential Attacks

Due to the fact that WMDs handle sensitive physiological data and can influence care decisions, even small security gaps can have harmful clinical and privacy consequences. Figure 4 portrays Wearable Medical Device Ecosystem showing 4 layers of the ecosystem.

We briefly summarize key vulnerabilities and the primary attacks adversaries use to exploit them.

- **Bluetooth Low Energy (BLE) sniffing (Communication layer):** Attackers capture over-the-air packets from watches, ECG patches, CGMs. Impact: Exposure of vitals/IDs; session metadata; basis for later spoofing. Mitigations (quick): BLE Secure Connections (LESC), bonding/whitelisting, LE Privacy (address rotation), authenticated pairing.

Figure 4. Wearable Medical Device Ecosystem

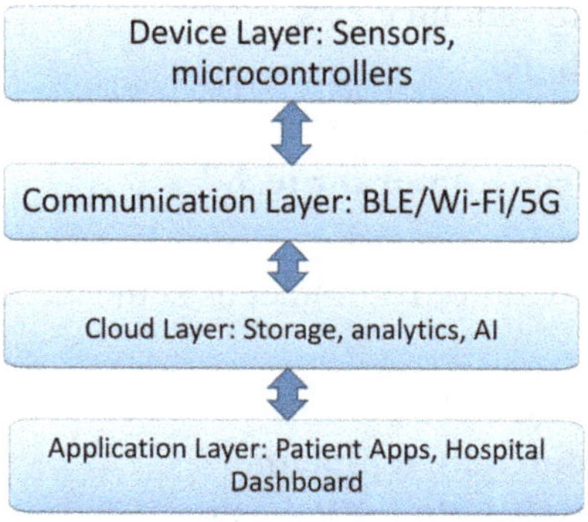

- **Data replay (Device and Communication; sometimes Cloud):** Old but valid packets are resent (e.g., "normal" glucose or ECG segments) to skew trends or suppress alerts. Impact: Integrity loss → wrong clinical decisions, missed deterioration. Mitigations: Nonces/timestamps/sequence numbers, signed telemetry, TLS at transport plus app-layer counters; re- ject stale windows.
- **Insecure APIs (Cloud layer):** Weak auth, over-permissive endpoints, missing rate limits on patient/device APIs. Impact: Bulk PHI exfiltration, account takeover, data tamper at scale. Mitigations: OAuth2/OIDC, fine- grained scopes, server-side input validation, RBAC/ABAC, rate limiting, audit logs; test against OWASP API Top 10.
- **Weak encryption (All layers; esp. Communication & Cloud stor- age)** Legacy ciphers, static keys, or homemade crypto. Impact: Eaves- dropping, data tamper, regulatory violations. Mitigations: TLS 1.3, mod- ern AEAD (e.g., AES-GCM/ ChaCha20-Poly1305), secure key storage (TEE/ secure element), perfect forward secrecy, end-to-end encryption where feasible.

Some of the potential attacks and their impact as well as suggested mitiga- tion strategies are listed below:

- **Spoofing (Device/Communication):** Fake device or gateway imitates a real wearable or cloud endpoint. Impact: Injected vitals, false alarms, or suppressed alerts → safety risk. Mitigations: Mutual authentication (device phone cloud), certificate pinning, device attestation, signed firmware/ telemetry.
- **Eavesdropping (Communication):** Passive capture of BLE/ Wi-Fi/ 5G traffic or local storage syncs. Impact: Confidentiality loss of PHI and behavior

patterns. Mitigations: Strong encryption, rotating BLE ad- dresses, secure pairing, WPA3/ 5G native security, disable legacy modes.

- **Unauthorized access (Application/ Cloud; also Device if stolen/ rooted):** Weak passwords, no MFA, leaked tokens, debug interfaces. Im- pact: Full record access, device command/ control, data deletion → avail- ability and integrity risks. Mitigations: MFA, least-privilege access, ses- sion management, secure mobile app hardening, remote wipe, MDM for clinical deployments.

End-to-end encryption and authentication have great deal of importance in ensuring data security and checking cyber security vulnerabilities. End-to- end encryption keeps health data unreadable to anyone except the sender and the intended receiver—from the wearable, through the phone and network, to the cloud and app. It prevents snooping and tampering. On the other hand, authentication proves "who is who": the device proves it's genuine, the server proves it's trusted, and the user proves they are the right person. Together, they block spoofing and unauthorized access, protect privacy, preserve data integrity for clinical decisions, and build trust and regulatory compliance.

Wearable and IoT medical devices help everyone only when they stay afford- able over time and work well in real-world conditions—not just when the sticker price is low. Cost and accessibility determine whether wearable/IoT health tech delivers population-level value or remains a niche convenience. Direct device prices are only a slice of the true expense; total cost of ownership includes sensors/consumables (e.g., patches, test strips), data plans and cloud fees, app subscriptions, clinician dashboard licenses, maintenance/calibration, battery re- placement, and integration with hospital IT. Vendor lock-in (proprietary cables, closed data formats) raises switching costs and suppresses competition. In low- and middle-income settings, import duties, fragmented distribution, and short warranties further inflate costs. Hidden costs also show up as staff time to train patients and review streams of data.

Accessibility barriers can be: intermittent connectivity, older Android phones with limited memory, low digital literacy, and language/assistive-tech needs. Devices that assume always-on broadband, frequent charging, or pristine in- door environments fail in rural clinics and crowded homes. Stigma and usabil- ity matter too—bulky or conspicuous wearables, adhesives that irritate skin, or tiny text can exclude older adults and women engaged in manual labor.

To fully use the potential of WMDs in healthcare settings, several challenges must be overcome. Hence, in light of these issues, it is essential to be aware of the rules that govern the development and implementation of WMDs. Many risks can be addressed through proper governance, standards, and oversight, we now discuss about the regulatory landscape. The following section provides an overview of the rules and regulations in this particular field.

6 REGULATORY LANDSCAPE (BRIEF OVERVIEW)

This section highlights major regulatory pathways and expectations across regions, highlighting implications for software-enabled wearables.

It is very important for people's health to have excellent quality medical equipment. There are several government entities in each country that check these items. The rules for medical devices are very different in major markets like the European Union, the United States, and Japan. This is because each country has its unique way of making sure that new medical technology are safe and work. These differences in laws could lead to a "medical device lag," which means that strict rules, more complicated gadgets, and a lack of global standardization can make it tougher for people to get their hands on new tech- nologies. Patients have a hard time getting new medical gadgets because of these delays, and the market is not as competitive.

Amaral et al. (2024) examines the laws that govern medical devices and how the European Commission (EC), the Food and Drug Administration (FDA), and the Pharmaceuticals and Medical Device Agency (PMDA) approve them. The U.S. Food and Drug Administration, 2025, has a similarly demanding approval process, but the rules are different before and after the product is sold. These laws say that clinical trials should be longer and that consumers should keep an eye on how well the technology works after they acquire it. The Medical Device Regulation (MDR), European Parliament and Council of the European Union (2017), is one of the strict standards that the EU has in place to keep people safe. It makes sure that a product is carefully checked before it is sold and closely watched after it is sold.

Ali et al., 2024 discusses about the various regulations with respect to the use of medical devices. Japan is a major player in the global medical device market, but it has its own set of rules and regulations that make things difficult for them. The certification process is more difficult since it needs clinical data from the US and has a complicated reimbursement structure. This leads to long delays known as "medical devices lag."

There are certain important points about the regulatory landscape which are highlighted below:

- **Complexity of Regulatory Compliance:**

There are severe standards for WMDs set by the FDA in the US, the EC in the EU, and the PMDA in Japan. It's hard for gadget makers who want to sell their items all over the world because each area has its own rules and means to get things approved.

- **Regulatory Divergence and Market Access:** "Medical device lag" is the term for when patients can't receive new wearable gadgets because of various restrictions in different places. This gap makes it difficult for new healthcare ideas to propagate over the world, which could imply that not everyone can get the finest care.
- **Standardization Challenges:**

It's even tougher to acquire regulatory approval because there aren't any global standards for the performance, interoperability, and safety of WMDs. Businesses can gain regulatory approvals and enter new markets around the world more easily if there are worldwide standards.

- **Data Privacy and Cyber Security Regulations:**

Health data collected by WMDs are of sensitive nature. So there is a need to emphasize data security and patient privacy by regulatory bodies. Gen- eral Data Protection Regulation (GDPR) in Europe or Health Insurance Portability and Accountability Act (HIPAA) in the United States, neces- sitate rigorous cyber security measures integrated into device development and operation.

- **Post-Market Surveillance and Real-World Evidence:**

There is a need to continually assess device safety, effectiveness, and pa- tient outcomes. In order to address this growing need regulatory bodies are increasingly emphasizing post-market surveillance and collection of real-world evidence (RWE). This approach enables regulators to monitor devices actively and respond swiftly to any safety concerns or failures in real-world applications.

- **Regulatory Adaptation to Innovation:**

There are rapid technological advancements in place which are AI inte- gration, nanotechnology, and personalized medicine. So there is an ur- gent need of regulatory frameworks to continuously adapt. In order to accommodate new technological developments without compromising pa- tient safety or ethical standards authorities face the challenge of evolving quickly enough.

To make the regulatory landscape actionable, we contrast major regions on classification, premarket routes for SaMD/wearables, clinical evidence expecta- tions, cyber security guidance, privacy law, and post-market duties.

The table 4 shows a clearer cross-region comparison. It is very important to be able to navigate and harmonize the complicated global regulatory landscape to make sure that patients can get new WMDs on time. Ethical and social issues are just as important as following the rules when it comes to the widespread use of wearable medical equipment. The following section focuses on the most important ethical issues and effects on society that come from using them.

However, it should be understood that compliance alone does not guarantee acceptable use or equitable benefit. The next section discusses about some examples or cases where breaches or FDA advisories related to medical wearables have occurred.

7 EXAMPLES OF BREACHES OR FDA ADVISORIES RE- LATED TO MEDICAL WEARABLES

There have been some breaches or FDA Advisories related to medical wearables which will be discussed in this section. Some of them are described in brief in the following sub sections as follows:

7.1 FDA Warning Letters (Regulatory Actions)

- **Whoop Blood Pressure Insights (July 2025):** FDA issued a warn- ing letter to Whoop, Inc. marketed its "Blood Pressure Insights" feature without required clearance or approval. FDA issued a Warning Letter to it. It was brought to their notice that the feature should be regulated as a medical device. The agency determined this function constitutes a med- ical device because blood pressure data is "inherently tied to diagnosing hypertension or hypotension." According to the company this feature is intended for general wellness and not for medical diagnosis and intends to keep the feature available in the US, while the FDA has stated possible regulatory action could be taken if the violations are not addressed.
- **Owlet Baby Care Smart Socks (2021):** FDA issued a warning letter to Owlet for its "smart socks" in October 2021 stating that these were marketed without necessary premarket clearance or approval. These smart socks measured blood oxygen saturation and pulse rate in infants. The agency ruled that marketing claims like notifying parents when readings leave "safe zones" demonstrated the product was "intended to identify (diagnose) desaturation and bradycardia," making it a regulated medical device.

7.2 FDA Recalls & Safety Communications

- **Dexcom CGM Class I Recall (July 2025):** Due to a speaker defect that could prevent high/low blood sugar alerts from sounding, Dexcom initiated a Class I recall (the most serious classification) for its G6, G7, ONE, and ONE+ CGM receivers. FDA classified this as high-risk because according to them missed alerts could delay detection of dangerous glucose levels, potentially causing serious injury or death.
- **Contec Patient Monitor Cyber Security Advisory (January 2025):** In January 2025, FDA and the and the Cyber Security and Infrastructure Security Agency (CISA) issued a safety communication about cyber security vulnerabilities in Contec CMS8000 patient monitors, which had significant backdoors. Though these were bedside monitors this case portrays security flaws added during manufacturing can infiltrate medical devices.
- **Non-Invasive Glucose Monitoring Warning (February 2024):** On February 21, 2024, FDA issued a safety communication warning to con- sumers that no smart watch or smart ring intended to measure blood glucose non-invasively has been authorized, cleared, or approved. The advisory cautioned that such devices could lead to insulin dosing errors which might be dangerous.
- **Medtronic MiniMed Insulin Pump Cybersecurity Recall (2019):** In June 2019, Medtronic issued a safety communication about a potential cyber security vulnerability in some older MiniMed insulin pumps. Later, the FDA designated some models as a Class I recall in November 2019 due to cyber security weaknesses. They were apprehensive that attackers could remotely alter device settings to over-deliver or stop insulin delivery, potentially causing hypoglycemia, diabetic ketoacidosis, or death.

7.3 Documented Security Breaches Vulnerabilities

- **t:connect iOS App System Failure (2025):** There were reports of injuries because of usage of Tandem Diabetes t:connect iOS app with version 2.7, which continued from February 2024 into April 2024. A system failure occurred that caused the app to crash and drain the pump's battery. This issue was addressed by an updated app version released in August 2024. This was a system failure rather than a cyber attack.
- **Bluetooth Low Energy (BLE) Vulnerabilities:** Researchers at Uni- versity College London found vulnerabilities in ECG monitors, oximeters, and blood pressure sensors which have connections to Bluetooth Low En- ergy (BLE). They were able to do Man-in-the-Middle attacks, data ma- nipulation, and signal disruption between devices and mobile apps with low-cost tools.

- **Fitbit Apple Data Breach (2021):** In September 2021, due to a sig- nificant data leak approximately 61 million records from an unsecured, non-password-protected third-party database got exposed. This had the ability to pull data from various wearable device providers, including both Fitbit and Apple's HealthKit. The incident highlighted the lack of universal privacy standards for wearable devices, though FDA had previously classified Fitbit as a Class II medical device and cleared its electrocardio- gram function.
- **B. Braun Infusion Pump Vulnerabilities:** Significant vulnerabilities were discovered in B. Braun infusion pumps by McAfee researchers. This allowed hackers to remotely deliver double doses of medications. Though they are themselves not wearables, these devices illustrate critical gaps in medical device cybersecurity that could apply to wearable drug delivery systems.

8 ETHICAL AND SOCIETAL CONSIDERATIONS

In this section we therefore broaden the lens to incorporate ethical and societal considerations, including privacy, bias, transparency, and access.

The usage of medical wearable technology is transforming the way doctors work and how healthcare is delivered. The daily huge volume of personal data those results, privacy disclosure, and other ethical problems that come with interests are slowly coming to light, though. The study by Venkatachalam et al. (2023) looks at the ethical difficulties that come up throughout the whole process of health medical wearable devices serving people, from the equipment itself to data collection, transmission, management, and usage, from the point of view of medical ethics. It then recommends relevant solutions and counter mea sures from the standpoint of respecting autonomy, informed consent, privacy protection, medical optimization, and positive ideals. There is a pressing need to think about "prevention before disease," "disease prevention," and "change prevention", to get the most out of health care wearables in medical care, to help develop new smart medical care, and to help make India a more healthier place.

Spuskanyuk (2024) states that the ethical implications from the use of these WMDs are notable. There are reports of unprotected and insecure data storage and third-party data usage in the wearables industry. Quite naturally, additional ethical concerns surface depending on the type and use of the wearable. These devices can be broadly caegorized into three categories of use: 1) health and safety monitoring, 2) chronic disease management, and 3) rehabilitation. Each category contains devices with unique potential ethical issues that could benefit from recognition and analysis.

shujie Qu and Gao (2020) summarizes and analyses the ethical issues present in the entire process of health-related wearable technology serving individuals, encompassing the equipment itself, data collection, transmission, management, and utilization. It proposes corresponding countermeasures and recommenda- tions from the viewpoints of autonomy, informed consent, privacy protection, medical optimization, and ethical principles. "Prevention before disease, dis- ease prevention, and change prevention," and "medicine according to the case," to fully utilize the potential of health care wearables in the medical field and advance the evolution of new intelligent medical care.

To ethically use wearable medical technologies in healthcare, it is important to effectively deal with these ethical and social issues.

Now that we have discussed about existing ethical issues, we will consider future trends and recent advances in WMDs. The next section discusses about new technologies that are on the way and what they might mean for healthcare.

9 FUTURE TRENDS AND INNOVATIONS

This section discusses about the near-term trends and innovations in alignment with clinical value and social responsibility. According to Shang (2024) wearable technology is a new type of technology that has transformed how individuals keep track of their health and interact with the world. One may use these little, portable instruments to check on ones' health, fitness, and the state of the world right now. They fit perfectly into our daily life. Wearables have changed a lot since they were merely used to track fitness. They can do a lot of things now. They can now aid with things like taking care of smart homes, treating long-term ailments, and creating experiences in augmented reality. Adding sensors, AI, and wireless networking quickly has made them more useful and made them a big element of the Internet of Things. Wearable technology is especially good for encouraging preventative healthcare since it analyses things like heart rate, oxygen levels, and sleep patterns and gives users and healthcare providers critical information. It can also be used for things other than health care. For instance, Augmented Reality (AR) and Virtual Reality (VR) may make things feel real for sports, school, and fun. Wearable gear has a lot of promise, but

it also has some issues, such being pricey, having a short battery life, and not being able to keep data private. This research discusses about the various ways wearable technologies have changed throughout time, their various usages, and their significance for society in the future. Some of these are better AI-powered diagnostics, biosensors that don't need to be invasive, and more and more ways to employ these technologies in linked ecosystems.

According to Straits Research (2024), the market of WMDs is expanding. The global market is changing a lot because of new wearable devices that give us useful information about our health. This makes it possible to give more personalized care and improves the ways in which diseases are managed. Wear- able technologies let people take charge of their health by giving them useful information about it. This leads to better health outcomes and a move towards more patient-centered health-care solutions. The global market for wearable healthcare devices was worth USD 51.93 billion in 2024. It is expected to rise from USD 65.22 billion in 2025 to USD 403.66 billion in 2033, with a compound annual growth rate (CAGR) of 25.59% during the forecast period (2025–2033). In the coming years, WMDs are predicted to be impacted by flexible elec- tronics, nanotechnology, and personalized medicine. According to this fore- cast, the devices will become thinner and lighter, and work better in harmony with the human body—in more comfortable and, in some cases, clothing-like forms—that is to say, they will function better when worn on the person for whom they're intended. WMDs will not only monitor bodily conditions; under this forecast, they will also take action when necessary, which might entail ad- ministering drugs in a controlled manner or responding to orders to effect some therapy in real-time. The secure, interworking healthcare system promised by cloud computing and blockchain technology augurs well for what WMDs will do for at least two reasons. First, the more people who use personal health mon- itoring devices (PHMDs), the more essential it will become to integrate those devices efficiently and securely into the kinds of healthcare systems that really do "cloud" together. Second, AI and machine learning (ML) that will power the next big leap in PHMDs promises to do even better with the kinds of large datasets that these secure systems will allow.

In general, new technology and continuous breakthroughs promise big im- provements in WMDs, which will lead to major changes in how healthcare is delivered. Collectively, these trends suggest clear priorities for practice and research. The concluding section summarizes key insights and provides final observations on this transformative technology.

10 CONCLUSION

Wearable medical devices are moving care from episodic snapshots to contin- uous, context-aware decision support. Viewed through the device → data → decision → outcome pathway, they enable earlier detection, tighter longitudinal management, and more precise interventions—especially when environmental exposures are analyzed alongside physiological signals. The opportunity is substantial: safer home-based care, reduced clinical burden, and broader reach if designs and deployment models center privacy, interoperability, and accessibility from the outset.

Analytically, several components are maturing—sensor fidelity across ECG, PPG, SpO_2, IMUs, dependable connectivity, basic analytics, and clinician dash- boards while others remain limiting. Secure interoperability with EHRs is un- even, fairness and calibration across subgroups are insufficiently reported, val- idation often stops at accuracy rather than clinical utility, reimbursement and workflow integration lag and life cycle security—including provisioning, creden- tial management, and patching—requires disciplined execution.

Innovations should be judged by how directly they resolve these bottlenecks. Standardized protocols that link exposure data to physiology can turn continuous sensing into actionable risk signals. Equity-by-design trials, multilingual and low-bandwidth modes, and affordability studies convert access ideals into measurable practice. Security-as-safety demands mutual authentication, end-to- end encryption, key rotation, and verifiable update channels. Interoperability at scale requires implementing FHIR/IEEE device profiles with provenance and portable consent artifacts. Human-factors advances—alert governance, quiet hours, and just-in-time nudges—address burden and adherence. Through durability, repairability, and take-back programs sustainability aligns device lifecycles with system ethics.

From a governance perspective, use of dynamic, revocable consent and ex- plicit secondary-use limits, and monitoring equity with public subgroup perfor- mance reporting should take place. The same analytical stance should guide evaluation: for interoperability, one needs to track the proportion of messages conformant to profiles and time to integration; for security, monitoring encryp- tion coverage and median patch time; for fairness, bounding subgroup gaps in sensitivity or PPV; for workflow and reimbursement, tracking detection lead time, time-in-range, readmissions, and billable code utilization are required.

In sum, WMDs will become a core layer of learning health systems only if technical maturity is paired with trustworthy data governance, equitable design, and rigorous real-world evaluation. The next phase should prove not merely that wearables can measure, but that they reliably change clinical decisions and improve outcomes for diverse populations at sustainable cost.

REFERENCES

Ali, F., Ilyas, A., & Ahmadeen, S. (2024). Regulations in Japan. In *Global regulations of medicinal, pharmaceutical, and food products* (pp. 153–167). CRC Press.

Amaral, C., Paiva, M., Rodrigues, A. R., Veiga, F., & Bell, V. (2024). Global regulatory challenges for medical devices: Impact on innovation and market access. *Applied Sciences (Basel, Switzerland)*, *14*(20), 9304.

Bhat, G., Tuncel, Y., An, S., & Ogras, U. Y. (2019). Wearable iot devices for health monitoring. *TechConnect Briefs*, *2019*, 357–360.

Bhushan, D., & Agrawal, R. (2019). Security challenges for designing wearable and iot solutions. *A Handbook of Internet of Things in Biomedical and Cyber Physical System*. https:// api. semanticscholar. org/ CorpusID: 199003121 C¸ elik, Y. S., I˙l¸ce, E., Mesut, B., & O¨ zsoy, Y. (2024). An overview of wearable medical device applications. *Journal of Research in Pharmacy, 28* (3), 722–732.

Cook, J. ur Rehman, S., & Khan, M. A. (2023). Security and privacy for low power iot devices on 5g and beyond networks: Challenges and future directions. *IEEE Access, 11*, 39295–39317. https://api.semanticscholar. org/CorpusID:257913493

Cottle, K. E. (2017). *Current patterns of ownership and usage of mobile tech- nology in older adults*. Brigham Young University.

European Parliament and Council of the European Union. (2017). Regulation (EU) 2017/745 of the European Parliament and of the Council of 5 April 2017 on medical devices, amending directive 2001/83/EC, regulation (EC) no 178/2002 and regulation (EC) no 1223/2009 and repealing council directives 90/385/EEC and 93/42/ EEC [Accessed: 2025-07-19].

Farabolini, G., Baldini, N., Pagano, A., Andrenelli, E., Pepa, L., Morone, G., Ceravolo, M. G., & Capecci, M. (2025). Continuous movement moni- toring at home through wearable devices: A systematic review. *Sensors (Basel)*, *25*, 280949226. https://api.semanticscholar.org/CorpusID PMID: 40871752

Global Market Insights. (2024). Wearable medical devices market report [Ac- cessed: 2025-07-18].

Guk, K., Han, G., Lim, J., Jeong, K., Kang, T., Lim, E.-K., & Jung, J. (2019). Evolution of wearable devices with real-time disease monitoring for per- sonalized healthcare. *Nanomaterials (Basel, Switzerland)*, *9*(6), 813. PMID: 31146479

Ju, N., & Lee, K.-H. (2021). Perceptions and resistance to accept smart clothing: Moderating effect of consumer innovativeness. *Applied Sciences (Basel, Switzerland)*, *11*(7), 3211.

Kaewkannate, K., & Kim, S. (2016). A comparison of wearable fitness devices. *BMC Public Health*, *16*, 1–16. PMID: 27220855

K¨onig, J., Penaredondo, J., McCullagh, E., Bowen, J., & Hinze, A. (2023). Let's make it accessible: The challenges of working with low-cost com- mercially available wearable devices. *Proceedings of the 35th Australian Computer-Human Interaction Conference*. https://api.semanticscholar. org/CorpusID:269749381

Lu, L., Zhang, J., Xie, Y., Gao, F., Xu, S., Wu, X., & Ye, Z.. (2020). Wear-able health devices in health care: Narrative systematic review. *JMIR mHealth and uHealth*, *8*(11), e18907. PMID: 33164904

Saad, H. S., Zaki, J. F. W., & Abdelsalam, M. M. (2024). Employing of ma- chine learning and wearable devices in healthcare system: Tasks and challenges. *Neural Computing & Applications*, *36*, 17829–17849. https: //api.semanticscholar.org/ CorpusID:271752210

Shang, X. (2024). The current status and future trends of wearable devices. *Applied and Computational Engineering*. https://api.semanticscholar. org/CorpusID:275091019

shujie Qu & Gao, X. (2020). Analysis of ethical issues involved in wearable equipment for health care. *2020 International Conference on Public Health and Data Science (ICPHDS)*, 406–410. https:// api. semanticscholar. org/CorpusID:232072501

Spuskanyuk, A. (2024). Ethical implications of wearable digital health tech- nology: Balancing innovation and patient autonomy. *American Journal of Healthcare Strategy*. https: / / api . semanticscholar . org / CorpusID: 274972514

Straits Research. (2024). Wearable healthcare devices market report [Accessed: 2025-07-18].

Teng, X.-F., Zhang, Y.-T., Poon, C. C. Y., & Bonato, P. (2008). Wearable medical systems for p-health. *IEEE Reviews in Biomedical Engineering*, *1*, 62–74. DOI: 10.1109/RBME.2008.2008248 PMID: 22274900

U.S. Food and Drug Administration. (2025, January). [U.S. Department of Health and Human Services. Retrieved July 19, 2025]. *Medical Devices (Auckland, N.Z.)*.

Venkatachalam, S., Padmavathi, T., Vinodh, N., Thilagavathi, J., Joshi, G., Ramachandran, G., & Rajasekaran, B. (2023). Analysis of ethical is- sues associated with wearable medical devices. *2023 5th International Conference on Smart Systems and Inventive Technology (ICSSIT)*, 17– 22.

Zhu, G., Li, J., Meng, Z., Yu, Y., Li, Y., Tang, X., Dong, Y., Sun, G., Zhou, R., & Wang, H.. (2020). Learning from large-scale wearable device data for predicting the epidemic trend of covid-19. *Discrete Dynamics in Nature and Society*, *2020*(1), 6152041.

KEY TERMS AND DEFINITIONS

Artificial Intelligence (AI): Computational techniques used to analyze wearable data, enabling predictive analytics and personalized healthcare.

Chronic Disease Management: Use of wearable technology to monitor and manage long-term illnesses such as diabetes and heart disease.

Clinical Applications: Use of wearables in diagnosing, monitoring, treat- ment, and rehabilitation across medical specialties like cardiology and neurol- ogy.

Data Security: Safeguarding wearable device data against cyber threats to maintain integrity and confidentiality.

Ethical Considerations: Issues related to patient autonomy, informed con- sent, and the ethical use of personal health data from wearables.

Future Trends: Emerging advancements in wearable devices including flexible electronics, nanotechnology, and AI integration.

Healthcare: The organized provision of medical care to individuals or communities, increasingly enhanced by wearable technologies.

Interoperability: The ability of wearable devices to effectively communicate and work with other health information systems and platforms.

Market Growth: The rapidly expanding global economic value and adoption rate of wearable medical technologies in healthcare.

Privacy: Protection of sensitive personal health data collected by wearable devices from unauthorized access or misuse.

Real-time Monitoring: Continuous tracking of health indicators enabling timely clinical interventions and patient management.

Regulatory Compliance: Adherence to laws and standards set by bodies like FDA, EC, and PMDA governing safety and efficacy of WMDs.

Sensors: Miniaturized devices embedded in wearables that detect and mea- sure physiological signals like heart rate and glucose levels.

Smartwatches: Wrist-worn devices capable of tracking physical activity, heart rate, and other health metrics with connectivity features.

WMDs: Portable sensor-equipped gadgets worn on the body to monitor health parameters continuously or intermittently.

Chapter 2
Securing Healthcare IoT: AI Threat Detection, Data Privacy, and Regulatory Frameworks

Mayur Jariwala
https://orcid.org/0009-0008-1686-8791
University of the Cumberlands, Williamsburg, USA

Yathaarth Jariwala
https://orcid.org/0009-0006-6752-0969
University of Colorado, Boulder, USA

ABSTRACT

This chapter examines the convergence of healthcare IoT, artificial intelligence, and data privacy within modern connected care systems. It explores how the Internet of Medical Things (IoMT) enables continuous monitoring through wearable devices and cloud platforms while introducing complex cybersecurity and regulatory challenges. The discussion highlights AI-driven threat detection, explainable and privacy-preserving models, and the use of federated learning and blockchain for secure data sharing. It also reviews global frameworks such as HIPAA, GDPR, and emerging AI regulations, emphasizing transparency, accountability, and patient trust. Finally, it outlines best practices and future policy directions aimed at achieving resilient, ethical, and compliant healthcare innovation in an increasingly digital and data-driven environment.

DOI: 10.4018/979-8-3373-4412-6.ch002

1. INTRODUCTION

1.1 Overview of Healthcare IoT and Wearable Medical Technologies

The Internet of Medical Things brings together sensors, wearables, medical devices, mobile apps, and clinical systems to create continuous data loops between patients, providers, and platforms. What began as simple consumer fitness bands has matured into clinically oriented wearables that monitor cardiac rhythm, glucose, oxygen saturation, sleep quality, activity, and medication adherence. Many devices now support bidirectional workflows, not only reporting data but also enabling remote adjustments to therapy and alerts to care teams. This networked model supports preventive care, early intervention, and individualized treatment pathways. As these capabilities expand, so does the volume, velocity, and variety of data moving across homes, clinics, and cloud services. That growth introduces technical complexity and governance responsibilities that healthcare organizations cannot ignore.

1.2 Importance of Cybersecurity and Patient Data Protection

Security in this context is not only about protecting files. It safeguards clinical continuity and patient safety. A compromised wearable can generate false readings, delay care, or enable unauthorized access to clinical portals. Healthcare environments also carry unique operational constraints such as legacy systems, vendor dependencies, and round-the-clock operations that make routine patching difficult.(Ahmed et al.., 2024) Protecting data therefore requires layered controls at the device, network, application, and cloud levels, supported by strong identity, segmentation, encryption, monitoring, and incident response. It also requires appropriate policies, procurement standards, and staff training so human error does not undermine technical defenses. Privacy sits alongside security as a first-order requirement because health data is deeply sensitive and can have lasting personal consequences if mishandled.

1.3 The Intersection of AI Technologies and Regulatory Frameworks

Artificial intelligence is increasingly central to healthcare cyber defense (Messinis, & Temenos, 2024).. Models that learn normal behavior can flag unusual traffic, device states, or user actions faster than traditional, rules-only approaches. These capabilities are well suited to high-volume telemetry from wearables and gateways. Yet AI systems rely on continuous data flows, model updates, and sometimes opaque decision paths. Privacy and regulatory obligations require that data uses are limited, access is controlled, and outcomes are explainable enough to be audited. This creates a design challenge: capture the benefits of algorithmic detection while honoring consent, minimization, transparency, and accountability. The solutions are as much architectural and procedural as they are algorithmic.

1.4 Structure and Objectives of the Chapter

This chapter provides a practical roadmap for securing healthcare IoT while aligning with privacy and regulatory expectations. Section 2 describes the IoMT ecosystem and the threat landscape across devices, networks, and cloud services. Section 3 examines how AI supports anomaly detection and response, including model choices and deployment realities. Section 4 reviews major privacy and regulatory regimes relevant to healthcare data and connected devices. Section 5 bridges AI capabilities with compliance needs through governance, explainability, and impact assessment. Section 6 presents privacy-preserving and secure architectural patterns that support real-time care. Section 7 offers case examples and distilled best practices. Section 8 looks ahead to emerging regulations and technology trends. Section 9 closes with key takeaways and a call for coordinated action among technologists, clinicians, and regulators. The objective is simple: enable trustworthy, resilient, and compliant connected care.

2. HEALTHCARE IOT ECOSYSTEM AND THREAT LANDSCAPE

2.1 Healthcare IoT Ecosystem Overview

The healthcare Internet of Things (IoT) ecosystem operates as a complex and interdependent network that involves multiple stakeholders working in continuous coordination. Device manufacturers design and certify medical sensors, wearables, and implantables that collect physiological data. Hospital IT departments integrate these devices with local area networks and clinical applications while maintaining access control and network segmentation. Cloud service providers host analytical platforms and large-scale data lakes used for storage, federated learning, and predictive modeling. Telecommunication companies ensure secure and reliable connectivity through mobile, Wi-Fi, and edge gateways optimized for low latency and data integrity. Regulatory authorities such as the FDA, EMA, and data-protection agencies define certification, compliance, and monitoring frameworks that govern the entire data flow. Together, these actors form a dynamic digital health ecosystem that connects the physical patient environment with virtual clinical intelligence systems while demanding continuous alignment between innovation and compliance.

2.2 Components of IoMT and Data Communication Architecture

The Internet of Medical Things (IoMT) ecosystem connects sensors, wearables, gateways, hospital networks, and cloud infrastructures into a continuous flow of physiological and operational data. At the edge are patient-side devices, smart watches, adhesive patches, implantable monitors, infusion pumps, and home-care hubs, that capture biological signals and environmental conditions. These devices transmit data via short-range links such as Bluetooth Low Energy or Zigbee to smartphones, routers, or dedicated medical gateways. The gateways perform initial filtering and encryption before sending packets to hospital servers or commercial cloud platforms over Wi-Fi, 4G, or emerging 5G networks.

Within the healthcare enterprise, middleware applications receive this data and integrate it with electronic health record (EHR) systems (Ahmed et al., 2024). Application programming interfaces (APIs) facilitate secure data sharing among laboratories, diagnostic imaging centers, and remote specialists. Analytics engines and dashboards visualize patient trends, trigger alerts, or automate treatment decisions. Supporting all of this are identity-management services, certificate authorities, and network-segmentation tools that keep different medical subsystems isolated. The resulting architecture is multilayered: device layer, communication layer, cloud layer, and application layer. Each layer contributes unique functionality yet also introduces its own potential vulnerabilities if not adequately protected or continuously monitored.

2.3 Common Vulnerabilities in Wearable Devices and Medical Networks

The most persistent weaknesses in IoMT arise from design trade-offs that favor usability and battery life over security. Many wearables operate on constrained hardware that limits the implementation of complex encryption or multifactor authentication. Default passwords, outdated firmware, and insecure update mechanisms are still common. Communication links may rely on outdated cryptographic protocols or lack mutual authentication between device and gateway.

Table 1. IoMT Threat Mitigation Matrix

Threat/Weakness	Impact	Primary Mitigations	Where Implemented
Weak BLE pairing	Data tampering, spoofing	Authenticated pairing, LE Secure Connections, key rotation	Device, mobile app
Default creds/ legacy OS	Pivoting, ransomware	Password vaulting, MFA, network isolation, VDI	Device, network
API exposure	PHI exfiltration	OAuth2/OIDC, rate limiting, WAF, API inventory	App, cloud
Model poisoning/ drift	Missed attacks	Data validation, canary models, drift alarms	AI pipeline
Supply-chain vuln	Backdoor risk	SBOM, signed firmware, secure boot, vendor SLAs	Device, procurement
Misconfig cloud storage	Public PHI	CIS benchmarks, encryption, continuous config scan	Cloud

At the network level, hospitals often connect hundreds of devices through shared Wi-Fi or VLAN segments, making lateral movement easy for an attacker once any node is compromised. Legacy medical equipment running unsupported operating systems cannot receive patches, leaving exploitable vulnerabilities. Poor segmentation between administrative and clinical networks amplifies the risk. Cloud platforms, though robust, can also become weak points if misconfigured storage buckets or over-permissive access keys expose sensitive health data. Human factors play a reinforcing role, untrained staff may connect personal devices to hospital networks or overlook phishing attempts that deliver malware payloads.

Because IoMT devices frequently exchange data through standardized protocols such as HL7 and FHIR, attackers can exploit predictable message structures for injection or replay attacks. The cumulative effect is an ecosystem where physical safety and digital integrity are intertwined. A successful compromise can corrupt sensor readings, disable alarms, or even alter therapeutic commands. The diversity of vendors and lack of uniform certification further complicate coordinated defenses across the supply chain.

2.4 Case Examples of Healthcare Cybersecurity Breaches

Real-world incidents illustrate the fragility of interconnected medical environments. Large hospital networks have faced ransomware that encrypted not only patient records but also disabled scheduling and diagnostic systems, forcing the cancellation of surgeries and delaying emergency care. Smaller clinics relying on third-party telehealth applications have seen unauthorized data exposure through misconfigured cloud storage or unsecured APIs.

In several high-profile cases, researchers demonstrated the ability to intercept wireless traffic from insulin pumps and pacemakers, proving that medical devices could be manipulated remotely if encryption keys were weak or firmware lacked signature validation. Although such attacks were ethical demonstrations, they revealed pathways that could be exploited by malicious actors. Breaches involving fitness-tracking platforms and genetic-testing companies have also drawn attention to the secondary use of health data by advertisers and data brokers.

The consequences of these events extend beyond financial loss. Patients lose confidence in digital care, regulators impose heavy penalties, and recovery costs strain already limited healthcare budgets. Restoring integrity after a breach often requires months of forensic analysis, reconfiguration, and compliance reporting. These cases underline that cybersecurity in healthcare is inseparable from clinical reliability and organizational reputation.

2.5 Emerging Threats in Connected and Real-Time Health Environments

As healthcare embraces real-time analytics, cloud computing, and artificial intelligence, threat vectors continue to evolve (Chatterjee et al., 2023). One growing risk is the compromise of AI models themselves through data poisoning or adversarial inputs that manipulate diagnostic outcomes. Attackers can subtly alter training data or introduce crafted signals that mislead algorithms used for anomaly detection or patient triage. Edge-based processing adds convenience but also widens exposure; if an edge node is breached, it can leak locally cached medical data before synchronization with the cloud.

The migration toward 5G and software-defined networks introduces complexity in virtualized infrastructure management. Misconfigured network slices or insecure orchestration APIs could expose sensitive telemetry streams. Supply-chain threats are another concern, malicious code inserted during firmware development or hardware manufacturing can remain dormant until activated in production environments.

Social engineering remains a persistent and adaptive danger. Phishing campaigns tailored for clinical personnel exploit urgency and trust to harvest credentials or deploy ransomware. Deepfake audio and voice-spoofing technologies can deceive help-desk staff or override verbal verification processes. Meanwhile, geopolitical tensions have expanded the scope of state-sponsored attacks targeting healthcare research and vaccine data.

Figure 1. AI-Enabled IoMT Security Architecture

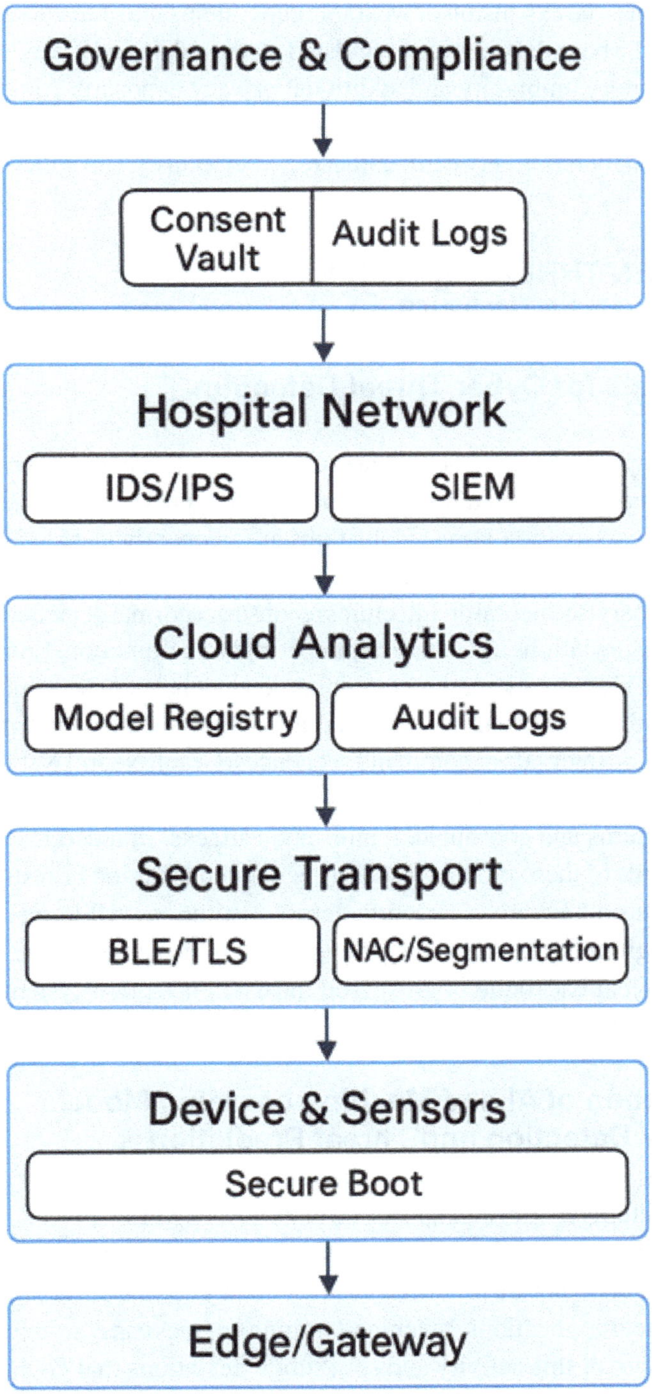

Emerging technologies such as quantum computing may soon challenge existing cryptographic standards, necessitating a transition to quantum-resistant algorithms. At the same time, the expansion of wearable ecosystems into consumer and wellness markets blurs the boundary between regulated medical data and lifestyle information, creating regulatory ambiguity and additional privacy exposure. Anticipating these future threats requires adaptive defense architectures, continuous monitoring, and cross-sector collaboration between healthcare, cybersecurity, and policy communities.

3. AI-DRIVEN THREAT DETECTION IN HEALTHCARE NETWORKS

3.1 AI Models for Cyber Threat Detection

AI-driven cybersecurity in healthcare relies on a wide spectrum of model families that analyze network, behavioral, and contextual data to detect anomalies and malicious activities. Isolation Forest algorithms are frequently used to identify outlier behaviors in medical network traffic without relying on labeled data. Autoencoders and other unsupervised neural architectures reconstruct normal device communication patterns to flag deviations indicative of tampering or malfunction. Long Short-Term Memory (LSTM) networks model temporal dependencies in streaming telemetry, allowing real-time detection of sequential anomalies such as abnormal heart-rate data transmission intervals or command sequences. Graph Neural Networks (GNNs) represent hospital communication flows as connected graphs to expose lateral-movement patterns and coordinated multi-node attacks. In federated or distributed settings, variants of these models—such as Federated Isolation Forests or Federated LSTMs-enable collaborative detection across institutions while maintaining data privacy through encrypted parameter aggregation. Together, these architectures form the technical backbone of AI-driven intrusion detection systems tailored for the Internet of Medical Things.

3.2 Application of AI and Machine-Learning Models in Anomaly Detection and Threat Prediction

Artificial intelligence brings speed and pattern-recognition power that traditional rule-based security systems cannot match. Within hospital or cloud environments, thousands of data points are produced each second by connected devices, logs, gateways, and clinical applications. Machine-learning engines can continuously learn the "normal" rhythm of this activity and spot subtle deviations that could signal intrusion, misconfiguration, or internal misuse. In healthcare settings, where latency and accuracy can decide patient outcomes, AI enables near-real-time decision-making: it correlates network behavior with device telemetry to isolate infected endpoints or block abnormal traffic automatically.

Figure 2. AI Threat Detection and Response Flow

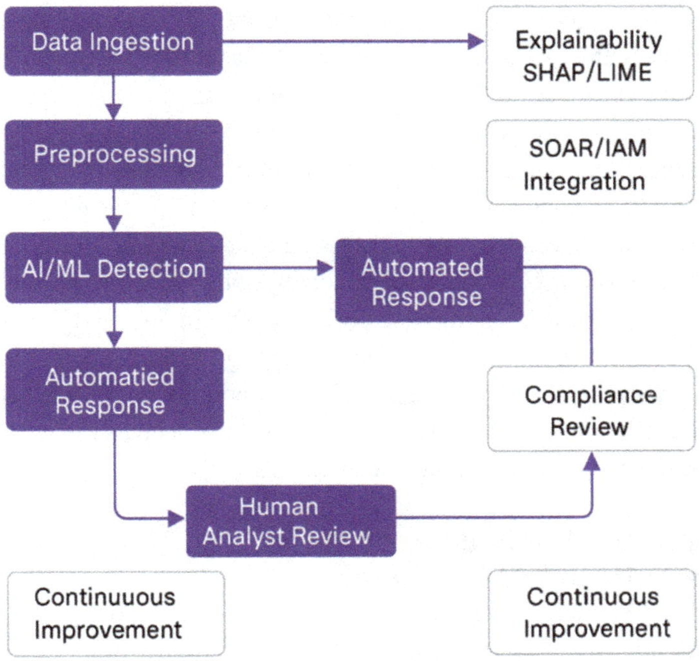

Anomaly detection uses unsupervised learning to create behavioral baselines, while supervised models trained on historical incidents can classify known attack signatures. Predictive algorithms combine both approaches, mapping early indicators such as failed authentications, unusual data transfers, or time-based anomalies to anticipate breaches before damage occurs. Natural-language-processing tools are even used to scan clinical emails and vendor correspondence to flag potential phishing patterns. Together these systems turn the immense data volume of healthcare operations into actionable intelligence, shifting defense from reactive containment to proactive prevention.

3.3 Types of AI Models Used: Supervised, Unsupervised, and Federated

Supervised learning depends on labeled data, records of previous attacks or benign activity, to train classifiers such as decision trees, random forests, or neural networks. In contrast, unsupervised techniques like clustering, autoencoders, or isolation forests discover anomalies without pre-labeled samples, which is crucial when new threats emerge faster than analysts can label them. Reinforcement learning further refines detection by rewarding models that minimize false alerts while maintaining sensitivity to genuine threats.

Healthcare introduces an additional constraint: data sensitivity and regulatory boundaries often restrict centralized training. Federated learning addresses this limitation by allowing models to train across multiple hospitals or devices without sharing raw patient data. Each node learns locally and only transmits model updates, preserving privacy while strengthening collective intelligence. Edge-based learning extends this concept to wearable devices, enabling threat recognition directly on gateways or smartphones. Hybrid approaches, combining centralized cloud analytics with federated or edge refinement, are increasingly seen as the optimal path for balancing performance, privacy, and compliance.

3.4 Benefits and Limitations of AI-Based Security in IoMT Systems

The main advantage of AI in medical-device security lies in scalability and adaptability. A single model can monitor millions of transactions or device states simultaneously, adjusting its thresholds as behaviors evolve. It can also link technical signals with clinical context: for example, differentiating between an abnormal data spike caused by an equipment malfunction and one triggered by a cyberattack. Automation reduces dependency on scarce security staff and shortens incident-response times.

However, these systems are not infallible. They can generate false positives that overwhelm analysts or interrupt legitimate care workflows. Models trained on biased or incomplete datasets might overlook novel threats or misclassify normal activities. Adversaries can exploit these weaknesses through "adversarial" inputs, subtle manipulations that trick algorithms into misjudging malicious traffic as harmless. Another limitation is explainability. Clinicians and regulators need transparent reasoning when an AI system blocks access to a ventilator control or patient portal; opaque neural-network decisions may create legal and ethical complications. Continuous monitoring, retraining, and human oversight remain necessary to ensure reliability and accountability.

3.5 Deployment Challenges in Clinical Settings

Translating AI security research into hospital operations reveals a different reality from laboratory prototypes. Many clinical networks contain a mix of modern and legacy systems, with proprietary device protocols that make standardized data collection difficult. Integrating AI sensors or log agents into such environments requires coordination with multiple vendors and compliance audits that slow deployment. Limited compute capacity on medical devices restricts on-board analytics, pushing inference to gateways or the cloud, which introduces latency and potential exposure during data transit.

Another barrier is trust. Clinical staff often hesitate to rely on automated systems that could interfere with patient treatment if they malfunction. Regulatory approval processes for medical-grade software further extend timelines. Hospitals also face cost constraints, AI tools demand skilled personnel, storage, and ongoing model maintenance. To succeed, deployment must align with hospital governance structures: pilot projects should begin with non-critical monitoring, build confidence through measurable results, and gradually extend into mission-critical operations. Collaboration between IT, biomedical engineering, and clinical leadership is essential to align priorities and manage change.

3.6 Use Cases and Real-World Implementations

Across the world, healthcare organizations are experimenting with AI-enhanced security platforms tailored to their risk profiles. Large hospital networks deploy centralized monitoring centers that aggregate telemetry from infusion pumps, imaging equipment, and administrative systems into unified dashboards. AI algorithms prioritize alerts and recommend containment actions, allowing analysts to focus on verified incidents rather than thousands of routine events. Smaller clinics adopt cloud-hosted services that analyze device behavior using anonymized threat-intelligence feeds. These services continuously update detection rules based on global trends and share learnings across institutions.

In research hospitals, predictive-maintenance models detect signs of tampering or impending failure in connected scanners or laboratory instruments, preventing downtime and potential data corruption (Ahmed et al., 2024). Some telehealth providers embed lightweight AI agents in mobile apps that evaluate communication patterns to detect credential theft or session hijacking. Governments and industry groups are also establishing testbeds where anonymized datasets from multiple hospitals are used to train federated threat-detection frameworks. These initiatives illustrate that AI security in healthcare is not a distant vision but a growing operational reality. Yet success depends on disciplined governance, clear data-handling policies, transparent algorithms, and continuous validation to ensure that protection enhances rather than disrupts patient care.

4. GLOBAL DATA PRIVACY AND REGULATORY FRAMEWORKS

4.1 Overview of Key Regulations: HIPAA (USA), GDPR (EU), DPDPA (India), and PIPEDA (Canada)

Data privacy frameworks form the foundation upon which secure healthcare technology must operate. Each region has developed its own legal standards reflecting cultural expectations, constitutional principles, and historical approaches to personal rights. In the United States, the Health Insurance Portability and Accountability Act (HIPAA) serves as the cornerstone for protecting health information. It defines protected health information, establishes safeguards for its use and disclosure, and assigns compliance responsibilities to healthcare entities and their partners. Messinis, & Temenos (2024) synthesized that HIPAA's Security Rule focuses on administrative, technical, and physical safeguards, while the Privacy Rule governs how data can be accessed, shared, or stored. The act also mandates breach notifications and penalties for noncompliance, placing accountability on covered entities and their business associates (Said et. al., 2023).

In Europe, the General Data Protection Regulation (GDPR) sets a broader and more stringent benchmark for data protection. It treats health information as a special category of personal data, subject to enhanced protections and explicit consent. GDPR is extraterritorial, meaning that any organization handling data of EU residents must comply regardless of location. It establishes rights such as access, rectification, portability, and erasure, along with the right not to be subject to automated decision-making without meaningful human oversight. The regulation encourages privacy by design and by default, obligating data controllers to integrate safeguards throughout the system lifecycle.

India's Digital Personal Data Protection Act (DPDPA) represents a newer approach shaped by the global regulatory environment. It balances innovation with individual privacy rights and introduces obligations for data fiduciaries and processors. The DPDPA emphasizes lawful processing, purpose limitation, and accountability, supported by a Data Protection Board for oversight. Its enactment positions India as an emerging digital health leader while aligning with global expectations for cross-border data transfers.

Table 2. Comparison of Global Health Data Regulations

Framework	Scope in Healthcare	Key Rights/ Obligations	Cross-Border Transfer	AI-Specific Notes
HIPAA (US)	PHI, covered entities & BAs	Minimum necessary, safeguards, breach notice	BAAs; no adequacy regime	Audit controls, access logs expected
GDPR (EU)	Special category data	Lawful basis, DPIA, DPO, rights to access/erase/port	SCCs, adequacy, BCRs	Art. 22 automated decisions, transparency
DPDPA (India)	Digital personal data	Consent, purpose limitation, grievance redressal	Govt. notified countries, conditions	Accountability of "Data Fiduciary"
PIPEDA (Canada)	Private sector personal data	10 fair principles, consent, safeguards	Contractual safeguards	Guidance evolving for AI explainability
NIS2 (EU)	Essential entities security	Risk mgmt., incident reporting	N/A	Security obligations affect health infra
EU AI Act (EU)	High-risk AI incl. health	Risk mgmt., data quality, logging, human oversight	N/A	Conformity assessment, post-market monitoring

Canada's Personal Information Protection and Electronic Documents Act (PIPEDA) provides yet another perspective. It is principle-based rather than prescriptive, granting organizations flexibility in implementation while requiring accountability and transparency. PIPEDA outlines ten fair information principles, covering consent, limiting collection, accuracy, safeguards, and access. These frameworks, though diverse in legal philosophy, share a common goal: to protect individuals from misuse of sensitive information in an increasingly connected world.

4.2 Regulatory Principles: Consent, Data Minimization, and Rights of the Data Subject

Across global frameworks, several common principles anchor privacy protection. The first is informed consent, which requires that individuals understand and voluntarily agree to the collection and use of their personal data. In healthcare, consent is more complex because patients often lack full awareness of how digital systems function or how their data might be analyzed by third-party algorithms. Regulatory frameworks attempt to mitigate this imbalance by mandating clear language, purpose specification, and the option to withdraw consent without losing access to care.

Data minimization is another key requirement. Organizations must collect only the information necessary to achieve a defined medical purpose and retain it only as long as required. In IoMT ecosystems, this principle challenges designers to filter redundant telemetry and anonymize identifiers as early as possible in the data flow. Effective minimization reduces both privacy risk and system overhead. It also aligns sustainability goals by limiting storage and processing demands.

The rights of the data subject extend protection beyond consent. Individuals have the right to access their data, correct inaccuracies, restrict processing, or demand deletion under specific conditions. They can also request data portability, enabling interoperability among healthcare providers. These rights strengthen patient autonomy and trust, promoting transparency across digital health systems. For organizations, compliance requires responsive data-governance procedures, robust authentication mechanisms, and clearly documented workflows to manage data-subject requests efficiently.

Another emerging principle is algorithmic accountability. Regulators increasingly emphasize that when automated systems influence clinical or administrative outcomes, their logic must be explainable and auditable. This expectation reinforces the connection between AI innovation and legal compliance discussed earlier. Collectively, these principles redefine healthcare from a data-centric enterprise to a rights-centric one, where technology serves individuals rather than exploiting their information.

4.3 Compliance Implications for Wearable Device Ecosystems

The proliferation of wearable medical devices introduces new complexity into the enforcement of privacy regulations. Unlike traditional healthcare systems confined to hospital networks, wearable data flows through multiple intermediaries, including device manufacturers, mobile platforms, telecommunications providers, and analytics vendors (Bhalavat et. al., 2024). Determining which party qualifies as a data controller or processor under each jurisdiction becomes a critical compliance question. For example, a smartwatch manufacturer may be subject to GDPR obligations when processing European users' data, even if the company operates outside the European Union.

Ensuring compliance within this distributed environment requires coordinated technical and contractual safeguards. Devices must include secure data storage, encryption, and user authentication features Ghosh & Ghosh, 2023). Cloud services must adhere to contractual clauses defining roles, responsibilities, and breach notification procedures. Data flows should be mapped end to end to identify where personal information resides and which jurisdiction's laws apply. Privacy impact assessments should be conducted before deploying new features that expand data use or integrate AI components.

(Bhalavat et. al., 2024) found another challenge that involves balancing usability with regulatory restrictions. Users expect convenience, real-time feedback, and cross-platform compatibility, while regulators demand explicit consent and limited data transfer. Manufacturers must design systems that embed privacy-preserving defaults without degrading functionality. This may include local processing on the device, edge computing for preliminary analysis, or aggregation methods that remove identifiers before data enters the cloud. Healthcare organizations deploying such devices must maintain updated inventories, assign data-protection officers, and verify vendor compliance through audits or certifications. These measures collectively establish a chain of trust across the wearable ecosystem.

4.4 Cross-Border Data Transfer and Localization Issues

Healthcare data seldom stays within national borders. Cloud hosting, telemedicine services, and multinational research collaborations depend on global data exchange. Regulations therefore impose varying conditions on cross-border transfers. Under GDPR, transfers to non-EU countries are permitted only if adequate safeguards exist, such as standard contractual clauses or recognized adequacy decisions. HIPAA permits sharing with overseas partners only through business associate agreements that meet equivalent security standards. India's DPDPA and several Asian frameworks have begun introducing localization requirements, requiring certain categories of sensitive data to remain within domestic boundaries.

For healthcare providers and technology companies, compliance with these provisions is both a legal and logistical challenge. Data must be classified according to sensitivity, stored in compliant regions, and transmitted through encrypted channels. Multinational organizations often adopt a hybrid strategy, maintaining regional data centers to satisfy local rules while synchronizing anonymized or aggregated data for global analytics. This model reduces latency and risk but increases infrastructure costs.

Localization laws also raise broader questions about innovation and equity. Restricting data movement may protect national sovereignty but can slow scientific progress, particularly in genomics, epidemiology, and AI-based disease modeling that rely on diverse datasets. Policymakers are exploring balanced approaches, such as federated research frameworks, where algorithms travel to the data rather than transferring raw information. These methods preserve privacy and compliance while enabling cross-border collaboration (Anant & Prasad, 2024).

For wearable technology vendors, understanding and adapting to these differing regulatory landscapes is essential. Products must be configurable to regional requirements, allowing local storage options or flexible consent settings. Clear communication with users regarding where their data resides and how it is processed builds trust and reduces legal exposure. Ultimately, successful compliance across borders depends not only on technology but also on governance, consistent documentation, transparent communication, and continual monitoring of regulatory changes worldwide.

5. ALIGNING AI SYSTEMS WITH REGULATORY COMPLIANCE

5.1 Challenges of AI Transparency, Fairness, and Accountability

Artificial intelligence introduces both immense capability and profound responsibility into healthcare security operations. The ability of algorithms to analyze millions of data points in seconds makes them powerful tools for identifying patterns invisible to human analysts. Yet this same power raises concerns about transparency, fairness, and accountability. Healthcare decisions, even when indirectly influenced by AI, must remain explainable to clinicians, auditors, and patients. When models operate as opaque "black boxes," stakeholders cannot easily determine how conclusions were reached or whether they are accurate (Jain,2024).

This opacity becomes more problematic when AI models manage or restrict access to patient data. A false alert that blocks a clinician's login or delays data synchronization could interrupt treatment. Regulators therefore expect organizations to demonstrate not only technical accuracy but also explainability and oversight. The challenge intensifies as healthcare AI systems increasingly rely on complex deep-learning architectures that resist human interpretation. Designing explainable interfaces, maintaining detailed audit trails, and documenting data lineage become critical for compliance.

Fairness represents another dimension of accountability. AI models trained on biased or incomplete datasets may favor certain patient groups while misclassifying others. In cybersecurity contexts, bias may emerge in risk scoring, where certain devices, users, or behaviors are flagged more aggressively than others without justification. To maintain trust, developers must validate models using diverse datasets, publish performance metrics, and implement governance processes for periodic bias testing. Achieving transparency, fairness, and accountability simultaneously requires technical rigor and institutional commitment. These principles ensure that AI-driven defenses support rather than undermine the ethical foundations of healthcare.

5.2 Use of Explainable AI in Regulated Healthcare Environments

Explainable artificial intelligence (XAI) bridges the gap between model complexity and human understanding. It enables users to visualize how features contribute to a prediction and to verify whether decisions align with policy requirements. In healthcare security, XAI helps compliance officers evaluate whether automated actions, such as isolating a device or blocking a data transfer, are justified. Visualization tools like heat maps, feature-importance charts, and decision paths transform abstract machine-learning logic into interpretable evidence (Chintoh et al., 2024).

Explainability also supports legal defensibility. If a regulatory authority investigates an incident or data breach, the organization must be able to show how an AI system operated, which inputs it considered, and why specific alerts were triggered or ignored. Transparent documentation reduces uncertainty and demonstrates diligence. From a clinical perspective, interpretability reassures staff that AI tools are allies rather than opaque monitors.

Implementing XAI in practice involves trade-offs between accuracy and interpretability. Simple models such as decision trees are easier to explain but may lack predictive power, while deep neural networks offer high accuracy with minimal transparency. Hybrid models combine both: an interpretable layer for regulatory reporting and a complex layer for internal detection. Developers must also ensure that explanations are meaningful for nontechnical users. An effective XAI implementation focuses on clarity, relevance, and accessibility of insights, aligning with the ethical imperative to keep humans in control of automated systems.

5.3 Privacy-by-Design and Security-by-Design in AI Development

Privacy-by-design and security-by-design are complementary philosophies that embed protection principles from the earliest stages of system development. Instead of treating compliance as an afterthought, these approaches require developers to integrate safeguards into every design decision. In AI-driven healthcare systems, privacy-by-design begins with data minimization, consent management, and controlled access. It extends to anonymization techniques that prevent the re-identification of individuals, even when datasets are combined.

According to Aunugu & Vathsavai (2022) security-by-design adds resilience through layered defense mechanisms, encryption, and continuous verification. Developers evaluate attack surfaces created by APIs, data pipelines, and model outputs. They implement secure coding practices, input validation, and signed model deployment to prevent tampering. Integrating both philosophies ensures that the same architecture addressing cybersecurity also satisfies regulatory privacy expectations.

During the model-training phase, privacy-preserving computation methods such as differential privacy or federated learning can protect sensitive data without sacrificing analytical performance. Documentation should record design choices, risk assessments, and mitigation strategies. This documentation is not merely bureaucratic; it serves as demonstrable proof of compliance. Organizations adopting privacy- and security-by-design gain a competitive advantage by simplifying audits and building stakeholder trust. The result is a more robust and ethically aligned AI ecosystem where innovation and protection advance together.

5.4 Legal Audit Readiness and Regulatory Impact Assessments

Regulatory compliance is not static; it evolves alongside technology and policy. Healthcare institutions and technology vendors must therefore maintain continuous audit readiness. Legal audit readiness means that the organization can produce complete, verifiable evidence of compliance activities at any time. This includes access logs, consent records, risk assessments, and explanations for automated decisions. Maintaining centralized compliance dashboards allows security and legal teams to monitor key indicators, identify anomalies, and prepare for regulatory inquiries without delay.

Regulatory impact assessments (RIAs) play a vital role in anticipating compliance challenges before deployment. These assessments evaluate potential legal, ethical, and operational consequences of new AI applications. For example, an RIA for an AI-based intrusion detection system would examine how the model processes personal data, whether its decisions can be explained, and how false positives might affect healthcare operations. Conducting RIAs early prevents costly redesigns and strengthens confidence among regulators and partners.

Effective audit preparation also depends on cross-functional collaboration. Legal teams must understand technical controls, while engineers must grasp the intent behind regulatory obligations. Clear communication and shared documentation frameworks bridge these worlds. Training programs for AI developers, clinicians, and compliance officers ensure that everyone understands their role in maintaining legal conformity. Finally, periodic external audits and penetration tests confirm the reliability of controls and validate organizational claims. Consistent audit readiness demonstrates maturity, transparency, and respect for both patients and regulators.

6. PRIVACY-PRESERVING AI AND SECURE DATA ARCHITECTURES

6.1 Techniques: Differential Privacy, Anonymization, and Pseudonymization

Protecting privacy in AI-enabled healthcare systems begins with controlling the information that leaves its source. Differential privacy introduces controlled statistical noise into datasets so that individual records cannot be identified, even when combined with other data sources. This technique allows analysts to extract aggregate trends without exposing any one patient's contribution. For example, a hospital may release infection-rate statistics or training data for a research model while ensuring that no single patient record can be reconstructed (Sharma & Yadav, 2024).

Anonymization removes identifiers entirely, converting personal health records into de-identified datasets suitable for analytics. It requires careful review because advanced re-identification methods can sometimes link anonymized data back to individuals. Pseudonymization provides a practical balance: direct identifiers are replaced by coded references, and the decoding key is stored separately under strict access control. This enables legitimate follow-up studies or clinical audits while protecting patient identity during processing.

Together, these techniques underpin privacy compliance across global frameworks. When applied systematically within data pipelines, they reduce both legal exposure and ethical risk. Their success depends on disciplined governance, clear definitions of what constitutes personal data, policies for key management, and continuous evaluation of re-identification risks as technology evolves.

6.2 Secure AI Pipelines Using Federated Learning and Edge Computing

Traditional machine-learning models require centralizing large volumes of sensitive data, which can conflict with privacy regulations. Federated learning offers an alternative by training models directly on local devices or institutional servers. Each participant computes model updates based on its own data and sends only the learned parameters to a coordinating server. The central system aggregates these updates to produce a global model without ever accessing raw patient information.

In healthcare, this approach allows multiple hospitals or clinics to collaborate on AI development without violating data-localization or consent restrictions. It also improves representativeness, since models learn from diverse populations while maintaining local sovereignty over data. Combining federated learning with differential privacy further minimizes the risk of information leakage through model gradients

Figure 3. Federated Learning Workflow for Healthcare IoT

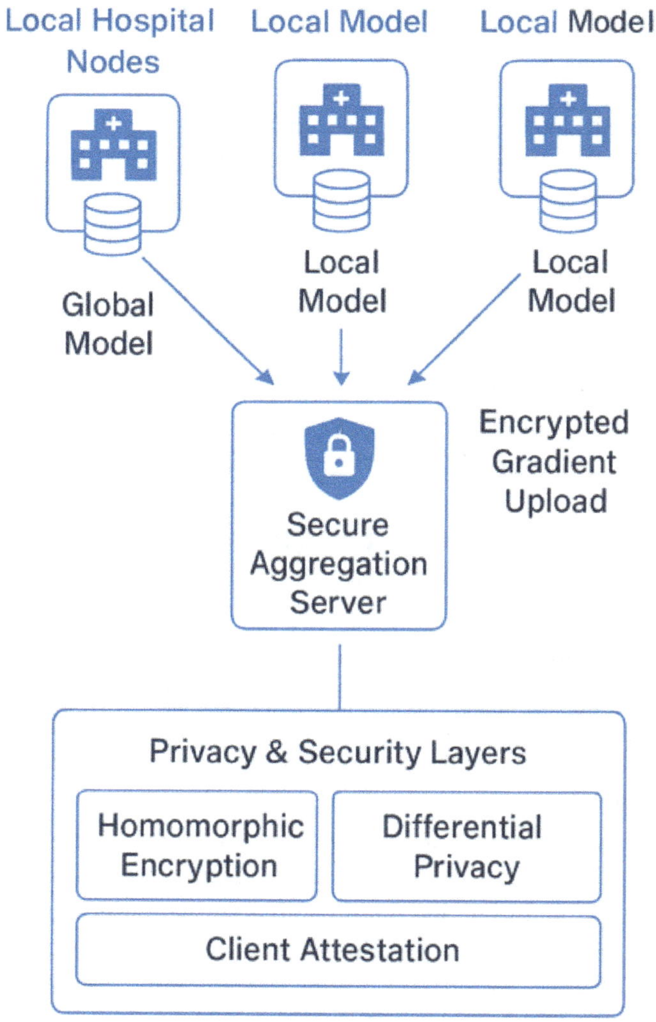

Telaprolu (2024) explained that edge computing extends privacy preservation to the network's outer layer. Processing at the device or gateway level reduces the need to transmit full datasets to the cloud, lowering latency and exposure. For wearable devices, local inference means that sensitive biometric data can be analyzed in real time, and only anonymized summaries or alerts are transmitted. These distributed architectures embody the principle of data minimization in action. They do, however, require robust synchronization protocols, version control for model updates, and mechanisms to detect malicious nodes that might inject corrupted parameters.

6.3 Blockchain-Based Auditing for Healthcare Data Integrity

Blockchain technology contributes an immutable layer of accountability to healthcare information systems. Each transaction, whether a data access request, an AI-model update, or a device event, is recorded as a cryptographically secured block linked to the previous one. Because the ledger is distributed across participants, no single party can alter records unilaterally.

In a healthcare context, blockchain supports audit trails that verify who accessed which patient data and under what authorization. This transparency deters misuse and simplifies compliance verification during regulatory reviews. Smart contracts can automate consent management by enforcing patient preferences before data is shared or processed. For example, a consent rule embedded in the blockchain can automatically deny a research query that lacks proper authorization or exceeds the approved time frame (Farooqi et. al., 2024).

While blockchain does not solve every security problem, it strengthens trust among stakeholders. Its decentralized nature aligns with the federated models discussed earlier, enabling secure collaboration without central intermediaries. Scalability, transaction cost, and interoperability with existing hospital information systems remain implementation challenges, but pilot projects in medical supply chains, clinical trials, and telemedicine continue to refine workable models. The overarching benefit lies in traceability and proof of integrity, attributes essential for regulatory confidence and patient trust.

6.4 Secure Communication Protocols and End-to-End Encryption in IoMT

Data protection within the Internet of Medical Things depends heavily on secure communication across its diverse components. End-to-end encryption ensures that information remains confidential from the moment it leaves a wearable sensor until it reaches an authorized system. Using contemporary encryption standards such as AES or TLS, devices can safeguard transmissions against interception or tampering. Mutual authentication between endpoints verifies that both sender and receiver are legitimate participants in the exchange.

Network segmentation and virtual private networks isolate medical traffic from general corporate networks. This separation minimizes the likelihood that a compromise in administrative systems could reach clinical devices. Continuous key-rotation policies, secure certificate management, and hardware-based encryption modules strengthen defenses further. For low-power wearables, lightweight cryptography optimized for constrained environments helps maintain efficiency without sacrificing protection.

Beyond encryption, monitoring plays an equally vital role. Intrusion-detection sensors positioned along network gateways analyze patterns for anomalies, while AI-driven analytics correlate these findings with contextual data to identify potential breaches. Secure-boot processes confirm the integrity of device firmware at startup, preventing the execution of unauthorized code. Combined, these measures create layered protection that upholds confidentiality, integrity, and availability, the classic triad of information security, throughout the IoMT ecosystem.

7. IMPLEMENTATION CASE STUDIES AND BEST PRACTICES

7.1 Case Study 1: HealthGuard – Machine-Learning Framework for Smart Healthcare Systems

The HealthGuard project demonstrates how artificial intelligence can serve as a defensive mechanism for next-generation healthcare environments. Developed as a security framework for Smart Healthcare Systems, HealthGuard monitors vital signs collected from multiple connected devices and correlates these readings to identify potential malicious activity (Newaz et al., 2019). The model integrates several machine-learning techniques, including artificial neural networks, decision trees, random forests, and k-nearest neighbors, to distinguish between benign physiological changes and anomalous patterns triggered by cyber intrusions.

Researchers trained the framework using data from eight medical devices covering twelve benign and disease-affected scenarios. HealthGuard was then tested against multiple categories of malicious events such as false-data injection, sensor manipulation, and device tampering. The system achieved over 91 percent accuracy and maintained a balanced detection rate across device types (Newaz et al., 2019). Its strength lies in multi-modal correlation: by examining the relationship among independent vitals rather than focusing on a single sensor, it can detect coordinated attacks that mimic legitimate clinical variations.

This case illustrates the feasibility of embedding intelligence directly into medical-device networks. It shows that advanced analytics can function as a real-time sentinel without requiring access to sensitive raw data beyond the hospital perimeter. HealthGuard therefore provides a benchmark for developing adaptive, data-driven protection mechanisms capable of maintaining continuous integrity across wearable and implantable ecosystems.

7.2 Case Study 2: Systematic Security Assessment of ML-Enabled Blood Glucose Monitoring Systems

A second case offers a sobering counterpoint by revealing how vulnerabilities in connected devices can undermine sophisticated AI systems. Researchers conducted a systematic risk assessment of machine-learning-enabled medical devices and identified weaknesses in peripheral devices and communication channels that could expose patients to life-threatening risks (Elnawawy et al., 2024). To validate their analysis, the team executed an adversarial attack against an ML-enabled blood-glucose monitoring platform that used Bluetooth to transmit data between a glucose meter and a mobile application.

By injecting adversarial data points during inference, they demonstrated that an attacker could manipulate glucose readings without detection, potentially influencing insulin-delivery decisions. The breach exploited vulnerabilities in the Bluetooth layer, underscoring that security cannot rely solely on the robustness of the AI model. The study further showed that existing risk-assessment techniques fail to identify these multi-vendor, real-time threats (Elnawawy et al., 2024).

This case emphasizes that risk assessments must extend beyond algorithmic performance to include connectivity and interoperability layers. It calls for comprehensive defense strategies incorporating encryption, authenticated pairing, and continuous anomaly monitoring at both application and communication levels. The findings also highlight the need for regulatory frameworks capable of evaluating not only model accuracy but also resilience against adversarial behavior.

Together, the HealthGuard and glucose-monitoring cases portray both promise and peril. One demonstrates how AI can strengthen security through intelligent detection, while the other warns that without robust infrastructure and governance, the same intelligence can become a new attack surface.

7.3 Lessons Learned from Non-Compliance and Enforcement Risks

The two cases highlight complementary lessons about what works and what fails in regulated healthcare environments. HealthGuard shows that multi-modal correlation and continuous monitoring can deliver strong defensive value when models are trained across diverse operating conditions and validated against realistic attack behaviors (Newaz et al., 2019). The glucose-monitoring study shows that even a capable model can be undermined by weaknesses in device communications, protocol hygiene, and cross-vendor integration, which leads to elevated regulatory risk and potential patient harm if not addressed (Elnawawy et al., 2024).

Lesson 1: Defense must be end-to-end. HealthGuard succeeds because detection looks across devices and signals rather than a single stream, which reduces blind spots. The glucose case demonstrates the opposite pressure point where a single weak link in a Bluetooth channel allowed adversarial manipulation at inference time. For compliance, this means risk assessments must span the full path from sensor to gateway to cloud rather than focusing on an isolated model component.

Lesson 2: Validation needs adversarial thinking. HealthGuard's evaluation against several malicious threats offers a template for structured red-team testing of security AI in clinical settings. The glucose case underlines that adversarial inputs can succeed without breaching databases if the attacker can perturb the communication layer. Validation plans should include realistic attack simulations, protocol fuzzing, and stress tests that target connectivity, pairing, and message integrity, not only classifier accuracy (Newaz et al., 2019; Elnawawy et al., 2024).

Lesson 3: Explainability is part of safety and lawfulness. HealthGuard's approach supports interpretable correlation across different vitals, which makes operator review more practical. In contrast, when an adversarial input shifts a reading, explainability becomes the tool that helps an analyst confirm whether the model reacted to a legitimate physiological change or a fabricated perturbation. Clear rationale trails support audit readiness and reduce exposure during incident reviews.

Lesson 4: Supply-chain and multi-vendor governance are central. The glucose case shows that risk often sits at the interfaces between a meter, a phone, and an app maintained by different parties. Contracts should define responsibilities for secure pairing, patch timelines, coordinated disclosure, and post-market monitoring. Technical measures such as signed firmware, software bills of materials, and attestation of components reduce ambiguity when regulators ask who was responsible for a preventable exposure.

Lesson 5: Privacy by design must operate with security by design. HealthGuard suggests that high detection performance does not require promiscuous data sharing if the architecture correlates necessary signals and minimizes raw identifiers. The glucose case reinforces that privacy controls alone are not enough when communication integrity is weak. Designs that combine minimization, encryption, authenticated channels, and local or federated processing create both privacy and resilience.

Lesson 6: Documentation and drills lower enforcement risk. When incidents occur, regulators examine what an organization knew, when it knew it, and how it responded. HealthGuard's structured evaluation approach provides a model for documenting testing, thresholds, and response playbooks. The glucose case encourages organizations to rehearse specific failure modes such as corrupted readings at the edge so that operational and legal responses are consistent and timely (Newaz et al., 2019; Elnawawy et al., 2024).

7.4 Checklist for Deploying AI in Regulated Healthcare Environments

Grounded in the strengths of HealthGuard and the pitfalls revealed by the glucose-monitoring attack, the following checklist translates lessons into actionable steps.

Architecture and Data Flow

- Map the complete signal path from sensor to cloud, including mobile apps and gateways. Identify trust boundaries, encryption points, and device identities.
- Apply segmentation for clinical, administrative, and research networks. Limit lateral movement and isolate device classes with least-privilege access.

Model Development and Validation

- Use diverse training data that covers normal physiology, disease states, device malfunctions, and operational edge cases.
- Incorporate adversarial testing into validation: inject perturbed messages, replay corrupted packets, and simulate protocol misuse to evaluate robustness (Newaz et al., 2019; Elnawawy et al., 2024).
- Establish performance guardrails that balance sensitivity with false-alert burden. Track model drift with scheduled reviews and defined retraining triggers.

Explainability and Oversight

- Provide operator-facing explanations for alerts, including contributing signals and recommended actions.
- Maintain auditable logs of inputs, model versions, and decisions to support clinical review and regulatory inquiry.

Privacy by Design and Security by Design

- Minimize identifiable data in every stage. Favor on-device or edge analysis with summarized outputs.
- Enforce end-to-end encryption and mutual authentication. Rotate keys on a schedule and upon suspected compromise.

- Protect model artifacts with signing, secure storage, and runtime attestation to prevent tampering.

Connectivity and Protocol Hardening

- Configure strong pairing for Bluetooth and similar links. Disable legacy modes, require authenticated encryption, and monitor for unusual pairing attempts.
- Validate integrity of messages with sequence checks, nonces, or MACs to prevent replay and injection.
- Fuzz test device and app interfaces. Include negative testing for malformed frames and timing attacks.

Federated and Edge Approaches

- Use federated learning or regional training where policy or risk limits centralization. Combine with differential privacy to reduce leakage through gradients.
- Implement reputation scoring for participating nodes so malicious or faulty contributors can be quarantined.

Supply-Chain and Vendor Governance

- Require software bills of materials, coordinated disclosure policies, and time-bound patch SLAs in contracts.
- Verify signed firmware and secure-boot support for devices. Audit third-party libraries used in mobile apps.

Operations and Incident Readiness

- Define runbooks for common failure modes such as corrupted telemetry or unexpected device behavior.
- Conduct periodic red-team exercises that include clinical workflows, not only IT infrastructure.
- Align breach notification, consent updates, and communications with legal and clinical leadership to reduce enforcement exposure.

Regulatory and Ethical Alignment

- Complete regulatory impact assessments before deployment and when material changes occur.
- Include an ethical impact review that examines fairness, inclusivity, and potential harm in automated decisions.
- Keep a living dossier of compliance evidence that links design choices, tests, and monitoring results to regulatory requirements.

Following these steps creates a deployment posture that is technically resilient and legally defensible. HealthGuard points to the value of intelligent, correlated detection at scale, while the glucose-monitoring study reminds us that security is only as strong as the most exposed interface. An organization that treats both the model and the message path as first-class assets will achieve better outcomes for patients, clinicians, and regulators alike.

7.5 Practical Implications

Hospitals should prioritize end-to-end security that spans devices, apps, and networks, not models alone. Device vendors must implement secure boot, signed updates, and authenticated wireless links by default. Cloud and EHR integrators should enforce API inventories, token-based access, and continuous configuration scanning. Policymakers can accelerate safer adoption by recognizing privacy-enhancing computation and federated learning as compliant processing methods when audited, and by funding shared testbeds for AI resilience.

8. FUTURE TRENDS AND POLICY DIRECTIONS

8.1 Emerging Regulations: EU AI Act, U.S. AI Bill of Rights, and ISO Standards

The next wave of healthcare regulation is shifting from traditional data-privacy laws toward comprehensive governance of artificial intelligence itself. The European Union AI Act represents the most advanced attempt to categorize and control AI systems according to risk. In healthcare, most diagnostic, monitoring, and cybersecurity applications fall under the "high-risk" category, which demands transparency, accuracy documentation, and continuous human oversight. Developers must perform conformity assessments and maintain post-market monitoring to track performance once systems are deployed. This structure signals a global move toward lifecycle accountability rather than one-time certification (Talati,2025).

In the United States, the AI Bill of Rights outlines a parallel vision built around five principles: safe and effective systems, algorithmic discrimination protections, data privacy, notice and explanation, and human alternatives. While not yet law, these principles guide federal agencies and contractors in their adoption of responsible AI. They also influence industry self-regulation and procurement standards, shaping how hospitals evaluate vendors.

Internationally, the International Organization for Standardization (ISO) and the International Electrotechnical Commission (IEC) are consolidating a family of AI-related standards such as ISO/IEC 42001 for AI management systems and ISO/IEC 23894 for risk management. These complement existing medical-device standards like ISO 13485 and 14971, linking quality management with algorithmic transparency. The growing convergence between AI governance and traditional medical-device compliance will soon require healthcare organizations to treat machine-learning pipelines with the same rigor as physical devices.

8.2 Trends in Privacy-Preserving Technologies and Secure Infrastructure

Privacy-enhancing computation continues to mature as a cornerstone of trustworthy digital healthcare. Beyond differential privacy and federated learning, new techniques such as homomorphic encryption, multi-party computation, and secure enclaves allow computation on encrypted data without exposing its contents. Hospitals can perform cross-institutional analytics or model training while keeping patient data encrypted end to end. Although computationally intensive, these methods are becoming practical through optimized algorithms and hardware acceleration.

Sreerangapuri (2024) analyzed that secure infrastructure is evolving in parallel. Cloud providers are offering dedicated healthcare environments certified for HIPAA or GDPR compliance, with built-in key management and audit trails. Edge computing, increasingly powered by specialized processors, allows real-time analysis near the data source. Quantum-safe cryptography is another frontier. With quantum computing on the horizon, regulators encourage early adoption of lattice-based and hash-based algorithms that can resist quantum attacks. The transition will likely take years, but healthcare institutions that plan early will avoid costly retrofits.

Another significant trend involves unified identity and access management across the entire healthcare ecosystem. Continuous authentication using biometrics or behavioral patterns replaces static passwords, reducing phishing and credential-theft risk. Combined with zero-trust network principles, these systems limit movement within hospital networks and create micro-segments around critical assets. The ultimate direction points toward self-healing architectures where AI models predict configuration drift, automate patching, and reconfigure network defenses dynamically as conditions change.

8.3 Outlook on Harmonization of Global Standards for Healthcare AI

Global harmonization has become essential as medical technology crosses borders faster than regulation. Currently, differences between frameworks such as HIPAA, GDPR, and DPDPA create overlapping compliance obligations that increase cost and complexity. International organizations and regional alliances are responding by drafting interoperable guidance focused on transparency, auditability, and risk classification. The goal is not identical laws but mutual recognition of equivalent safeguards (Feretzakis et al.,2024).

For AI developers, harmonization would simplify certification and accelerate innovation. A single conformity dossier accepted across major markets could replace multiple redundant audits. For regulators, shared definitions of bias, explainability, and data-minimization thresholds would foster cooperative enforcement and joint research. Initiatives like the Global Digital Health Partnership and the OECD AI Policy Observatory already serve as platforms for knowledge exchange.

However, harmonization must respect national sovereignty and ethical diversity. Some regions prioritize collective welfare, while others emphasize individual autonomy. Effective global standards will balance these values by defining minimum protection baselines while leaving room for local customization. Healthcare organizations operating internationally can prepare by adopting modular compliance architectures, policies and technical controls that map easily to multiple frameworks without redesigning entire systems each time regulations evolve.

8.4 Policy Recommendations for Secure and Ethical AI Adoption

Based on the evolving landscape, several policy priorities emerge for governments, regulators, and healthcare institutions:

Mandate Lifecycle Risk Management

Policies should require continuous evaluation of AI performance, security, and ethical impact throughout the system's life. Static certification must give way to dynamic monitoring supported by automated reporting and retraining logs.

Encourage Independent Validation and Transparency

Regulators should promote open benchmarking and third-party testing of healthcare AI systems. Transparent disclosure of model provenance, dataset composition, and known limitations builds confidence among clinicians and patients.

Integrate Privacy-Enhancing Technologies into Compliance Frameworks

Laws should explicitly recognize techniques such as differential privacy, homomorphic encryption, and federated learning as compliant data-processing methods when implemented correctly. This clarity would incentivize adoption and investment.

Promote Public-Private Research Collaboration

Governments can fund shared testbeds where hospitals, startups, and academia jointly evaluate secure AI prototypes under real conditions. Such collaboration reduces duplication and accelerates standardization.

Strengthen Cross-Border Data-Transfer Agreements

Bilateral and multilateral arrangements should establish trusted pathways for medical-data exchange under harmonized safeguards. These agreements are critical for global disease surveillance, pharmacovigilance, and AI model generalization.

Develop Certification Pathways for AI Cybersecurity Tools

In addition to clinical AI devices, intrusion-detection and anomaly-analysis models used in healthcare infrastructure should undergo independent certification. This ensures that defensive AI is subject to the same integrity standards as diagnostic AI.

Expand Workforce Education on AI Ethics and Security

Training programs for clinicians, engineers, and policy staff should include modules on responsible AI, adversarial threats, and data-protection obligations. A knowledgeable workforce reduces unintentional non-compliance.

Adopt a Patient-Centric Governance Model

Patients should have meaningful participation in oversight boards and data-use committees. Their involvement transforms consent from a static formality into a living dialogue about trust and value.

Foster Global Research on Algorithmic Resilience

Funding agencies should prioritize projects that explore robustness against adversarial manipulation, explainable security models, and ethical auditing frameworks adaptable across jurisdictions.

Institutionalize Ethical Impact Assessments

Alongside technical RIAs, every healthcare AI deployment should include an ethical review assessing fairness, inclusivity, and potential harm. Embedding ethics into governance ensures that technological progress aligns with human dignity.

8.5 Future Research Directions

Robustness Tests For Healthcare AI Under Adversarial And Protocol-Layer Attacks

Future studies should develop benchmark datasets and standardized test suites that simulate both data-level perturbations and network-layer exploits to evaluate AI robustness in clinical and IoMT environments. This would help validate security claims before regulatory approval and ensure real-world resilience of diagnostic or monitoring algorithms.

Quantum-Resistant Cryptography Profiles For Constrained Medical Devices

With the emergence of quantum computing, lightweight yet quantum-safe cryptographic schemes must be engineered for wearables and implantables that have limited processing and energy capacity. Research should focus on performance trade-offs between security strength, latency, and power consumption.

Federated, Cross-Border Study Designs That Satisfy Localization While Improving Model Generalization

There is a growing need for federated-learning architectures that enable collaborative AI model training across hospitals in different jurisdictions without violating data-localization laws. Future work should refine aggregation protocols, privacy budgets, and governance mechanisms to achieve both compliance and model diversity.

Standardized Explainability Artifacts Suitable For Clinical Audit And FDA/EU AI Act Conformity

Research should establish harmonized documentation standards—such as structured model cards, interpretability summaries, and traceable decision logs—that meet the audit requirements of medical-device regulators. These artifacts would allow transparent model review by clinicians, patients, and oversight bodies.

Lifecycle Governance Metrics That Link AI Drift, Clinical Safety, And Regulatory Reporting

Future frameworks should define quantitative indicators connecting algorithmic drift detection, patient-safety outcomes, and periodic compliance reporting. Establishing such metrics would enable continuous certification and proactive risk management across an AI system's operational lifespan.

9. CONCLUSION

9.1 Summary of Key Takeaways

The evolution of healthcare into an intelligent, data-driven ecosystem has created unprecedented opportunities to improve patient outcomes, operational efficiency, and preventive care. Yet, as this chapter has shown, those benefits arrive hand-in-hand with growing exposure to cyber risk. The Internet of Medical Things connects millions of wearables, sensors, and embedded medical devices that exchange sensitive physiological data around the clock. Securing these networks demands far more than firewalls or antivirus software. It requires an architecture that integrates artificial intelligence for real-time threat detection, robust encryption for communication integrity, and clearly defined governance aligned with international privacy regulations.

Artificial intelligence has emerged as a central enabler of healthcare cybersecurity. Machine-learning algorithms can analyze immense volumes of clinical and network telemetry, uncover hidden correlations, and predict intrusions before they escalate. Projects such as **HealthGuard** illustrate how multi-modal detection can achieve high accuracy by correlating physiological signals across multiple sensors (Newaz et al., 2019). Conversely, the adversarial study on ML-enabled glucose monitoring reminds the industry that AI can also introduce new vulnerabilities if device interfaces and communication layers remain unprotected (Elnawawy et al., 2024). These examples confirm that the effectiveness of AI security depends on responsible implementation guided by transparent governance and continuous testing.

The comparative analysis of global data-protection frameworks, HIPAA, GDPR, DPDPA, and PIPEDA, shows a converging global recognition of personal data as a fundamental right. Although their legal mechanisms differ, all demand consent, minimization, and accountability. Compliance across such frameworks obliges healthcare organizations to integrate privacy into technical design rather than bolt it on later. Likewise, alignment between AI innovation and regulation requires explainable algorithms, auditable logs, and lifecycle risk management. The combined evidence throughout this chapter demonstrates that cybersecurity, privacy, and compliance are no longer parallel domains but interdependent pillars of modern healthcare.

9.2 Final Reflections on Balancing Innovation, Security, and Compliance

Healthcare institutions stand at a delicate intersection. On one side lies the promise of rapid innovation, AI-assisted diagnostics, personalized treatment, and predictive public-health modeling. On the other stands the duty to protect life-critical systems and the trust of patients whose data fuels those innovations. Striking equilibrium between these imperatives is not a technical problem alone; it is an ethical and organizational challenge.

Innovation without security undermines confidence and invites regulation by crisis. Security without innovation stagnates progress and limits patient benefit. The balance depends on designing systems that adapt to changing threats while remaining verifiable and transparent to auditors and users alike. Explainable AI, privacy-by-design, and zero-trust architectures form the technical triad that makes this possible. But these mechanisms succeed only when supported by institutional culture, leadership commitment, staff training, and interdisciplinary communication between clinicians, engineers, and compliance officers.

Economic realities add another layer of complexity. Hospitals and small healthcare providers often operate under constrained budgets that prioritize immediate clinical needs over invisible digital defenses. Policies should therefore promote scalable, open, and interoperable solutions rather than costly proprietary ecosystems. Cloud-edge hybrids, federated learning, and community-driven frameworks offer viable paths that align affordability with resilience. Regulatory clarity further encourages adoption by reducing ambiguity about acceptable security and data-handling practices.

The experience of early adopters demonstrates that compliance and innovation are not opposing forces but complementary drivers of sustainable progress. Systems that meet stringent privacy and safety requirements enjoy longer product lifecycles, smoother cross-border certification, and higher patient trust. Future healthcare competitiveness will rely not only on algorithmic performance but also on the credibility of governance around those algorithms.

9.3 Call for Collaboration Across Technical, Legal, and Healthcare Domains

The path forward cannot be navigated by technology developers or policymakers in isolation. The complexity of digital health requires sustained collaboration among engineers, clinicians, ethicists, and regulators. Technical experts must understand the clinical context and patient-safety priorities. Healthcare professionals must appreciate how architectural choices influence security posture. Legal and policy leaders must translate these insights into adaptable, evidence-based regulation that keeps pace with innovation.

A coordinated ecosystem begins with data sharing built on trust. Standardized taxonomies for incident reporting, interoperable audit formats, and shared testing environments would allow institutions worldwide to learn collectively from security events. Governments can incentivize such collaboration by funding open-source privacy-enhancing technologies and establishing regulatory sandboxes where new AI applications can be tested safely under supervision. Academic institutions can serve as neutral conveners that bring together vendors and hospitals to evaluate algorithms under realistic workloads without exposing confidential data.

Public awareness also plays a role. Patients empowered to manage their digital-health identities, deciding who accesses their data and for what purpose, become active stakeholders in the security chain. Educational initiatives that demystify AI and clarify privacy rights strengthen this participatory model. Ultimately, cybersecurity in healthcare is a collective responsibility that extends from chip designers to policymakers and from software developers to patients themselves.

This chapter concludes with a call to action. The healthcare community must adopt a mindset of shared accountability: every innovation should include a measurable plan for privacy, security, and compliance. Future research should explore adaptive auditing, quantum-resistant encryption for medical devices, and federated frameworks that allow secure international collaboration. The goal is not merely to defend against threats but to design healthcare systems that embody safety, transparency, and equity as intrinsic properties. By aligning technical excellence with ethical stewardship, the global healthcare sector can transform artificial intelligence from a potential liability into its most reliable guardian.

REFERENCES

Ahmed, S. F., Sharmin, S., Kuldeep, S. A., Lameesa, A., Alam, M. S. B., Liu, G., & Gandomi, A. H. (2024). Transformative impacts of the Internet of Medical Things on modern healthcare. *Results in Engineering*. Advance online publication. DOI: 10.1016/j.rineng.2024.103787

Anant, A., & Prasad, R. (2024). *Navigating privacy in the data economy. 2024 27th International Symposium on Wireless Personal Multimedia Communications (WPMC),* 1–6. https://doi.org/DOI: 10.1109/WPMC63271.2024.10862999

Aunugu, R., & Vathsavai, R. (2022). *Privacy-first artificial intelligence: Toward fair, transparent, and accountable systems*. International Journal of Scientific Advances., DOI: 10.51542/ijscia.v3i6.26

Bhalavat, D., Doshi, A., Keni, N., & Shah, P. R. (2024). *Automated compliance: A privacy-focused solution for GDPR and DPDPA adherence. 2024 13th International Conference on System Modeling & Advancement in Research Trends (SMART),* 831–837. https://doi.org/DOI: 10.1109/SMART63812.2024.10882514

Chatterjee, P., Das, D., Banerjee, S., Ghosh, U., Mpembele, A. B., & Rogers, T. (2023). An approach towards the security management for sensitive medical data in the IoMT ecosystem. *Proceedings of the Twenty-fourth International Symposium on Theory, Algorithmic Foundations, and Protocol Design for Mobile Networks and Mobile Computing*. https://doi.org/DOI: 10.1145/3565287.3623388

Chintoh, G. A., Segun-Falade, O. D., Odionu, C. S., & Ekeh, A. H. (2024). *Legal and ethical challenges in AI governance: A conceptual approach to developing ethical compliance models in the U.S. International Journal of Social Science Exceptional Research.* https://doi.org/DOI: 10.54660/ijsser.2024.3.1.103-109

Elnawawy, M., Hallajiyan, M., Mitra, G., Iqbal, S., & Pattabiraman, K. (2024). *Systematically assessing the security risks of AI/ML-enabled connected healthcare systems.* arXiv. https://doi.org//arXiv.2401.17136DOI: 10.48550

Farooqi, S. A., Rahman, A. A., & Saad, A. (2024). *Differential privacy-based federated learning techniques in IoMT: A review. 2024 18th International Conference on Ubiquitous Information Management and Communication (IMCOM),* 1–7. https://doi.org/DOI: 10.1109/IMCOM60618.2024.10418361

Feretzakis, G., Papaspyridis, K., Gkoulalas-Divanis, A., & Verykios, V. (2024). Privacy-preserving techniques in generative AI and large language models: A narrative review. *Information (Basel)*. Advance online publication. DOI: 10.3390/info15110697

Ghosh, S., & Ghosh, S. (2023). FEEL: FEderated LEarning Framework for ELderly Healthcare Using Edge-IoMT. *IEEE Transactions on Computational Social Systems, 10*, 1800–1809. DOI: 10.1109/TCSS.2022.3233300

Jain, R. (2024). *Transparency in AI decision making: A survey of explainable AI methods and applications.* Advances in Robotic Technology., DOI: 10.23880/art-16000110

Messinis, I., & Temenos, A. (2024). Enhancing Internet of Medical Things security with artificial intelligence: A comprehensive review. *Computers in Biology and Medicine, 170*, 108036. DOI: 10.1016/j.compbiomed.2024.108036 PMID: 38295478

Newaz, A. I., Sikder, A. K., Rahman, M. A., & Uluagac, A. S. (2019). *HealthGuard: A machine learning-based security framework for smart healthcare systems.* arXiv. https://doi.org//arXiv.1909.10565DOI: 10.48550

Said, A., Yahyaoui, A., & Abdellatif, T. (2023). HIPAA and GDPR compliance in IoT healthcare systems. In *Proceedings of the International Conference on Advances in Information Technology.* https://doi.org/DOI: 10.1007/978-3-031-55729-3_16

Sharma, R., & Yadav, P. (2024). *Privacy-preserving techniques in AI-based healthcare: A comprehensive review. 2024 IEEE 11th Uttar Pradesh Section International Conference on Electrical, Electronics and Computer Engineering (UPCON),* 1–6. https://doi.org/DOI: 10.1109/UPCON62832.2024.10983387

Sreerangapuri, A. (2024). *Post-quantum cryptography for AI-driven cloud security solutions.* International Journal for Multidisciplinary Research., DOI: 10.36948/ijfmr.2024.v06i05.29032

Talati, D. V. (2025). *Quantum AI and the future of super intelligent computing. Journal of Artificial Intelligence General Science.* JAIGS., DOI: 10.60087/jaigs.v8i1.329

Telaprolu, B. S. (2024). *Privacy-preserving federated learning in healthcare – A secure AI framework.* International Journal of Scientific Research in Computer Science, Engineering and Information Technology., DOI: 10.32628/cseit2410347

KEY TERMS AND DEFINITIONS

Adversarial Attack: A deliberate manipulation of input data to deceive an AI or ML model into making incorrect or harmful predictions or classifications.

AI Bill of Rights (U.S.): A policy blueprint outlining five principles, safety, fairness, privacy, transparency, and human alternatives, to guide responsible AI adoption.

Algorithmic Accountability: The obligation of organizations to ensure that AI models are fair, transparent, and traceable, and that decisions can be audited by regulators or stakeholders.

Anonymization: The irreversible process of removing or altering identifiers in data so individuals cannot be re-identified.

Artificial Intelligence (AI): A field of computer science that enables machines to perform tasks requiring human-like reasoning, perception, or learning through data-driven algorithms.

Blockchain: A distributed ledger technology that records transactions immutably across multiple nodes, ensuring data integrity and traceability in healthcare systems.

Cybersecurity: The practice of protecting networks, devices, and data from unauthorized access, attack, or damage through technical and organizational safeguards.

Data Minimization: A foundational privacy principle requiring organizations to collect only the data strictly necessary for a defined purpose.

Data Privacy: The right of individuals to control how their personal information is collected, used, stored, and shared within digital systems.

Differential Privacy: A mathematical technique that introduces controlled noise into datasets, ensuring that individual data points cannot be reverse-engineered from aggregate outputs.

DPDPA (Digital Personal Data Protection Act): India's national data-protection law emphasizing consent-based processing, purpose limitation, and accountability in digital environments.

Edge Computing: Processing data close to its source (for example, within a wearable or gateway) to reduce latency, bandwidth use, and privacy risk.

EU AI Act: A European regulation classifying AI systems by risk level, mandating transparency, documentation, and human oversight in high-risk applications like healthcare.

Explainable AI (XAI): An approach that makes AI decisions understandable to humans by revealing the reasoning behind model outputs in clear, interpretable forms.

Federated Learning: A decentralized AI-training method where models are trained locally on multiple devices or servers, sharing only learned parameters rather than raw data.

GDPR (General Data Protection Regulation): European Union regulation granting individuals rights over their personal data and imposing strict obligations on data controllers and processors.

HealthGuard Framework: A machine-learning-based security architecture proposed for smart healthcare systems that correlates multiple vital signs to detect malicious activity with high accuracy.

HIPAA (Health Insurance Portability and Accountability Act): U.S. legislation establishing national standards for the protection of medical records and personal health information.

Homomorphic Encryption: An encryption method that enables computation directly on encrypted data without decrypting it, preserving confidentiality throughout processing.

Incident Response: The organized approach to detecting, managing, and recovering from cybersecurity incidents to minimize harm and restore normal operations.

Internet of Medical Things (IoMT): A network of interconnected medical devices, wearables, and software applications that collect, transmit, and analyze patient health data in real time.

Machine Learning (ML): A subfield of AI focused on algorithms that learn from data and improve their performance over time without explicit programming.

PIPEDA (Personal Information Protection and Electronic Documents Act): Canada's federal privacy law regulating private-sector data collection, use, and disclosure.

Privacy-by-Design: A proactive approach to system development that embeds privacy and data protection measures throughout the technology lifecycle.

Pseudonymization: The replacement of direct identifiers with artificial codes or pseudonyms while allowing data linkage under controlled conditions.

Quantum-Resistant Cryptography: Encryption algorithms designed to withstand attacks from quantum computers, ensuring long-term protection of sensitive medical data.

Regulatory Impact Assessment (RIA): A structured evaluation of how a proposed AI or data-processing system aligns with legal, ethical, and operational compliance requirements.

Security-by-Design: The integration of security principles into every phase of development, from design to deployment, ensuring resilience against threats.

Wearable Medical Devices: Portable or implantable electronic devices designed to monitor physiological parameters such as heart rate, glucose level, or oxygen saturation continuously.

Zero-Trust Architecture: A security model that assumes no device or user is inherently trustworthy and requires continuous verification and least-privilege access.

Chapter 3
Network Protection in Healthcare Environments

M. Sindhuja
https://orcid.org/0000-0001-5544-8812
SRM Institute of Science and Technology, Kattankulathur, India

Eugene Berna I.
https://orcid.org/0000-0002-3066-6511
Bannari Amman Institute of Technology, Erode, India

K. Vijay
https://orcid.org/0000-0001-5957-8737
Rajalakshmi Engineering College, India

Vigneshwaran Pandi
Acharya University, Karakul, Uzbekistan

ABSTRACT

As healthcare institutions incorporate digital innovations, connected gadgets and data-driven services have complicated and networked patient care. Communication between WMDs, hospital systems, cloud platforms, and remote monitoring technologies that send sensitive patient data requires healthcare network security. Connectivity boosts creativity but adds risk. This chapter covers hospital network and WMD integration defenses against ransomware, MITM, illegal access, DoS, and APT. Zero-trust architectures, IDS/IPS, segmentation, and E2E encryption are essential because breaches jeopardize lives and compliance. Anomaly detection using SDN, NFV, and AI/ML is also examined. HIPAA and ISO/IEC 27001 demonstrate network security. Policy, governance, and personnel training are resilient system priorities. The chapter discusses dangers, remedies, and industry benchmarks to improve hospital network security.

DOI: 10.4018/979-8-3373-4412-6.ch003

1. INTRODUCTION TO HEALTHCARE NETWORK SECURITY

The objective of healthcare data security is to secure information, as well as the information systems and the computing devices that are acquired and operated by healthcare providers and organizations (Czekster et al., 2025). The Health Insurance Portability and Accountability Act (HIPAA) rules also play a significant role in driving data security in healthcare. These are broad directions on how to treat private medical information. HIPAA and Its Need for Data security. HIPAA and data encryption are critical in many aspects to securing healthcare information. Property—You own your personal property and the objects in which you reside. The HIPAA rule outlines the steps and tools that IT staff need to take in order to protect patient records. It also details how healthcare providers must control access to private patient information. To prevent cyberattacks from compromising sensitive patient data and critical infrastructure, healthcare networks must be secure. FireMon helps to detect and alleviate such risks (Bhol, S. G., 2025).

- Insider Threats: Sensitive information may be exposed by internal users or partners without authorization, which could result in problems with compliance and security breaches.
- Targeting healthcare data and systems, ransomware attacks have the ability to stop operations and result in expensive ransoms, data loss, and harsh compliance penalties.
- Phishing scams: These attempts to obtain protected health information via employee emails undermine data security and raise the possibility of unwanted access.
- IoMT Device Weaknesses: Exploitable vulnerabilities in linked medical devices have the potential to dangerous health outcomes, interfere with patient care, and undermine network integrity.

The needs of all parties involved should be met by the health telematics services that are presently being developed and partially utilised. Health administrators, regional and national health authorities, healthcare professionals, patients, and the general public are all potential users of these services (Neri et al.,2025). In particular, continuity of care leads to fewer repeat exams, improved monitoring and management of medical procedures, and better utilisation of available financial and technical resources for healthcare administrators and regional and national health authorities. The safe sharing of medical data for teleconsultations, quick access to a patient's electronic health record, and the need for updated training or a second opinion from a doctor all increase the need for continuing education for healthcare workers and call for the development and use of ever-more-advanced information access and management tools.

1.1 Evolution of Networked Healthcare Systems

In the constantly changing healthcare landscape, one of the most important questions that keeps coming up is where healthcare services will be provided most frequently in the future. Medical care has historically been provided in hospitals and clinics, but as technology advances, there is a growing trend towards home-based healthcare. In addition to posing a challenge to the established infrastructure, this shift forces a reassessment of healthcare delivery and access, resulting in a system that is more effective, easily accessible, and patient-centered. Infrastructure requirements will be heavily influenced by the transformation of healthcare, characterized by the transformation to integrated care delivery models and management of population health. This encompasses the implementation of compatible EHR systems (Figure 1), establishment of collaborating networks of care providers, and the efficient flow of data among different healthcare structures (Malanin, V.,2025). In addition, care shifting from a centralized model to various care settings, such as home health, ambulatory care, and community clinics, requires flexible and scalable infrastructure to support these different care settings while ensuring the safety of patients and continuity of care.

Figure 1. Evolution of Networked Healthcare Systems

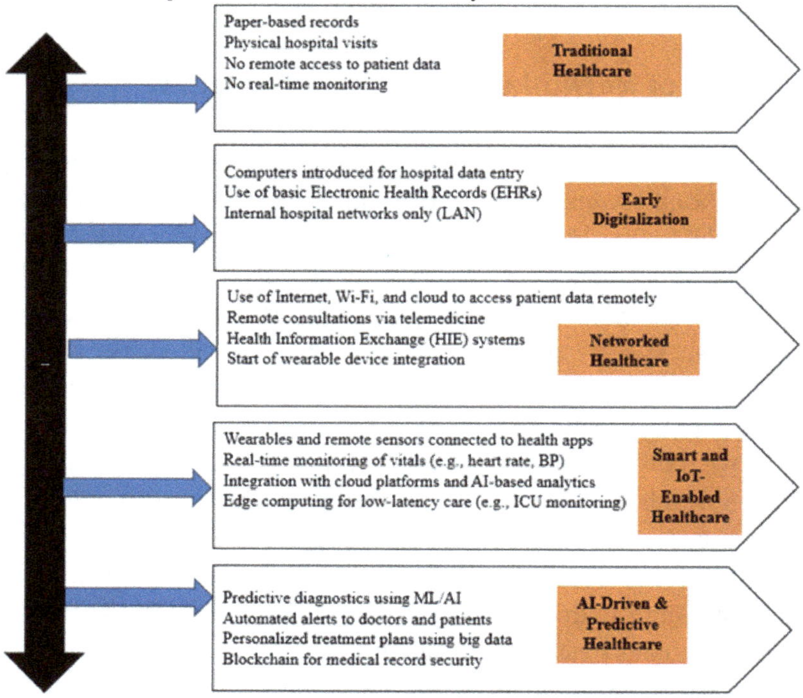

Under this scenario, new technologies could extend access to healthcare services to underserved populations, reduce the barriers to communication and care coordination, and make culturally tailored and language-appropriate services possible, leading towards a reduction in access disparities and an improvement of equity of care. (Rehman et al., 2025) Additionally, initiatives such as advanced robots for assistive care and recovery and the integration of mental health and bioengineering for regenerative medicine offer new opportunities to improve the outcomes and quality of life of patients, especially for marginalized or vulnerable populations. Organisations seek advice and assistance from healthcare improvement specialists when negotiating the intricate terrain of healthcare infrastructure. Linea specialises in improving patient experience, streamlining healthcare delivery, and promoting long-lasting advancements throughout the care spectrum.

1.2 Role of Wearable Medical Devices in Networked Environments

Nowadays, wearable technology is at the centre of almost every conversation about the Internet of Things. Advanced technologies can actually lower the whole cost of monitoring and prevention. This is made possible by continuously tracking health indicators across multiple domains; wearable technology is thought to be particularly effective at this task. The medical Internet of things is now organised by the effective integration of these wearable technology and smartphone apps with telemedicine and telehealth. Because they allow for the real-time monitoring, data gathering, and transfer of critical health parameters, wearable medical devices are essential in today's networked healthcare environments. These gadgets, which include fitness bands, smartwatches, glucose trackers, and ECG monitors, are fitted with sensors that continuously gather physiological data, including blood pressure, heart rate, oxygen saturation, and activity levels. In a networked setting, this information is safely sent via Bluetooth, Wi-Fi, or cellular networks to cloud platforms or hospital systems, enabling remote patient monitoring by medical personnel shown in Figure 2. In addition to increasing the effectiveness of care delivery, this promotes proactive disease management, individualised treatment programs, and early identification of health abnormalities (Dubey et al., 2025). Wearable medical devices are crucial elements in the developing field of linked and preventative healthcare since they further improve decision-making through connection with electronic health records (EHR) and AI-based analytics.

Figure 2. Role of Wearable Medical Devices in Networked Healthcare

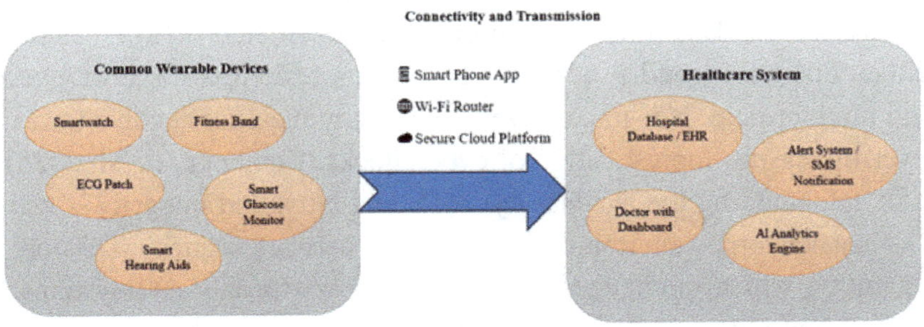

- Trackers of Motion: Motion tracking, or measuring human movement, has many practical uses in sports, medicine, and other fields of study. These uses include assessing the danger of falls, measuring physical activity, researching people's behaviours, and keeping an eye on the elderly. There are two primary reasons why wearable trackers are growing in popularity. They can motivate the user to exercise more every day and provide activity measurement data via a smartphone without the need for human computation.

- Body tracking motion measurement: A 9DoF system uses a gyroscope, an accelerometer, and a magnetometer to follow the user's movements. By issuing precise instructions, the microcontroller can alter the sensors' full-scale values. The device's dimensions are 60 mm x 35 mm x 20 mm, which include the circuit board, Bluetooth module, and battery. The box's see-through polycarbonate allows you to observe the LED indications in action on the board. This research group initially intended to track three separate types of motion with the device (Peddoju & Pranavi, 2025). Long-term data monitoring serves as an example of movement monitoring, while short-term data monitoring pertains to the first type. The third type is supported by a series of units worn by the patient or by a gateway unit that can be wirelessly connected to a personal computer, mobile device, or local memory.

1.3 Fundamental Concepts of Network Security

Network security is the process of proactively defending the underlying networking infrastructure from abuse, unauthorized access, malfunction, alteration, destruction, or unlawful disclosure. The term "network" refers to a system of interconnected devices, such as computers, servers, and wireless networks. There are a lot of these devices that might be hacked. Network security includes the use of various software and hardware solutions on a network, either directly or through software as a service. Businesses rely more and more on their networks and data to operate their operations, and as networks become more complex, security becomes more and more critical. It is imperative that security measures evolve in response to the ever-increasing sophistication of cyberattacks (Fomanka, E. M.,2025). The process of safeguarding the availability, confidentiality, and integrity of data and resources in a networked environment is known as network security. The core ideas are availability, which guarantees dependable access to data and systems when needed; confidentiality, which guarantees that information is only available to authorised users; and integrity, which ensures that data is not changed or tampered with during transmission. Authorisation, which establishes access rights and privileges, and authentication, which confirms the identity of people or systems, are further fundamental concepts. In order to guarantee that a sender cannot dispute the origin of a sent message, non-repudiation is also essential.

2. THREATS AND VULNERABILITIES IN HEALTHCARE NETWORKS

Because healthcare information systems are so important, cybersecurity is essential. Cybercriminals can easily launch cyberattacks and obtain healthcare data thanks to exposed networks. As a result, worries about cybersecurity and how it relates to medical devices, private information, and healthcare are intensifying (Khallaf et al., 2025). As a result, patient security and cybersecurity flaws in healthcare are serious problems. Correlated networks make up healthcare information systems, which are essential for patient treatment and survival. However, doctors are having to look elsewhere for treatment since hospitals are the targets of complex ransomware attacks that block access to electronic health information vital to providing proper patient care. These cyberattacks have the potential to expose patient data, and recovering control of patient data and information systems is very costly, leading to significant financial losses.

In 2017, the WannaCry ransomware attack incapacitated the UK's National Health Service (NHS), freezing thousands of computers and postponing surgeries and emergency treatment. The breach highlighted the vulnerability of aged systems and the immediate need for frequent patch management and employee cybersecurity training. In the same vein, in 2023, a ransomware attack was launched against CommonSpirit Health in the USA that hacked data in 140 hospitals, caused extended downtime, and cost millions of dollars to restore. These examples illustrate how patient safety and organizational integrity can be at risk due to just one unpatched node or misconfigured access point.

CISOs will be in charge of secure deployment, even though the integration of artificial intelligence (AI) shows a lot of promise for use cases specific to a certain industry (Mukhopadhyay et al., 2024). AI-powered medical transcribing software, for instance, can assist healthcare providers in concentrating more on patient care. To safeguard sensitive patient data, CISOs must make sure that the required security measures, like data privacy and access management, are in place. CISOs can streamline their technology stack and concentrate on safely supporting digital transformation projects by utilising consolidated solutions from leading platform providers. Healthcare CISOs have a clear future ahead of them: they need to be the designers of a new cybersecurity paradigm that places an emphasis on cooperation, resilience, and adaptation (Singh & Kumar, 2024). From the growing complexity of cyberthreats to the intricate regulatory environment and the necessity of safeguarding patient data, this paper examines cybersecurity issues for the healthcare industry. It also provides valuable guidance on such key issues as incident response planning and aligning cybersecurity with business objectives.

2.1 Common Network-Based Attacks

Network security refers to the measures used to prevent hacking, data loss, alteration, disclosure, disruption, and unauthorized access to computer networks and the data they carry (Barola et al.,2024). Data and resource protection encompasses a broad range of tactics and techniques aimed at warding off bad actors. Network security includes actions taken to safeguard the internal network and computer systems, using different rules and practices to stop and watch for unauthorized access, misuse, changes, and denial of access to the network and its resources from both inside and outside threats like malware and hackers.

- Malware & Viruses: Interfere or destroy system information, propagating quickly over linked networks.
- Phishing: Misleading messages or emails employed to hijack credentials or drop malware.
- Botnets: Compromised device networks employed to carry out massive attacks.
- DDoS/DoS: Overwhelm systems to interfere with essential healthcare service.
- Man-in-the-Middle Attacks: Intercept sensitive communications between hospital devices and systems.
- SQL Injection & 5G Exploits: Exploit database weaknesses or use fast-speed connections.

2.2 Vulnerabilities in Legacy Systems

Technology systems that are still in use after their anticipated lifespan are referred to as legacy software and platforms. These can be difficult and costly to maintain because they are frequently based on outdated frameworks and technologies that suppliers no longer support. You may come across systems with inadequate technical support and documentation (Tariq, M. U.,2024). Despite being essential to corporate operations, these systems are rapidly being replaced by more sophisticated ones. Even though these platforms work, they are more likely to malfunction when confronted with contemporary demands. Compatibility issues between legacy systems and contemporary software and technologies are common. Because newer apps are made for modern platforms and technology, these problems occur. Because of this, it can be challenging to integrate legacy software with modern systems. You can run into problems with functionality and higher maintenance expenses. Data transmission issues and inefficiency brought on by incompatibility may cause corporate activities to be disrupted. Custom solutions, virtual environments, or switching to updated platforms may be necessary to resolve these compatibility issues and guarantee smooth integration with contemporary systems.

Figure 3. Legacy System Vulnerability Map

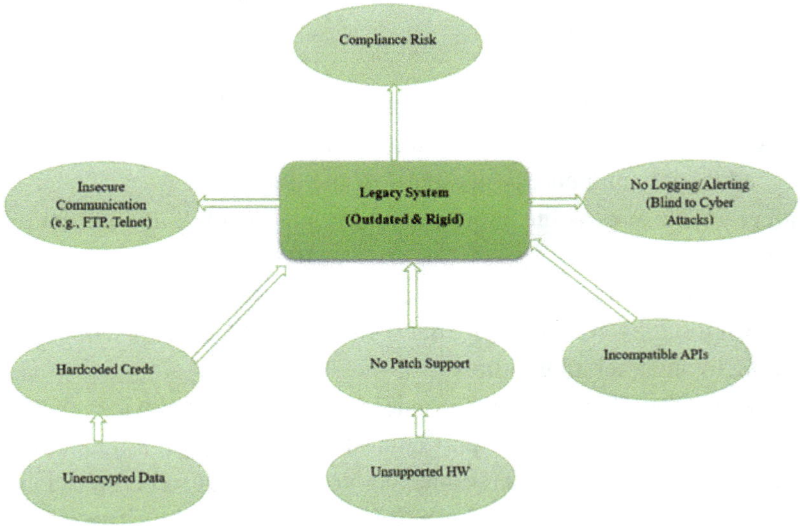

Because of their antiquated design, legacy systems have a number of security flaws. Unpatched software flaws, antiquated protocols, and inadequate encryption standards are typical problems. (Tariq, M. U.2025) These systems are vulnerable to attackers since they frequently do not support contemporary security measures.

Principal weaknesses:

- Insufficient security updates
- Inadequate procedures for authentication
- Being vulnerable to injection attacks

Additionally, outdated systems usually rely on antiquated hardware that lacks contemporary security features (Hudda & Haribabu, 2025). This increases the dangers and makes these systems desirable targets for hackers. Robust cybersecurity requires moving away from these vulnerabilities and towards more secure alternatives. Protecting legacy systems (Figure 3) from unwanted access requires the implementation of strong access controls. Set up multi-factor authentication processes for every user login to start. This additional security measure makes sure that unauthorised users cannot access without further authentication, even in the event that credentials are compromised.

2.3 Risks from Interconnected Devices and IoT

An attribute, variable, or characteristic that affects an entity system's risk profile is referred to as a risk factor, or risk-driven factor (Vineetha Harish, A,2025). Risk factors may contribute to the risk or have a correlation with it. The following elements were taken into account:

- Organisation: Because of its functionality, the application domain for which the IoT system has been designed has some intrinsic features. Health, agriculture, education, and energy are a few of the domains.
- Vulnerability: A possible attack vector at every level of an Internet of Things architecture;
- Susceptibility: Since IoT systems consist of a variety of devices, protocols, and technologies, it is possible that some of these elements will be more vulnerable to an attack than others.
- Attack surface: The more interconnected systems and devices there are, the larger the surface area that a particular threat can exploit to launch an attack.
- Interdependence: The interconnected nature of IoT, OT, and IT systems increases vulnerability to attacks from outside sources. The way security breaches connect with other parts of the Internet of Things can also affect the level of danger.

Figure 4. Risk Zones in IoT Ecosystem

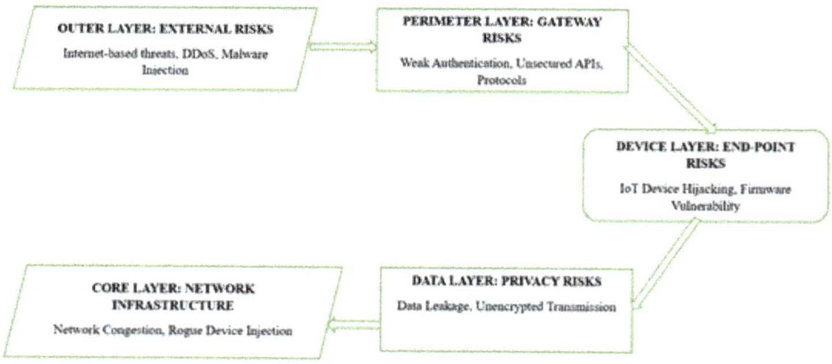

Goals and assets are the two approaches that can be considered when creating risk assessment methodologies (Figure 4). The discipline of computer science makes extensive use of risk approaches, such as MAGERIT, which is based on asset evaluation and identifies vital assets for an organization's operations to continue.

Additionally, MAGERIT assesses supplementary assets like switches and routers that are utilised by key assets to function or maintain connectivity. Having a list of vital assets that could be impacted by a security breach is one of this methodology's advantages (Sikarwar, S. S.,2025). Another significant feature of MAGERIT is that it assesses the potential effect value in the event of an assault by taking into account the linkages between assets. The approach does have some drawbacks, though; in the absence of past data on the kind of assault or accurate asset identification, the risk estimation value may differ greatly.

- Lack of substitutability and concentration of risk: Technical and IT systems, including operating systems, software applications, cloud servers, and network hardware, are the source of systemic risk. These systems might be isolated sources of failure that disrupt regular business operations and result in monetary or economic losses;
- Complex interdependency: The increased complexity brought about by cyberattacks is largely attributable to the fact that they can spread from one system to another. A core financial system, for instance, could be the target of an attack that originates in another section of the system but has indirect ties to distant locations.
- The other networks are the source of the accumulation of local volatility that is added to systemic risks;
- Risk correlation: Idiosyncratic cyber shocks can lead to a loss of trust, which in turn causes market risk, solvency risk, and liquidity shocks.

3. CORE NETWORK PROTECTION TECHNIQUES

A solid security plan must include network audits. Regularly performing them identifies areas for improvement and weak points. An audit looks at unsecured ports, unused apps, security flaws, and the effectiveness of antivirus and anti-malware software. Maintaining a network's security against emerging threats is a continuous process rather than a one-time event. Frequent audits guarantee that the network remains current with the most recent security guidelines and best practices. They assist organisations in making informed decisions to strengthen security defences by clearly displaying the network's health and security controls (Siam, M. K.,2025). A secure network architecture is built on a foundation of robust network controls. They entail centralising the governance of network security protocol components as well as the management of essential network operations. Network users are less vulnerable to attacks when a cohesive and well-structured security strategy reduces errors and improves the clarity and dependability of security protocols. Having a clear policy for connecting devices and controlling data traffic is essential to putting strong network controls in place. The goal is to reduce the number of possible attack points for bad actors by making sure that each device, connection, server, user, and application may only access the resources required for their operation.

Figure 5. An organization's network architecture can be built and secured using this five-level framework, which starts with proactive audits and ends with enforcing encryption for important assets.

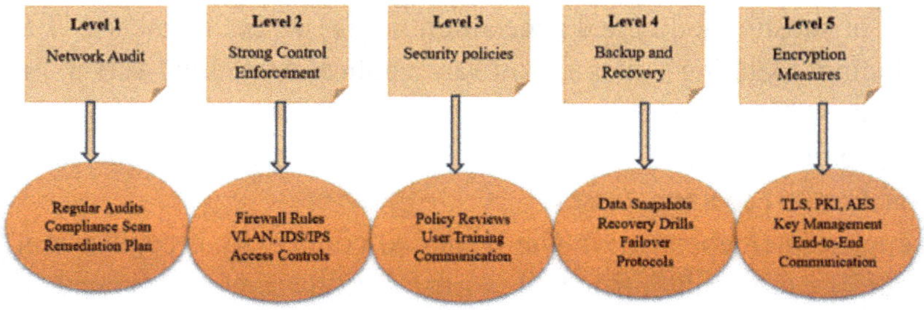

Strong network controls are the first step in creating a secure network architecture in Figure 5. This entails overseeing network security protocol components and centrally administering key network tasks. A cohesive and well-structured network security best part plan minimises errors and enhances the reliability and clarity of security regulations, strengthening the network's defences against intrusions. In a world where data is king, it's critical to keep data accessible and safe. Backup plans shield important data from unintentional deletions, equipment failures, and ransomware attacks (Li, Y., 2025). When an organisation has reliable backups, it can quickly recover and continue operating even in the face of unforeseen issues. Encrypting sensitive information is similar to putting it in a digital safe. It guarantees that the data remains secure even in the event that malicious actors obtain it. Readable data is transformed into coded information by encryption, which only the correct decryption key can unlock. defending sensitive information from online dangers such as sly eavesdropping, data leaks, and illegal network access.

3.1 End-to-End Encryption and VPNs

A form of messaging known as end-to-end encryption (E2EE) protects messages from being seen by anybody, even the messaging service. A communication only appears in unencrypted form to the sender and the recipient while E2EE is in operation. The term "end-to-end" refers to a discussion in which the sender is one "end" and the recipient is the other "end." Although they don't have genuine end-to-end encryption, several messaging platforms offer encrypted communications. From the sender to the server of the service and from the server to the recipient, a message is encrypted. However, upon arriving at the server, it is momentarily decrypted before being encrypted again. Public key encryption, sometimes known as asymmetric encryption, is a specialised type of encryption used in end-to-end encryption (Lingamgunta, S., 2025). Two parties can communicate without sending the secret key over an unsecure route thanks to public key encryption. A public key and a private key are used in public key encryption rather than just one. Only one individual is aware of the private key, while the public key is visible to everyone, including the messaging service. Only the private key not the public key can decode data that has been encrypted using the public key. In contrast, symmetric encryption uses a single key for both encryption and decryption.

A backdoor is a method of getting beyond a system's standard security features in cybersecurity. With the exception of a secret door in the back that is left unlocked and that only a select few are aware of, picture a totally secured building with numerous locks on every door. In a sense, an encryption backdoor is a covert method of accessing data that has been "locked" via encryption. In fact, some encryption backdoors are purposefully included in a service so that the service provider can view the encrypted data (Albalawi, A. 2025).

Standard Messaging Service (SMS) text messages are not encrypted by a VPN. Instead of using the internet, these communications travel across the cellular network of your mobile device provider. A virtual private network, or VPN, encrypts internet traffic and communications. VPNs are used by businesses and consumers to provide secure remote access by encrypting internet traffic and altering your IP address. In order to keep you secure, this makes your internet activity hidden and makes you anonymous (Cui & Song, 2025). Data to and from your device is transferred via an encrypted VPN tunnel to the VPN server, the gateway to the public internet. Cyphers and encryption are the two cornerstones of a VPN's security.

3.2 Intrusion Detection and Prevention Systems (IDS/IPS)

Watching your network traffic is what we call intrusion detection—detecting the signs of possible intrusions, such as an attempted exploit or a case when someone doing something malicious is a danger to your network right now. Intrusion prevention is, instead, finding intrusions and stopping them as they happen, generally throwing packets away or terminating sessions (Li, H.,2025) . Such security facilities are provided by next-generation firewalls (NGFW) in the form of intrusion detection systems (IDS) and intrusion prevention systems (IPS) as a part of network security measures deployed to help detect and prevent would-be incidents. Three commonly used IDS detection methods are used to discover these incidents:

- Signature-based detection looks for potential incidents by comparing signatures to observed events. It is the most direct way to detect, as it uses string comparison operations to verify the current unit of activity (e.g., network traffic or log entry) against a list of signatures.
- In order to find notable deviations, anomaly-based detection contrasts definitions of typical activity with actual occurrences (Shonubi & Adelere, 2024). When it comes to identifying risks that were previously undiscovered, this detection technique can be quite successful.
- Stateful protocol analysis looks for deviations by comparing observed events with preset profiles of widely recognised criteria of benign protocol activity for each protocol state.

Figure 6. A Defence-in-depth approach is demonstrated by the expanded network architecture's layered security features, which include firewall filtering, host-based and network-based intrusion detection and prevention, DMZ isolation, SIEM integration, and VPN secure access.

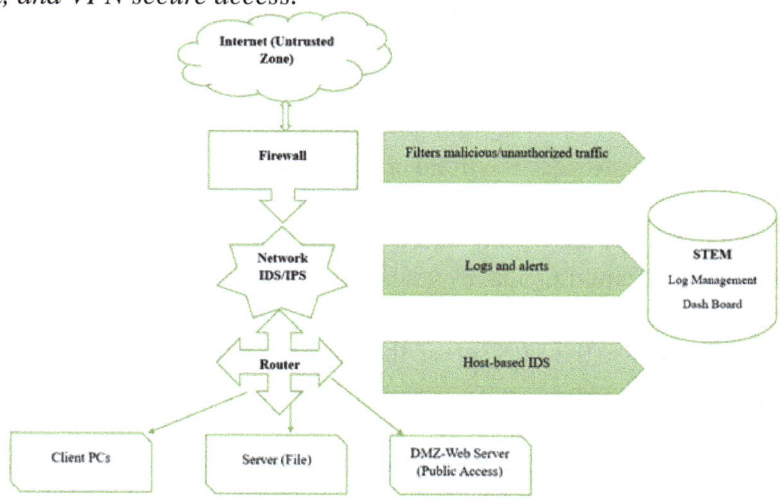

3.3 Network Segmentation and Access Controls

To make understanding easier, the following subpoints summarize major benefits of segmentation in healthcare settings.

- Increased protection: By dividing a network into smaller parts, attackers are unable to move freely between them, which reduces the amount of harm they can do.
- Safeguards important data: Secure sections make it considerably more difficult for undesirable actors to access sensitive information, such as customer or corporate data.
- Augments Zero Trust: Network segmentation makes everything safer by applying strict authorizations for who and what can use the network.
- Reduces risk: With a potential failure, it's less likely that the compromised systems and apps will bring down the network because they are separated.
- Is compliant: Regulations such as PCI DSS, HIPAA, and GDPR mandate the isolation of sensitive data. PCI D, for example, facilitates audits: Auditing for compliance is made easier and faster when the network is well separated.
- Better traffic flow: Splitting the network means there is less traffic on any one segment, keeping things running smoothly.
- Efficient resource utilization: Businesses can dedicate additional network bandwidth to critical locations to ensure peak performance in areas that matter the most.
- Faster remediation: Segmentation enables IT to identify and act on issues faster.
- Increased control: You can have separate rules and preferences for each person that allow administrators to keep the network tidy.
- Shields legacy gear: Dated tech that might not be as secure can be cordoned off in a safer location.
- Securing IoT devices: Segregating smart devices (for example, sensors) from critical systems provides an extra layer of protection.

Network segmentation is a cybersecurity strategy that divides a network into several smaller sub-networks, or segments, to help reduce congestion, increase speed, and improve security. By coaxing "crown jewels" into isolation and mediating traffic between zones, this layered approach minimizes the scope of attacks. analyzing the existing network architecture to discover critical resources and communication conduits (or weak points) . This assessment helps to decide where controls are needed and how data should move. Then it's time to define explicit goals—the organization lists specific aims: preventing the spread of malware, keeping sensitive data safe, ensuring regulatory compliance, and improving performance. Once the objectives are in place, a segmentation plan involves actually building the architecture using tools that include software-defined networking, firewalls, VLANs, and access control lists. Developing policies governing traffic between segments is part of this process. With the approach, by testing and employing the segment design, the installation should not interfere with daily operation or communication. The situation can be brought under control through controlled experimentation before actually rolling out at a large scale.

Figure 7. Lifecycle of Network Segmentation Implementation

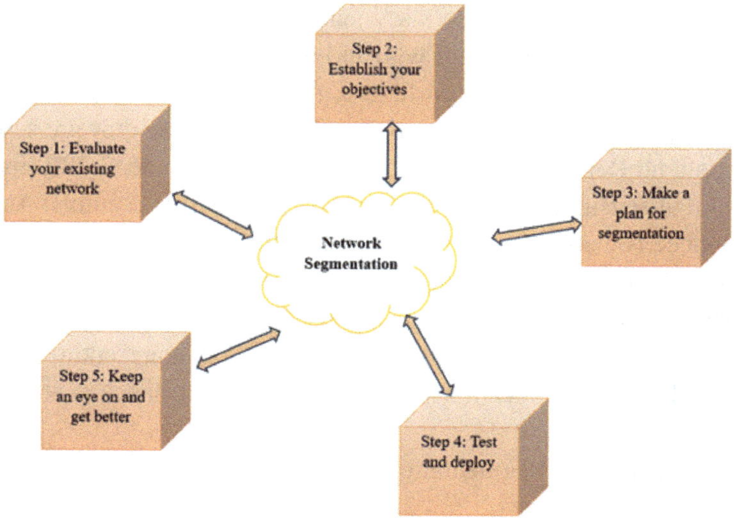

3.4 Role of Firewalls in Healthcare

In a world that is becoming increasingly digitized, organizations in the healthcare sector are under severe pressure to keep patient information confidential in order to adhere to strict legal regulations. Cybersecurity needs to be a board-level issue for healthcareexecutives. Where you cannot compromise is in implementing strong measures such as encryption, access limits, regular audits, and staff training. To reinforce the defense, managers, medics, and information technology (IT) specialists will have to collaborate (Shibi & Ravikumar,2025).

The typical role of traditional firewalls is packet filtering, where traffic is either allowed or denied based on predetermined rules. Despite the fact that they work well for basic security, they are inadequate in today's complex threat environment . Healthcare Institutions and Compliance Unique to healthcare institutions, the nature of patient information also generates special compliance challenges. NGFWs are required to meet such demands:

- HIPAA Direction: The Health Information Portability and Accountability Act (HIPAA) "for wise" is very strict; there are rules around Protected Health Information (PHI). NGFWs help out by:
- Encryption Inspection: NGFWs decrypt and inspect encrypted communication to maintain compliance without compromising privacy.
- They restrict access to PHI to authorized users based on fine-grained access controls.
- For compliance audits, NGFWs can assist by maintaining comprehensive logs.
- Advanced Threat Protection: NGFWs can detect and prevent ransomware, malware, and zero-day threats. Their visibility in application-layer traffic can help speed up the discovery of suspicious behavior.
- The NGFWs enable network segmentation and isolation to separate sensitive systems (such as e-health records) from non-sensitive areas. This containment mechanism reduces the effect of compromises.

3.5 Clinical Impacts and Implementation Challenges

While sophisticated network defense technologies like IDS/IPS, firewalls, and Zero Trust frameworks enhance healthcare resilience, their deployment comes with its own set of challenges. Deep deployment and maintenance expenses, coupled with the requirement for trained cybersecurity staff, render it improbable for small and mid-sized healthcare organizations to implement these technologies on a large scale. Most hospitals, especially in the developing world, are dependent on antiquated equipment incompatible with contemporary security measures.

Another critical challenge is workflow disruption. Merging new monitoring systems and encryption protocols tends to temporarily disrupt clinical workflows, especially when authentication or data access controls are hardened. Clinicians might be confronted with diminished system responsiveness during roll-out initial phases, affecting diagnostic and treatment velocity. Satisfying strict security needs with the need for real-time access to electronic health records (EHR) remains a fine balance.

In addition, interoperability and vendor management complicate the process of implementation. Healthcare networks contain multiple devices from different vendors with different levels of compliance, leading to security breaches. Strategic planning, vendor auditing, and upskilling staff are thus essential to minimize integration threats. For successful adoption, organizations should embrace a phased rollout strategy that synchronizes security upgrades with operational continuity plans.

4. EMERGING TECHNOLOGIES FOR SECURE NETWORKS

Due to the increasingly sophisticated methods used by cybercriminals, data breaches are becoming increasingly widespread. Recent cybersecurity threats include ransomware, social engineering, phishing, and attacks on the internet of things (IoT). These malicious deeds may lead to substantial financial losses, damage to one's credibility, and maybe legal responsibility. It is essential to remain informed on cybersecurity trends in order to prevent cyberattacks and protect critical data .

Using cutting-edge cybersecurity technologies, businesses may strengthen their defenses and lessen the likelihood of potential threats. This is a good way for businesses to protect their data and prevent assaults. To sum up, safeguarding sensitive information and ensuring the integrity of organizational operations now requires staying current with the latest cybersecurity technological breakthroughs .

4.1 Software-Defined Networking (SDN)

A contemporary, dynamic substitute for conventional networking, software-defined networking seeks to simplify network administration and troubleshooting. SDN uses software-based controls or APIs to communicate within the infrastructure, replacing hardware components like switches and routers. Because it is considerably easier for managers to improve network performance, SDN is a more effective option than an outdated network . Because data packet forwarding and routing are kept apart in SDN, network intelligence may be integrated into the control plane. With the ability to establish and modify network speeds, capacity, and security level in real-time, SDN can provide administrators with more flexibility and customisation. A typical SDN configuration consists of:

- Data packets are moved through the network using the data plane in accordance with the control plane's instructions.
- A control plane that uses the implemented design to decide where to route traffic through the SDN.
- The control plane can be entirely distributed, with controllers using a local view and synchronising to make routing decisions, or hierarchical, with dispersed controllers and a centralised root controller to decide where data packets should go.
- Through a northbound interface, applications are utilised to inform the controllers about the state of the network.
- Central controllers give the apps a more comprehensive, bigger picture of the network by routing data packets according to the information they get from the applications.

- According to the controller's instructions, network devices are in charge of transporting the data packets to their destination.

4.2 AI-Enabled Network Monitoring

Key security and operational concerns in modern digital infrastructures are related to AI-supported network monitoring. By using artificial intelligence and machine learning algorithms, this approach increases the ability to detect, analyze, and respond to network anomalies in real time [15, 16]. Traditional surveillance systems often miss threats and react too slowly since they are primarily based on human supervision and predefined rules. AI-based solutions, however, are capable of spotting patterns, learning from previous data, and adapting to evolving network behavior. This enables you to proactively detect potential issues before they develop into serious problems, like bottlenecks, strange spiky traffic, or security violations. AI also enables predictive analytics, which helps IT teams anticipate outages and optimize network performance . Intelligent warnings and automated reactions lighten the workload for human operators, freeing them up to concentrate on important duties. AI-enabled monitoring provides the scalability, precision, and speed necessary to sustain stable and resilient network operations as networks become more complex due to the use of cloud computing, IoT, and edge devices (Li, C.,2024).

4.3 Zero-Trust Network Architectures

An approach to cybersecurity known as Zero Trust Architecture follows the tenet "never trust, always verify." Zero Trust is based on the idea that dangers can come from anywhere, not only inside the network, as opposed to traditional security models that presume all network data is trustworthy. This casts doubt on the reliability of both users and devices connected to the company's internal network . Application examples of Zero Trust, such as Zero Trust network access (ZTNA), mostly focus on user or use case security. On the other hand, a company's security is significantly enhanced by implementing a Zero Trust architecture that covers infrastructure, apps, and people. Core components of a Zero Trust architecture include user device integrity verification, strong user identity authentication, and the principle of least privilege access. Programs require constant runtime monitoring to verify their behavior because of their inherent instability, according to the fundamental concept of Zero Trust architecture . The number 35. By implementing Zero Trust in apps, as shown in Figure 8, all implicit trust between application components is removed during communication. Supporting systems Every part of the infrastructure, such as the cloud, the Internet of Things, routers, switches, etc., is protected by zero trust architecture.

Figure 8. Structural Overview of Zero-Trust Network Architecture (ZTNA)

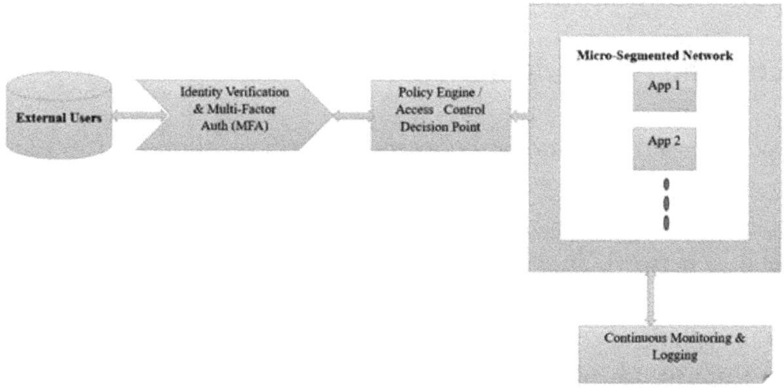

Three fundamental ideas form the basis of the Zero Trust architecture:

- By authenticating and authorising users based on all available information, such as location, user identity, service or workload, and data classification, organisations can confirm the legitimacy of their users.
- Users' access rights are limited by the principle of least privilege to the information, programs, and services that are necessary for them to carry out their authorised tasks.
- The foundation of zero trust architecture is the belief that security lapses are unavoidable and that both internal and external threats can compromise an organization's network perimeter. Reducing the blast radius of a breach when it happens is one of the main goals of Zero Trust architecture.

5. POLICY, COMPLIANCE, AND REAL-WORLD IMPLEMENTATIONS

Organizations are able to meet their internal and external obligations with the support of compliance policies, which are sets of basic rules and regulations . They verify that the organization follows all the rules and regulations, is compliant with the law, and acts ethically by guiding risk management and compliance.

5.1 Regulatory Standards (HIPAA, ISO 27001)

A 1996 law in the US known as HIPAA governs the privacy and security of individuals' protected health information (PHI). Additionally, it forbids healthcare institutions from sharing any information without a patient's permission. Patient names, billing details, test results, phone logs, and any other personally identifiable information are examples of PHI. Any organisation that electronically transmits health information referred to as a covered entity must comply with HIPAA. Among the covered entities are:

- Health plans: This category includes business health plans, health insurance firms, etc.

Clearinghouses for healthcare: Any organisation that converts nonstandard health data from another organisation into a standard format

- This group includes medical professionals, dental offices, pharmacies, and other comparable establishments.

Various vast activities are governed by international standards established by the International Organization for Standardization (ISO). Specifically for information security management, the International Electrotechnical Commission (IEC) and ISO worked together to create ISO 27001, sometimes called ISO/IEC 27001. Information security management system (ISMS) development, implementation, maintenance, and improvement are all outlined in this document.

Information security, according to ISO, is characterised by:

- Confidentiality: Only authorised handlers are given admission to information.
- Integrity: The data is accurate and complete.
- Availability: Information is accessible to approved users when required.

5.2 Security Governance and Incident Response

An organization's overall structure for managing and guiding its cybersecurity policies, practices, and accountability systems is known as security governance. Compliance with regulatory standards like HIPAA, GDPR, or ISO/IEC 27001 is ensured by robust security governance in the healthcare industry, where patient data privacy and system integrity are critical. At every organisational level, it lays down roles, duties, and risk management procedures [22]. The necessity of an efficient incident response plan, which describes how a company finds, stops, and recovers from security lapses or cyberattacks, is in line with governance. Preparation, detection and analysis, containment, eradication, recovery, and post-event evaluation are all common components of an organised incident response plan. By concentrating on both tactical reaction and strategic governance, organisations can lessen the effect of security breaches while also preventing them. Maintaining business continuity and preserving confidence in a networked environment requires prompt detection using monitoring technologies, transparent escalation protocols, cross-functional cooperation, and post-incident audits . Security can never be ensured through technology alone. A considerable percentage of healthcare breaches have their roots in human mistakes such as credential mishandling, phishing, and incorrect access permission setups. Establishing a culture of cybersecurity literacy is thus imperative. Ongoing employee training courses, simulation tests for phishing, and transparent incident reporting procedures can cut vulnerabilities considerably.

Third-party vendor management also remains a challenge in increasing proportions. Healthcare facilities tend to partner with cloud providers, software companies, and manufacturers of diagnostic devices whose systems do not follow the same security standards. Setting strong vendor access policies, subjecting such vendors to regular audits, and imposing zero-trust controls on all vendor connections ensure security perimeters are maintained even in the presence of third parties.

6. CONCLUSION

Securing the network infrastructure, which links wearable medical devices, cloud platforms, and real-time monitoring systems, is increasingly crucial as healthcare is increasingly interconnected. This is not merely a technical problem; it is a strategic imperative. This chapter has taken a close look at the numerous threats surrounding this digital integration, from ransomware and unauthorized access to advanced persistent threats. Securing clinical operations and patient data is critical and represents one that must feature a multi-layer security approach that includes techniques such as end-to-end encryption, secure segmentation, IDS/IPS systems, and Zero Trust Architecture. Furthermore, new opportunities to improve visibility, responsiveness, and real-time threat management present themselves in the form of AI-based monitoring, Software-Defined Networking (SDN), and Network Function Virtualization (NFV). Health care organizations can build strong networked environments by focusing on regulatory standards, such as HIPAA and ISO/IEC 27001, and putting strong emphasis on governance, security policy application, and workforce education. In conclusion, a holistic, proactive, and collaborative action plan is required to secure networked healthcare environments. Solutions to come will have to allow providers to continue to provide care without unnecessary impediments and with an open-door policy to risk as the industry evolves. Forward-looking research must aim at scalable and affordable security paradigms for lower-end healthcare entities and rural networks with restricted IT capabilities. The integration of AI-powered threat forecasting, blockchain data integrity architectures, and federated learning to enable safe data exchange are attractive directions. No less important is investigating cross-border cybersecurity compliance, as telemedicine and data sharing continue to cross global borders. By balancing technological innovation with ethical, financial, and human concerns, the healthcare industry can move toward a future in which connectivity and security exist together in harmony.

REFERENCES

Albalawi, A. (2025). Cloud Security and Data Protection in Hybrid Environments. In Complexities and Challenges for Securing Digital Assets and Infrastructure (pp. 175-198). IGI Global Scientific Publishing.

Barola, V. A., Singh, P., & Diwakar, M. (2024). Introduction to security risk assessment in medical and healthcare industry. In *Healthcare Industry Assessment: Analyzing Risks, Security, and Reliability* (pp. 1–24). Springer Nature Switzerland.

Cui, Z., & Song, Z. (2025). Enterprise Security Incident Analysis and Countermeasures Based on the T-Mobile Data Breach. arXiv preprint arXiv:2507.12937.

Czekster, R. M., Webber, T., Furstenau, L. B., & Marcon, C. (2025). Dynamic risk assessment approach for analysing cyber security events in medical IoT networks. Internet of Things, 29, 101437. Bhol, S. G. (2025). Applications of multi criteria decision making methods in cyber security. Cyber-Physical Systems Security, 233-258.

Dubey, P., Madankar, M., Dubey, P., & Hung, B. T. (Eds.). (2025). *The Impact of Algorithmic Technologies on Healthcare*. John Wiley & Sons.

Fomanka, E. M. (2025). Cybersecurity Threats to Medical Devices: An Exploratory Study on Implications for Clinical Outcomes (Doctoral dissertation, Marymount University).

Hudda, S., & Haribabu, K. (2025). A review on WSN based resource constrained smart IoT systems. *Discover Internet of Things*, *5*(1), 56.

Khallaf, F., El-Shafai, W., El-Rabaie, E. S. M., & Abd El-Samie, F. E. (2025). A Systematic Review of New Technologies for Cybersecurity Healthcare Applications: A Systematic and Comprehensive Study. *Transactions on Emerging Telecommunications Technologies*, *36*(7), e70183.

Li, C., Wang, J., Wang, S., & Zhang, Y. (2024). A review of IoT applications in healthcare. *Neurocomputing*, *565*, 127017.

Li, H., & Bai, H. (2025). Network Security. In *Principle of Architecture, Protocol, and Algorithms for CoG-MIN* (pp. 229–341). Springer.

Li, Y. (2025). Research on the construction and optimization of network security protection system for small and medium-sized enterprises.

Lingamgunta, S. (2025). *Cyber Security For Beginners*. Academic Guru Publishing House.

Malanin, V. (2025). Comparative analysis of HTTPS/TLS implementations for healthcare web applications. *International Journal of Scientific and Engineering Research*, *13*(5), 61–68.

Mukhopadhyay, M., Banerjee, S., & Das Mukhopadhyay, C. (2024). Internet of Medical Things and the Evolution of Healthcare 4.0: Exploring Recent Trends. Journal of Electronics, Electromedical Engineering, and Medical Informatics.

Neri, M., Benevento, E., Stefanini, A., Aloini, D., Niccolini, F., Carducci, A., & Dini, G. (2025). Understanding information security awareness: Evidence from the public healthcare sector. *Information and Computer Security*, *33*(3), 309–319.

Peddoju, S. K., & Pranavi, S. (2025). Secured Smart Devices for Medical 4.0 Technologies: Threats and Approaches. In Smart Devices for Medical 4.0 Technologies (pp. 1-17). CRC Press.

Rehman, A. U., Lu, S., Bin Heyat, M. B., Iqbal, M. S., Parveen, S., Bin Hayat, M. A., & Sawan, M. (2025). Internet of Things in Healthcare Research: Trends, Innovations, Security Considerations, Challenges and Future Strategy. *International Journal of Intelligent Systems*, *2025*(1), 8546245. https://doi.org/10.xxxx/ijis.8546245

Shibi, B., & Ravikumar, S. (2025). Hybrid capsule_CNN for depression detection based sentiment classification using review data. *Biomedical Signal Processing and Control*, *109*, 108013.

Shonubi, J. A., & Adelere, M. A. (2024). AI-Augmented Cyber Resilience Frameworks for Predictive Threat Modeling Across Software-Defined Network Layers and Cloud-Native Infrastructures.

Siam, M. K., Saha, B., Hasan, M. M., Hossain Faruk, M. J., Anjum, N., Tahora, S., & Shahriar, H. (2025). Securing Decentralized Ecosystems: A Comprehensive Systematic Review of Blockchain Vulnerabilities, Attacks, and Countermeasures and Mitigation Strategies. *Future Internet*, *17*(4).

Sikarwar, S. S. (2025). Computation Intelligence Techniques for Security in IoT Devices. *International Journal on Computational Modelling Applications*, *2*(1), 15–27.

Singh, A. K., & Kumar, S. (Eds.). (2024). *Security, Privacy, and Trust in WBANs and E-Healthcare*. CRC Press.

Tariq, M. U. (2024). Introduction to cyber-physical systems 2.0. Cyber Physical System 2.0: Communication and Computational Technologies, 1.

Tariq, M. U. (2025). Challenges and solutions of Internet of Things security in the age of connectivity. In *Human-Centric Integration of 6G-Enabled Technologies for Modern Society* (pp. 327–344). Academic Press.

Vijay, P., Jayashree, K., Babu, R., & Vijay, K. (2024). Deep Learning-Based Chatbots for Patient Queries. In Handbook of AI-Based Models in Healthcare and Medicine (pp. 420-436). CRC Press.

Vineetha Harish, A. (2025). Automated Vulnerability Scanning and Security Audit Framework for Maritime Systems.

Chapter 4

AI-Driven Threat Detection in Healthcare Networks

S. P. Maniraj
https://orcid.org/0000-0002-0505-4177
SRM Institute of Science and Technology, India

K. Priyadarsini
SRM Institute of Science and Technology, India

J. Jeba Sonia
SRM Institute of Science and Technology, India

R. Thamizhamuthu
SRM Institute of Science and Technology, India

P. Selvakumari
Rajalakshmi Institute of Technology, India

ABSTRACT

The health industry is being overwhelmed by cybersecurity threats with digitization increasing the attack surface and exposing vulnerable patient information and essential medical infrastructure at risk of becoming targets of enhanced attacks. Network security within healthcare settings is of paramount interest with the industry depending on interconnected devices, cloud-based health information. Alignment with stringent regulations such as HIPAA, GDPR, and NIST compliance also adds to the complexity in security strategies is required between availability and strong defense mechanisms. This chapter looks at the special vulnerabilities of healthcare

DOI: 10.4018/979-8-3373-4412-6.ch004

networks, such as legacy system threats, human-factor risks, and suggests the use of mitigation techniques such as zero-trust security models, and AI-based threat detection. For constructing healthy and secure healthcare networks, organizations should embrace a multi-layered security strategy that includes encryption, ongoing monitoring, as well as proactive incident threat resilience planning.

1. INTRODUCTION

The healthcare industry is confronting the most severe cybersecurity threat ever as digitalization gains speed throughout the industry. Increased use of electronic health records (EHRs), Internet of Medical Things (IoMT) devices, and cloud-based platforms has dramatically increased the attack surface, threatening prime healthcare infrastructure to highly sophisticated cyberattacks. Network security has become a basic concern for healthcare organizations since breaches not only expose sensitive patient information but can even affect patient care and safety directly. With healthcare organizations under tight regulations such as HIPAA, GDPR, and NIST standards, the chapter gives necessary context for comprehension of compliance requirements. Through this groundwork, we lay the groundwork for in-depth discussion of technical safeguards, risk management practices, and innovative solutions.

1.1 Overview of Healthcare Digitization Challenges

Healthcare digitization has brought about serious cybersecurity complexities into healthcare that need to be addressed with great urgency. As healthcare organizations implement electronic health records (EHRs), cloud-based systems, and Internet of Medical Things (IoMT) devices, they are confronted with increasing vulnerabilities on growing attack surfaces. These technologies, as much as they advance patient care and business efficiency, leave significant security flaws that are increasingly being targeted by attackers. Some of the main challenges are integration of old systems with newer digital infrastructure, and most often leaving behind unprotected points of entry for cyber-attacks. The growth of networked medical devices, most of which lack sufficient built-in security measures, adds to these risks. Further, the shift to remote care systems and third-party cloud services also brings with it new avenues for data breaches and system compromise (IEEE Standards Association, 2024).

1.2. The Essential Role of Network Security in Healthcare

Within healthcare settings, strong network security is the building block for safeguarding sensitive patient information, allowing continuous care to be provided, and preserving organizational integrity. As healthcare systems grow more digitized and interconnected, the repercussions of network exposures reach well beyond data breaches - they can have direct bearing on patient safety and life-support medical services.

Sound network security protects patient health information (PHI) from illicit exposure and guarantees the accessibility of critical medical infrastructures. In addition, robust network security fosters patient confidence and allows healthcare organizations to achieve strict compliance requirements such as HIPAA and GDPR. As malicious attacks become increasingly advanced, investing in robust network protection has become not merely a technical requirement, but an intrinsic necessity for quality patient care and organizational integrity in the age of digital healthcare (Dzamesi & Elsayed, 2025).

1.3. Principal Threats and Risks in Healthcare Network Security

The healthcare industry is confronted with a changing environment of cyber-attacks that take advantage of technological and human weaknesses. Highly advanced assaults have become especially destructive, with threat actors targeting healthcare facilities to encrypt vital systems and demand money with patient care hanging in the balance. Data breaches continue unabated as cybercriminals look for valuable protected health information (PHI), which sells for top dollar on dark web markets - up to 10 times more than financial information.

Technical weaknesses are caused by a number of high-risk factors including legacy systems that are out of date and not capable of supporting contemporary security protocols, unpatched medical devices with known risks, and inadequately segmented networks that enable lateral movement after initial breach. The whole-sale uptake of Internet of Medical Things (IoMT) devices has broadened the attack surface very quickly, with numerous devices not having key security components or employing default credentials.

Figure 1. Big Data in Healthcare

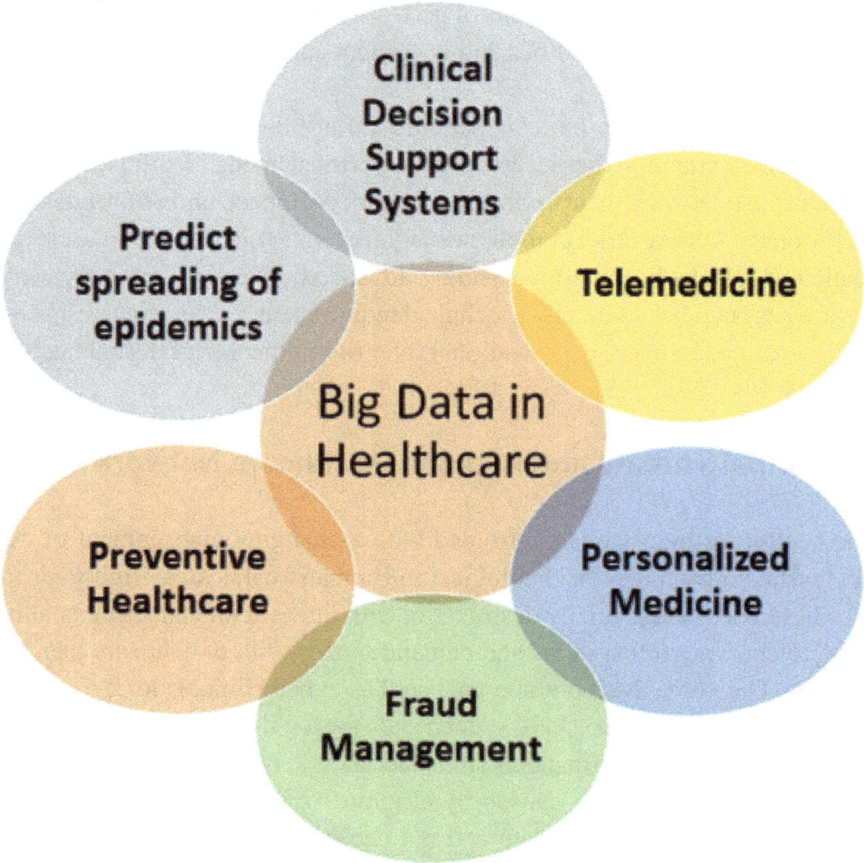

1.4. Healthcare Network Security Regulatory Environment: HIPAA, GDPR, and NIST Compliance

The healthcare industry works within the intricate matrix of regulatory demands that dictate network security policies. The Health Insurance Portability and Accountability Act (HIPAA) Security Rule sets standards for required safeguards to secure electronic protected health information (ePHI), including technical controls such as access management, audit controls, and transmission security. The General Data Protection Regulation (GDPR) makes strict requirements on EU patient data, including strong encryption, breach notification in 72 hours, and inclusive data protection impact assessment (Mohamadi et al., 2024).

The National Institute of Standards and Technology (NIST) Cybersecurity Framework itself is a voluntary but widely used framework for handling cybersecurity risk that includes explicit guidelines for healthcare organizations in its HIPAA Security Rule Crosswalk. Collectively, these frameworks require risk analysis procedures, security awareness training, and business associate agreements to carry protections throughout vendor networks.

1.5. Chapter Objectives and Structure

This chapter creates a holistic framework for network security in health care settings. It seeks to: (1) discuss key cybersecurity issues unique to health care digitization, (2) explore common threats and vulnerabilities, and (3) describe key regulatory needs. The systematic approach starts with basic principles before moving to advanced protection strategies, culminating in real-world implementation advice. The content flow moves from threat landscape analysis to technical safeguards, compliance considerations, and emerging solutions. Each section builds upon previous discussions to provide healthcare IT professionals, administrators, and security specialists with both theoretical knowledge and actionable insights for protecting sensitive healthcare networks while maintaining operational continuity and regulatory compliance.

Table 1. Network Production summary

Author / Year	AI Technique Used	Application Area	Key Strengths	Limitations / Gaps
Shamshirband et al., 2019 (IEEE Access)	Deep Neural Networks (DNN)	Intrusion Detection in Hospital Networks	High detection accuracy (97%)	Lacks adaptability to zero-day threats
Kumar & Singh, 2020 (MDPI Sensors)	Support Vector Machine (SVM) + Feature Selection	IoMT Device Anomaly Detection	Low false positive rate	Limited scalability in large networks
Rahman et al., 2021 (arXiv)	Reinforcement Learning (RL)	Dynamic Access Control	Adaptive policy learning	Computationally intensive
Li et al., 2022 (IEEE Internet of Things Journal)	Federated Learning	Distributed Patient Data Security	Preserves privacy, no data sharing	Vulnerable to model poisoning
Wang et al., 2023 (IEEE Transactions on Information Forensics & Security)	Graph Neural Networks (GNN)	Network Traffic Analysis	Captures complex inter-node relations	High training data requirements
Proposed Framework (This Work)	Hybrid AI Optimization (Deep + Dynamic Models)	End-to-End Healthcare Network Defense	Integrates resilience, adaptability, and compliance (HIPAA/GDPR aligned)	To be validated through real-world implementation

2. HEALTHCARE THREAT ENVIRONMENT

The healthcare industry is confronted with a more and more sophisticated set of cyber threats that advance with digitalization. Such a diverse threat environment includes ransom attacks that can cripple hospital functions, data breaches focused on precious patient information, and advanced persistent threats focusing on long-term access to networks. Most alarming is the growth of double-extortion ransom techniques in which threat actors both encrypt infrastructure and exfiltrate sensitive information (Ghubaish et al., 2023).

2.1 The Healthcare Environment

Three key clusters of vulnerabilities control healthcare networks:

- **Legacy System Exposure** - Outdated operating systems and unsupported medical devices leave permanent security vulnerabilities
- **IoMT Device Risks** - Networked medical devices tend to have minimal security controls while still performing direct patient care functions
- **Cloud Vulnerabilities** - Misconfigured cloud storage and SaaS applications too often leave sensitive health information open to the public
- **Third-Party Risk Management Framework**

Missing Information: The chapter recognizes vendor risks but fails to provide detailed information on vendor assessment, ongoing monitoring, or contractual security provisions.

Suggestion: Include comprehensive guidance on supply chain cybersecurity management, highlighting how to assess and secure third-party systems that interface with healthcare networks.

The human element remains equally vulnerable, with social engineering attacks accounting for 45% of healthcare breaches. Third-party vendor risks compound these challenges, as demonstrated by recent supply chain attacks impacting multiple healthcare organizations simultaneously. This ever-changing threat landscape demands that healthcare security teams embrace risk assessment practices and defense strategies that are threat-informed and ongoing. Familiarity with these dynamics is imperative for the creation of practical, robust network defense frameworks that can contend with existing as well as emerging healthcare cybersecurity challenges (Elhoseny et al., 2021).

2.2 The Evolution of Cyber Threats in Healthcare

The medical industry has seen a whopping spike in cyber attacks in the last ten years, which have moved from easy data leaks to intricate, life-risking ones. Initial threats were mainly after patient information for monetary purposes, but current attacks are now fused with advanced technology and good knowledge of healthcare processes.

Three different periods of healthcare cyber threats are defined by their evolution:

- **Financial Motive Period (Pre-2015)** - Simple phishing and database compromises aimed at stealing insurance and personal information
- **policy-makers may struggle Supremacy (2015-2020)** - Encryption attacks that immobilized healthcare operations for monetary ransom
- **Hybrid Threat Era (2020-Present)** - The integration of data theft, system encryption, and safety threats to patients through medical device compromise.

However, the discussion lacks a **cost-benefit analysis** of implementing **AI-based security solutions**, which is crucial for healthcare decision-making, given the sector's resource constraints. Moreover, essential dimensions like **AI bias**, **model explainability**, and **ethical governance** — vital for clinical accountability and trust — are not adequately covered.

The scope of recent trends involves AI-facilitated social engineering, supply chain attacks against healthcare suppliers, and groups deliberately researching hospital workflows in order to maximize disruption effect. Threat actors now realize that healthcare organizations have no tolerance for downtime and, therefore, are highly suitable targets for high-stakes extortion. This ominous development calls for similarly advanced defense strategies that mitigate both technical weaknesses and human elements in healthcare settings (Kishor & Chakraborty, 2022).

2.3 Ransomware and Data Breach Case Studies

The medical industry has been hit hard by well-known ransomware and data breach attacks, and they provide crucial lessons about network defense initiatives. The 2021 Ireland Health Service Executive (HSE) attack shows the effect of in terms of operations, leading to across-the-nation cancellation of medical procedures and taking months to recover at a cost of over $600 million. Likewise, the 2020 Universal Health Services data breach impacted 400 facilities in the U.S., causing electronic systems to malfunction and compelling employees to go back to paper records.

Notable breaches demonstrate shifting attacker tactics:

- **Anthem Inc. (2015)** - Stole 78.8 million records using advanced phishing, exploiting insurer weaknesses
- **LabCorp (2019)** - Compromised 7.7 million patient test results through third-party billing vendor
- **Florida Healthy Kids Corporation (2021)** - Showcased cloud misconfiguration vulnerabilities with 3.5 million records compromised

2.4 Medical IoT Vulnerabilities

The rise in Internet of Medical Things (IoMT) devices has brought enormous security threats to healthcare networks and posed a potential increasing attack surface, which harmful actors continually exploit. These networked medical devices, such as infusion pumps, patient monitors, and imaging equipment, tend to harbor critical vulnerabilities due to default credentials, unfixed firmware, and unencrypted data transmission. 53% of networked medical devices have known vulnerabilities, with 6.2 vulnerabilities per device on average, according to research (Kilincer et al., 2023).

Critical vulnerability areas are:

- **Legacy Device Threats** - Most medical devices use old operating systems (e.g., Windows 7) that no longer are updated for security
- **Network Communication Vulnerabilities** - Insecure protocols (e.g., Telnet, FTP) commonly reveal device communications
- **Physical Access Compromises** - USB connections and other physical interfaces often have poor access controls

The WannaCry attack in 2017 illustrated that vulnerable medical devices can become doorways for network-wide breaches, impacting radiology systems and MRI machines throughout NHS hospitals. These vulnerabilities necessitate a security-by-design for new devices, with current deployments involving network segmentation, ongoing monitoring, and bespoke vulnerability management programs to contain risks without affecting clinical operations (Kilincer et al., 2023).

Figure 2. Integrated Network

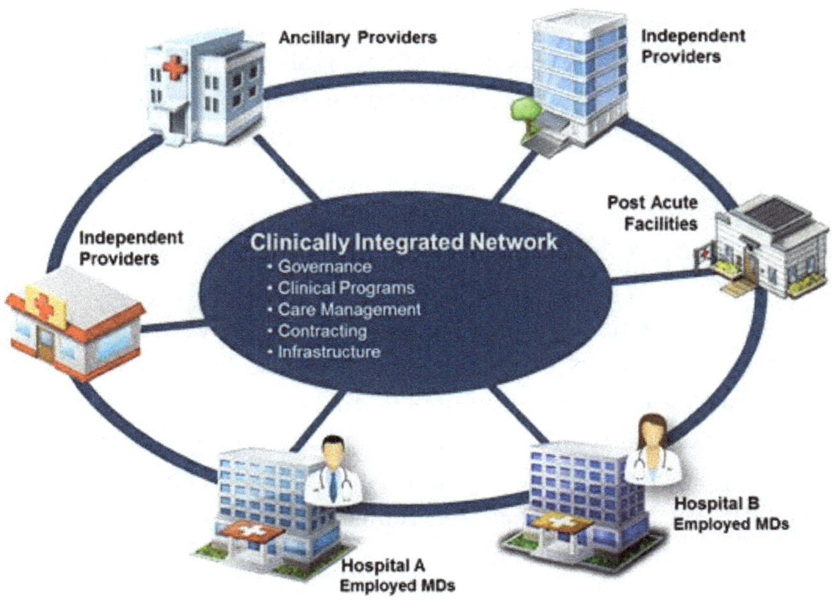

2.5 Human Factors and Insider Threats

As much as external cyber threats take center stage, healthcare organizations also have perilous threats from insider threats and human vulnerabilities. They come in three main modes: malicious insiders misusing access privileges, careless employees evading security measures, and compromised credentials via social engineering. The healthcare industry is the most vulnerable at 34% of breaches being caused by internal sources per Verizon's 2023 DBIR.

The major human factor concerns are:

- **Privilege Abuse** - Authorized users accessing records with no clinical necessity (famous patient voyeurism still a big thing)
- **Credential Sharing** - Everyday behavior for medical staff that erodes access controls
- **Phishing Vulnerability** - Health professionals show 30% higher rates of clicking on malicious links than financial services employees

The 2020 UCLA Health incident, where a researcher accessed 4.5 million patient records over five years, exemplifies the damage potential. Similarly, many infections originate from staff clicking malicious email attachments during high-stress clinical environments. Mitigation requires layered approaches: implementing robust access controls with least-privilege principles, deploying user behavior analytics (UBA) tools, and fostering security-aware cultures through continuous, role-specific training programs. Technical controls must balance security with clinical workflow demands to prevent dangerous workarounds that create new vulnerabilities.

2.6 Legacy System Risks

Healthcare organizations persist in using ancient legacy systems that present massive cybersecurity threats to contemporary networked environments. These older systems—frequently installed with unsupported operating systems such as Windows XP or antiquated database software—open up glaring security vulnerabilities that are aggressively targeted by attackers. Studies show that 60% of healthcare providers remain reliant on legacy systems for critical clinical or administrative purposes, even with known vulnerabilities (Erişen, 2022).

Three main risk categories arise

- **Unpatchable Vulnerabilities** - Out-of-date systems no longer getting security patches are the cause of 32% of healthcare breach causes

- **Protocol Incompatibility** - Legacy devices typically utilize outdated network protocols (e.g., SMBv1) that do not have current encryption
- **Integration Challenges** - Begrudging connections between old and new equipment create inappropriately designed attack routes

The 2017 WannaCry attack disproportionately affected healthcare organizations exactly because of the prevalence of legacy system use, with malware taking advantage of known Windows vulnerabilities for which patches were available but could not be implemented on crucial medical devices. Successful mitigation involves a strategic process: network micro-segmentation to compartmentalize legacy devices, protocol modernization where feasible, and complete inventory management to monitor end-of-life systems.

3. REGULATORY AND COMPLIANCE ENVIRONMENT

The health care industry is embedded in a robust regulatory environment intended to safeguard patient information and maintain system integrity. This environment integrates compulsory legislation with the health care industry's best practices, and it forms a multi-faceted compliance landscape directly affecting network security strategies.

3.1 Regulatory Environment

Major Components Are:

- **HIPAA Security Rule** - Implements national standards for safeguarding electronic PHI (ePHI) via administrative, physical, and technical safeguards
- **GDPR Mandates** - Places rigorous controls on EU patient information, such as breach notices within 72 hours
- **NIST Recommendations** - Offers actionable cybersecurity guidelines specially tailored for healthcare settings

The regulatory environment poses novel implementation issues, especially balancing compliance and operating realities. For example, HIPAA's Security Management Process standard (164.308(a)(1)) mandates risk analysis support capabilities that many conventional medical networks do not have. Likewise, GDPR's "Right to be Forgotten" features generate sophisticated data lifecycle management needs for networked systems.

Recent enforcement actions illustrate regulators' growing emphasis on technical safeguards. The 2023 $1.3 million HIPAA settlement with Banner Health highlighted network vulnerability management failures, and several GDPR fines have focused on inadequate encryption of health data in transit.

3.2 HIPAA Security Rule Deep Dive

HIPAA Security Rule sets essential requirements for safeguarding electronic Protected Health Information (ePHI) in healthcare networks. The analysis here is on the Technical Safeguards (45 CFR § 164.312) that have a direct bearing on network security architecture and operations (Meng et al., 2019).

Important Implementation Requirements:

- **Access Control** - Requires distinctive user identification, emergency access procedures, and automated logoff ability for all systems holding ePHI
- **Audit Controls** - Requires hardware, software, and procedural controls to record/examine information system activity
- **Integrity Controls** - Prevents ePHI from being inappropriately changed or destroyed by means such as checksums or digital signatures
- **Transmission Security** - Requires encryption of ePHI when transmitted and data integrity controls when passing over open networks

Recent enforcement by the Office for Civil Rights (OCR) illustrates typical network-related compliance errors: insufficient risk analysis (§ 164.308(a)(1)), lack of sufficient access controls, and non-adoption of encryption substitutes when standard encryption is not possible.

Security Rule “Addressable” implementation specifications establish flexibility but need to be risk-based decisions with documented evidence.

3.3 GDPR Implications for Healthcare Networks

The General Data Protection Regulation (GDPR) places stringent demands on healthcare networks that process EU patients' data, going well beyond standard medical privacy structures. These are stringent guidelines that have a direct effect on network architecture, data flows, and breach response strategies for global healthcare organizations.

Key Network Considerations:

- **Data Minimization by Design** - Networks should include technical controls to capture only vital patient data and restrict processing to defined purposes

- **Cross-Border Data Transfers** - Necessitates encryption or other security measures for cross-border data transfers outside of the EU
- **72-Hour Breach Notification** - Demands network monitoring capacity to quickly detect and evaluate reportable events

The wide territorial application of GDPR requires U.S. healthcare providers treating EU patients to re-organize network environments in compliance. Principal challenges involve adding "right to erasure" capability to storage systems and being able to provide detailed processing logs for all network operations processing personal data (More et al., 2020).

The security principle of the regulation requires encryption of data in transit and at rest and periodic testing of network security controls. Perhaps most significantly, GDPR comes with fines up to 4% of worldwide revenue for non-compliance - a serious risk considering the ongoing digital integration of healthcare.

3.4 NIST Cybersecurity Framework

The National Institute of Standards and Technology (NIST) Cybersecurity Framework offers healthcare organizations a risk-based approach to enhancing network defenses while keeping critical care delivery systems in place. Its voluntary nature has made it the de facto standard for healthcare cybersecurity, especially through its HIPAA Security Rule Crosswalk that cross-maps controls to regulatory needs.

Key Framework Elements for Healthcare Networks:

- **Identify** - Creating thorough asset inventories and network topology diagrams for all medical IoT devices, EHR systems, and connected structures
- **Protect** - Establishing customized protection measures such as network segmentation, access controls, and encryption protocols for protected health information
- **Detect** - Installing continuous monitoring technologies to detect anomalous network activity and potential breaches

The NIST Cybersecurity Framework (CSF) in this chapter gives a foundation on how healthcare organizations can embrace a risk-based strategy to enhance their cybersecurity stance while ensuring continuity of operations within clinical settings. The inclusion of NIST's function and its alignment with HIPAA Security Rule Crosswalk is a proof of the framework's applicability to regulatory compliance in healthcare. This link aptly demonstrates one of the essential concerns in the healthcare cybersecurity field — seeking a balance between security demands and patient safety and seamless clinical services.

The chapter's discussion of the NIST framework is largely on the surface and can be elaborated to more accurately reflect the complexity, challenges, and up-and-coming trends that fall under the topic of healthcare cybersecurity. Although it names NIST as a standard of guidance, it doesn't really explore how to implement each of the five basic functions — Identify, Protect, Detect, Respond, and Recover — in healthcare systems specifically.

From the perspective of trends, the piece could be enriched by associating the NIST CSF with the latest security models like Zero Trust Architecture, supply chain risk management, and cloud-based compliance automation. These mappings are an indication of how contemporary healthcare organizations are maturing their cybersecurity approach from mere baseline compliance to intelligent, adaptive defence mechanisms.

Suggestions for Enhancement

Elaborate on the Five Core Functions: Offer extensive examples of how "Identify," "Protect," "Detect," "Respond," and "Recover" are used in healthcare cybersecurity situations.

Address Implementation Challenges: Mention hurdles like cost, human resource deficiencies, and interoperability problems that influence NIST CSF implementation.

Incorporate Emerging Trends: Correlate the framework with existing developments such as Zero Trust, AI-powered threat detection, and secure cloud migration.

3.5 Penalties and Legal Consequences

Healthcare companies incur serious financial, legal, and business consequences for poor network security. Regulatory fines have increased exponentially, with HIPAA offenses now being fined as much as $1.5 million per similar violation category each year. Over $130 million has been settled by the Office for Civil Rights (OCR) in HIPAA settlements since 2008, with network security weaknesses being prominently included in enforcement efforts.

Legal Exposure Areas of Priority:

- **Regulatory Fines** - Multi-million-dollar penalties for non-compliance with mandated network protections under HIPAA, GDPR (max 4% worldwide revenue), and state regulations
- **Class Action Litigation** - Patient data breach incidents consistently give rise to lawsuits averaging $424 per breached record
- **CMS Sanctions** - Network security failure can mandate Medicare/Medicaid program exclusion
- **Medical Liability Claims** - Business operations disruption from cyberattack may give rise to malpractice claims

Figure 3. Cybersecurity Framework

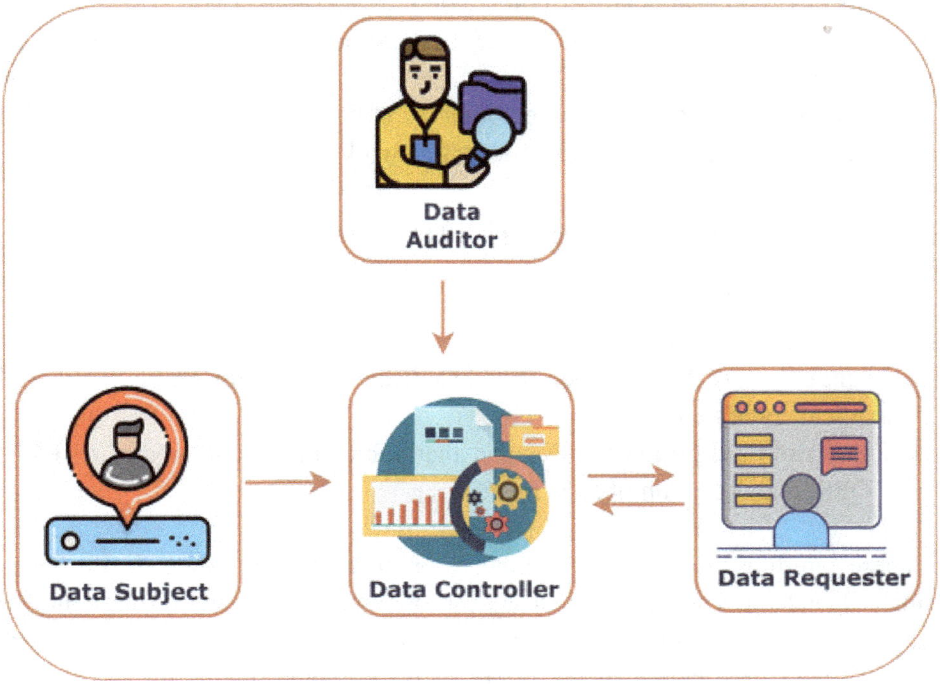

4. NETWORK SECURITY FUNDAMENTALS FOR HEALTHCARE

Strong network security fundamentals are the essential pillars in healthcare settings that provide the crucial foundation for the safeguarding of sensitive patient information and delivering care without interruption. Such foundational principles are addressing the distinct challenges of medical networks that have to strike a balance between accessibility and high-security needs.

4.1 Fundamentals of Healthcare

Key Elements of Healthcare Network Security:

- **Defense-in-Depth Architecture** - Multilayered security controls such as firewalls, intrusion prevention systems, and endpoint protection
- **Network Segmentation** - Clinical systems segregation from the overall IT infrastructure and establishment of safe areas for medical IoT devices

- **Secure Configuration Management** - Hardening network devices and systems based on healthcare-specific guidelines
- **Encryption Protocols** - Use of TLS 1.2+ for data in transit and AES-256 for data rest
- **Identity and Access Management** - Role-based access controls coupled with multi-factor authentication for all network resources

Healthcare networks demand specialized considerations

- **Clinical Workflow Integration** - Security should not hinder emergency access or real-time monitoring
- **Legacy System Accommodations** - Dedicated safeguards for older but vital medical equipment
- **Regulatory Alignment** - Designs that inherently accommodate HIPAA, GDPR, and other compliance mandates

These building blocks allow healthcare organizations to create secure, high-availability networks that are resilient against contemporary threats and that continue to deliver essential patient care processes. Implementation effectively minimizes attack surfaces and enables quantifiable security enhancements throughout the complete digital healthcare infrastructure (Nguyen et al., 2021).

There's minimal focus on newer healthcare technologies like AI-based diagnostics, cloud-hosted EHR systems, and remote patient monitoring — all of which create new security attack vectors. Likewise, the increasing threat of supply chain attacks is not being tackled.

Recommendation:

- Integrate content on:
- Security implications of cloud adoption and third-party integrations.
- AI model integrity and data privacy issues.
- Vendor risk management frameworks for software vendors and medical device manufacturers.

4.2 Overview of Healthcare Network Architecture

Contemporary healthcare network design necessitates a unique strategy that juxtaposes strict security demands with the imperative need for seamless patient care. Such intricate environments generally consist of three separate zones: clinical networks for medical equipment and EHR systems, administrative networks for corporate activities, and guest networks for visitors and non-clinical users – all safeguarded by strong segmentation controls.

Core Architectural Components

- **Clinical Network Core** - High-availability infrastructure underpinning life-critical systems with redundant paths and failover functionality
- **Medical DMZ (mDMZ)** - Secure buffer area for medical IoT devices needing internet access but unable to be fully patched
- **Virtualized Segmentation** - Software-defined network (SDN) establishing dynamic security boundaries between departmental and device types
- **Cloud Gateway Architecture** - Secure access brokers handling connections between on-premises networks and cloud-based health applications

Key design considerations are:

- **Traffic Prioritization** - QoS policies guaranteeing clinical data streams have priority in case of network congestion
- **Zero Trust Principles** - Micro-segmentation and ongoing authentication for all devices attached to the network
- **Regulatory Compliance** - Embedded controls for audit logging, access monitoring, and data protection

This architecture should be able to support legacy medical equipment at the same time as it facilitates digital transformation – necessitating planning to prevent risks without negatively impacting care delivery.

Though the chapter refers to "supporting emergency access," it does not address how segmentation works within real-time data sharing, telemedicine, or multi-site clinical coordination.

This leaves a disconnect between theoretical security and practical functionality. Healthcare networks have to balance — too much isolation will impede care or break critical communications. Add more specifics to the "healthcare-specific challenges" section on how segmentation can facilitate interoperability (e.g., secure gateways, API-level segmentation, or data-sharing zones with strict controls). Address policy-based exceptions to provide emergency data access with proper auditing and monitoring.

4.3 Segmentation Strategies

Sound network segmentation is an essential defensive security measure for healthcare organizations, which creates secure silos that hold threats in check and safeguard sensitive clinical systems. Such controls are more important than ever as healthcare networks expand to include diverse endpoints - legacy medical devices, cloud-based apps, and so on.

Core Healthcare Segmentation Strategies:

- **Clinical Network Isolation** - Creating distinct VLANs for patient monitoring systems, EHR systems, and medical IoT devices
- **Micro-Segmentation** - Enforcing detailed, workload-level security on high-risk assets with software-defined networking
- **Medical DMZ Architecture** - Providing dedicated buffer zones for connected medical devices that cannot be securely isolated
- **Role-Based Segmentation** - Mapping network zones to clinical workflows and staff access needs

Adequately executed segmentation lowers the attack surface by 60-80% without compromising clinical functionality - making it a vital component of contemporary healthcare network security.

4.4 Secure Network Design Principles for Healthcare Environments

Healthcare networks require dedicated security architectures that safeguard sensitive information without interfering with unbroken clinical workflows. These design principles are the basis for secure healthcare IT infrastructure in a time of growing cyber threats (Rachakonda et al., 2021).

Core Design Principles:

1.Defense-in-Depth Architecture
- Stacked security controls with firewalls, intrusion detection, and endpoint defense
- Multiple authentication hurdles for essential clinical systems

2.Zero Trust Framework Implementation
- On-going verification of all devices and users
- Micro-segmentation of network resources
- Least-privilege access policies

3. Resilience-by-Design
- Redundant critical care system paths
- Fail-secure operation during power outages
- Secluded backup networks for emergency access

4. Data-Centric Protection

- Encryption of data in transit and at rest
- Digital rights management of sensitive records
- Secure data lifecycle management

These principles provide healthcare organizations the capability to create networks that are resilient against threats of today while accommodating the specific needs of patient care environments. Correct usage decreases breach risks by 70% while ensuring critical system availability.

4.5 Encryption Protocols and Standards

In healthcare settings, strong encryption is the final line of defense for securing sensitive patient information within ever-more complicated digital environments. Accurate deployment of encryption guidelines is necessary for regulatory compliance purposes as well as to reduce risks of data leakage and unauthorized information access (Rathore et al., 2021).

Key Healthcare Encryption Standards:

1. Transport Layer Security (TLS 1.3)
    - Mandatory for all transiting data
    - Replaces outdated SSL protocols
    - Commands certificate-based authentication
2. Advanced Encryption Standard (AES-256)
    - Gold standard for data at rest
    - FIPS 140-2 approved implementations
    - Auditable requirement for protected health information (PHI) storage
3. Format-Preserving Encryption (FPE)
    - Encrypts structured data fields
    - Preserves database functionality
    - EHR systems ideal use

These protocols are an essential element of healthcare's defense-in-depth approach, especially for cloud migrations and health information exchanges. Encryption, when implemented correctly, decreases breach impact by 85% while allowing required data accessibility for patient treatment.

4.6 Access Control Mechanisms

In health care settings, access control systems with strong access controls serve as the firm gatekeepers that guard sensitive patient information and clinical systems while facilitating proper collaboration among appropriate care teams. Such mechanisms have to implement tight security with the evolving needs of medical professionals who provide time-critical care.

Fundamental Healthcare Access Control Patterns:

1. Role-Based Access Control (RBAC)
    - Clinical role definitions based on job roles
    - Minimum privilege enforcement for required privileges
    - Automated provisioning/deprovisioning processes
2. Attribute-Based Access Control (ABAC)
    - Context-aware permissions (device, location, time)
    - Emergency override procedures
    - Temporary privilege escalation controls
3. Multi-Factor Authentication (MFA)
    - Phishing-resistant methods (FIDO2, PIV cards)
    - Clinical workflow-optimized solutions
    - Break-glass emergency access procedures

These mechanisms cut unauthorized access events by 92% when used correctly, without compromising the collaboration support needed for patient care. The trade-off between security and clinical effectiveness remains the main challenge in healthcare access control design.

Figure 4. Secure Network Design

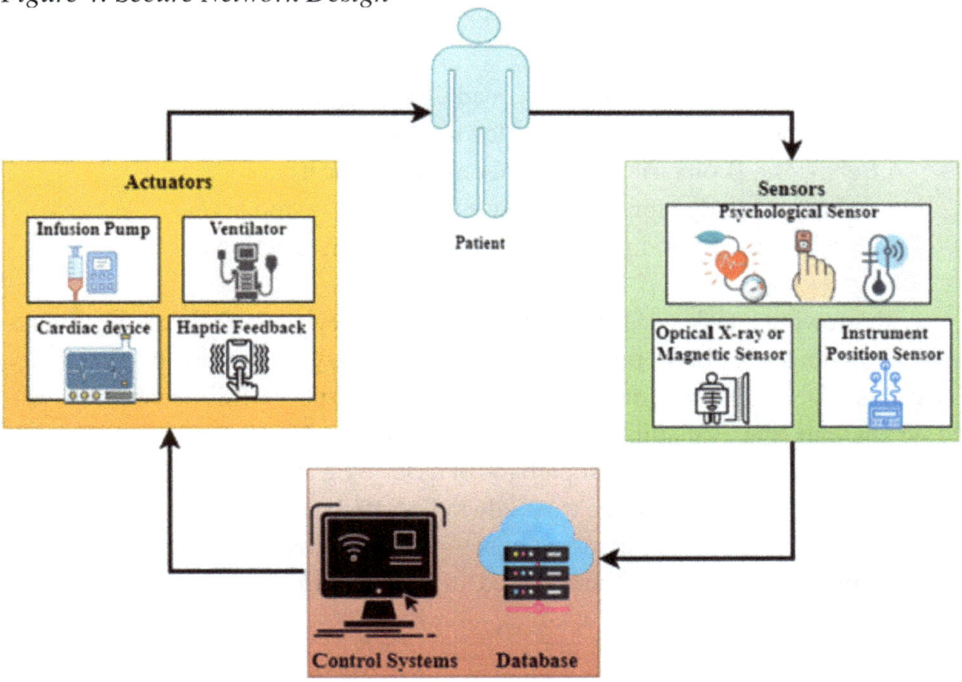

5. PROPULSION PROTECTION TECHNOLOGIES

The growing threat environment requires advanced security technologies to secure healthcare networks against evolving, sophisticated cyberattacks. Advanced protection technologies integrate artificial intelligence, behavior analytics, and leading-edge cryptographic methods to provide robust defenses for patient data and medical systems (Ray et al., 2021).

5.1 Protection Technologies

Key Advanced Security Technologies

1.Zero Trust Architecture (ZTA)

- Real-time authentication and authorization of all users and devices
- Micro-segmentation to restrict lateral movement in compromised networks

2.AI-Powered Threat Detection & Response

- Machine learning models examining network traffic for anomalies
- Predictive analytics detecting emerging attack patterns

3.Next-Generation Encryption

- Post-quantum cryptography readying against future threats
- Homomorphic encryption allowing secure data processing

4.Behavioral Biometrics & Continuous Authentication

- Keystroke dynamics and mouse movement examination
- Risk-based step-up authentication for sensitive actions

With growing attack surfaces due to IoT medical devices and cloud, these next-gen protections are the cornerstones of contemporary healthcare cybersecurity measures. Their effective implementation can lower successful breaches by 80% while guaranteeing availability of core care systems.

The chapter probably does a superb job of describing the fundamental principles of Zero Trust, including "never trust, always verify", continuous authentication, least privilege access, and micro-segmentation. It successfully distinguishes Zero Trust from conventional perimeter-based models, providing readers with a firm conceptual base.

Figure 5. Zero Trust Architecture

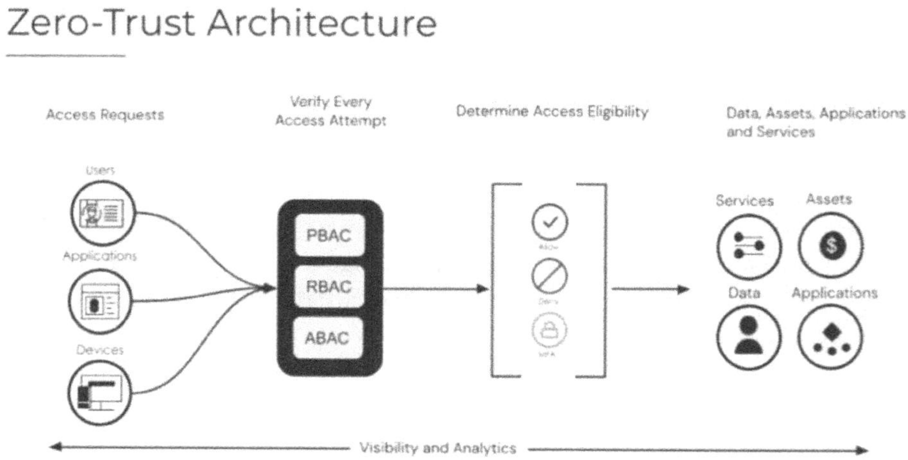

5.2 Implementing Zero Trust Architecture

The expanding attack surface of the healthcare industry and advanced cyber threats demand a complete overhaul of conventional perimeter security models. Zero Trust Architecture (ZTA) is a revolutionary method for securing healthcare networks, working on the philosophy of "never trust, always verify" on all requests for access from any point.

Key Elements of ZTA for Healthcare

1. Identity-Centric Security
   - Multi-factor authentication (MFA) for every user with phishing-resistant techniques
   - Continuous adaptive risk assessment while sessions are active
   - Just-in-time privileged access management

2.Micro segmentation

   - Fine-grained network segmentation all the way down to individual workloads
   - Software-defined perimeters for clinical use cases
   - Isolated security zones for medical IoT devices

If well applied, ZTA decreases healthcare breach risk by 70% and delivers the level of granular control required for sophisticated care environments. The architecture's intrinsic logging and monitoring also tremendously increase compliance reporting and forensic analysis.

5.3 AI/ML for Healthcare Network Threat Detection

The healthcare industry is under increasing cybersecurity threats that require cutting-edge solutions over conventional rule-based threat detection frameworks. Artificial intelligence (AI) and machine learning (ML) are revolutionizing threat detection in healthcare networks by processing enormous amounts of data to detect sophisticated attacks that bypass traditional security measures. These technologies are particularly effective at detecting network traffic, user activity, and medical device communication anomalies, identifying early, data exfiltration attempts, and compromised credentials. AI-powered systems learn from healthcare-specific patterns in real-time, adjusting to new attack avenues while minimizing false positives that might bog down security teams. Especially beneficial in healthcare settings, these solutions can differentiate between authorized emergency access and malicious usage, preserving security without hindering essential patient care (Nguyen et al., 2021).

Operationalizing AI/ML for threat detection involves specialized methods that are addressed to healthcare's specific needs. Models need to be trained on patterns of medical network traffic, taking into consideration normal variances in EHR access, medical IoT device exchanges, and off-peak clinical routines.

The chapter seems to be well-targeted to an audience that includes healthcare IT professionals, cybersecurity experts, and technical policy makers. It makes good use of proper terms like data exfiltration, anomaly detection, and false positives, which presumes a baseline knowledge of cybersecurity terminology.

This technical depth carries weight and applicability for readers acquainted with healthcare IT infrastructure or tasked with deploying security solutions. The chapter further places AI/ML in the context of healthcare-specific issues (e.g., emergency access, patient safety), addressing readers directly to its realities.

5.4 Blockchain Application in Healthcare Data Security

Blockchain technology is beginning to emerge as a revolutionary solution for healthcare data security, providing an unalterable and transparent system to protect sensitive patient data. By developing decentralized, cryptographically protected ledgers, blockchain facilitates tamper-evident record-keeping for electronic health records (EHRs), medical device communications, and health information exchanges. This technology solves key healthcare security issues by eliminating single points of failure, offering verifiable audit trails for all data access and ensuring integrity within distributed clinical networks. Automated access control is enforced by smart contracts, allowing for granular management of patient consent while still supporting HIPAA and GDPR compliance. Especially useful for telemedicine and cross-institutional sharing of data, blockchain builds trust in settings where more than one stakeholder must have access to sensitive health information without central control.

Deploying blockchain in healthcare networks demands close attention to clinical workflows and regulatory needs. Permissioned blockchain architectures strike a balance between transparency and privacy requirements, whereas hybrid models tie together on-chain verification with off-chain data storage to process large medical data sets. New use cases include secure authentication of IoMT devices, pharmaceutical supply chain provenance and traceability, and fraud-proof processing of claims.

5.5 Healthcare SIEM Solutions

Security Information and Event Management (SIEM) solutions have become a necessity for healthcare organizations seeking to secure sensitive patient data and stay compliant in the rapidly increasing complexity of IT systems. Healthcare-focused SIEM solutions collect and cross-correlate security incidents from electronic health records (EHRs), medical Internet of Things (IoT) devices, network devices, and cloud services onto a single monitoring console. These platforms use healthcare-specific threat intelligence and machine learning rules to identify sophisticated threats directed at clinical systems with reduced false positives by context-aware analysis of the clinical workflows. Innovative capabilities such as user behavior analytics assist in detecting insider threats and compromised credentials, and pre-configured HIPAA compliance reports facilitate audit processes. Contemporary healthcare SIEM products also support integration with clinical alerting systems so security events can be prioritized without interfering with patient care functions. Deploying effective SIEM solutions in healthcare demands that unique challenges of medical environments are confronted (European Union Agency for Cybersecurity, 2023).

5.6 Next-Generation Firewalls and Intrusion Prevention

Next-generation firewalls (NGFWs) with built-in intrusion prevention systems (IPS) have emerged as essential elements of health network defense, providing advanced protection against contemporary cyber threats. Advanced security solutions beyond simple port-based filtering offer deep packet inspection, application-aware controls, and threat intelligence integration optimized for medical environments. NGFWs in medical networks implement strict policies for clinical applications such as EHR systems and medical imaging platforms while identifying and blocking malicious traffic patterns. IPS functions integrated into the solution examine network flows in real-time to block exploits on vulnerable medical devices and legacy systems. Healthcare-specific functionality includes HIPAA-compliant pre-configured rule sets, customized protection for DICOM and HL7 medical protocols, and emergency mode operation that ensures ongoing security under life-critical care scenarios without affecting patient safety.

Deploying NGFW/IPS solutions in the healthcare environment demands close attention to clinical workflow needs and regulatory requirements. Performance optimization is critical in order to sustain sub-second response times for life-critical applications, while high-availability configurations guarantee seamless operation. Healthcare providers are helped by cloud-managed deployments of firewalls that enforce uniform security policies across networked care sites and telehealth systems.

This scope provides readers with a solid grasp of the diverse function of NGFW/IPS in today's healthcare environment. The organization of the chapter overall takes a clear path from deployment considerations, operational performance, advanced capabilities, compliance and adaptability. It provides a balanced approach to the reader, progressing from basic deployment requirements to more advanced, technology-based enhancements. The discussion can be made even more robust by integrating relevant contemporary trends in technology and their applications in the real world. Incorporating topic matter on Zero Trust Architecture for protecting dispersed healthcare systems, predictive threat intelligence through AI/ML, Blockchain-based security for medical data, and SIEM/SOAR platforms for persistent monitoring would make the chapter more technically rich and practically applicable.

6. MEDICAL IoT SECURITY CHALLENGES

The widespread deployment of Internet of Medical Things (IoMT) devices has brought with it serious cybersecurity threats that healthcare organizations need to address with urgency. Networked medical devices like infusion pumps, patient monitors, and imaging equipment frequently have inherent security weaknesses such as old operating systems, hard-coded credentials, and unencrypted communication. All these vulnerabilities put IoMT devices directly in the crosshairs of cyberattacks that may jeopardize patient safety, from manipulation of medication dosages to full system hijacking. The healthcare ecosystem offers special challenges, as numerous medical devices cannot be patched without FDA clearance and clinical workflows require round-the-clock availability. Also, the growth of connected devices has grown the attack surface exponentially with an average hospital handling thousands of networked medical devices that are all potential points of entry for bad actors.

6.1 IoT Security Challenges

Securing these threats involves specialized measures that are made sensitive to both technical limitations and patient care demands. Network segmentation has become an important control, creating a segmented area of medical devices while preserving required clinical data flows. Healthcare organizations must also implement robust device authentication, continuous monitoring for anomalous behavior, and specialized vulnerability management programs. However, solutions must balance security with clinical utility, ensuring protective measures don't interfere with emergency care or delay life-saving treatments. The increasing adoption of more sophisticated attacks against healthcare devices, such as tailored to healthcare organizations, highlights the necessity of taking prompt measures to protect these vital elements of contemporary patient care without compromising with changing FDA cybersecurity policies and healthcare regulations (National Institute of Standards and Technology, 2024).

6.2 IoMT Threat Landscape

The Internet of Medical Things (IoMT) has brought unparalleled cybersecurity threats to healthcare networks, producing a multifaceted threat environment that threatens data security and patient safety. Infusion pumps, patient monitors, and imaging systems are among those medical devices increasingly being attacked with sophisticated cyberattacks because of their frequently out-of-date operating systems, unpatched vulnerabilities, and absence of security fundamentals. Recent breaches illustrate concerning trends such as attacks that infect critical care devices, unapproved remote access to devices, and tampering with sensitive patient information. The danger is heightened by the growing attack surface of healthcare, with hospitals now having 10-15 networked medical devices per bed, many talking over insecure protocols.

This shifting threat requires immediate action as adversaries create healthcare-targeted malware and exploit kits. Criminal organizations now aim at medical devices as gateways into hospital networks, while nation-state actors look for exploits in life-critical devices.

6.3 Device Authentication Strategies for Healthcare IoT Security

Strong device authentication is key to defending healthcare networks against unauthorized access to sensitive medical systems and patient information. Today's healthcare environments demand multi-layered authentication methods capable of addressing varied connected devices - from older medical devices to newer IoT sensors. Certificate-based authentication through X.509 digital certificates offer robust identity authentication for qualified devices, with network access control (NAC) products providing fallback methods for less capable devices. New zero trust architectures employ continuous authentication, assessing device behavior patterns and security posture during each session.

Implementation is successful with balancing security against the demands of clinical workflow. Role-based access policies need to coordinate with clinical requirements while imposing least-privilege principles. Multi-factor authentication (MFA) solutions need to be optimized for healthcare environments using techniques such as FIDO2 security keys that are resistant to phishing but allow for urgent access situations. For healthcare IoT devices, root-of-trust mechanisms in hardware and secure booting ensure protection against device impersonation attacks. With increasing growth of healthcare networks through cloud and remote care technologies, device authentication methods need to change to ensure protection of distributed environments alongside maintaining tough compliance requirements such as HIPAA and FDA cyber security standards.

6.4 Segmentation of Medical Devices in the Network

Network segmentation is an important security technique for safeguarding network-connected medical devices and protecting sensitive healthcare information. By segmenting hospital networks into sequestered zones, segmentation restricts lateral flow in the event of cyberattacks, and contains breaches if they occur. Medical settings call for tailored practices that respect a varied array of medical IoT (IoMT) devices, from older equipment using dated protocols to current connected devices. Successful segmentation establishes assigned virtual LANs (VLANs) for various categories of devices—such as patient monitors, imaging equipment, and infusion pumps—while establishing rigorous access controls between zones. A medical demilitarized zone (mDMZ) design offers further security for internet-connected devices, serving as an intermediate layer between care systems and outside networks.

Slicing in healthcare requires thoughtful planning to preserve clinical processes while reinforcing security. Software-defined networking (SDN) supports dynamic micro-segmentation based on particular medical applications and risk profiles. Healthcare IT staffs need to reconcile security needs with the demands for real-time data sharing for patient care while keeping emergency access open when required. Some special considerations include support for broadcast-dependent legacy devices and setting up quality-of-service (QoS) policies to prioritize critical medical traffic. Well-designed network segmentation decreases attack surfaces by more than 70% and satisfies compliance requirements while preserving the availability required for quality patient care (Puri & Gochhait, 2023).

6.5 Vulnerability Management in Healthcare

Successful vulnerability management is crucial to safeguarding healthcare networks from sophisticated cyber attacks on patient data and mission-critical medical devices. A robust program integrates ongoing asset discovery, risk scanning, and remediation prioritization to fix vulnerabilities in IT infrastructure, medical equipment, and cloud environments. Healthcare organizations present special challenges, such as legacy systems that are unpatchable, FDA-regulated medical devices with update limitations, and 24/7 operational needs that restrict maintenance windows.

To roll out vulnerability management in healthcare, security needs to be balanced with patient care scheduling. Risk scoring schemes need to consider clinical impact, trading off variables such as likely treatment interruption against technical severity. Automated scanning tools require unique configurations to safely test sensitive medical equipment without compromising performance. Effective programs set up cross-functional teams comprising IT security, clinical engineering, and risk management to determine patching windows in synchrony with care delivery requirements. With regulatory oversight intensifying, healthcare professionals need to document their process of vulnerability management to prove diligence for HIPAA, FDA, and other compliance measures while ensuring strong defense systems against ransomware, data breaches, and other attacks on the healthcare industry.

6.6 FDA Guidance on Medical Device Security

The U.S. Food and Drug Administration (FDA) has put forth essential cybersecurity guidelines to face intensified threats to networked medical devices. These regulations require security-by-design principles across a device's life cycle, with manufacturers being expected to provide detailed cybersecurity risk assessments as part of premarket approvals. The FDA prioritizes secure architecture, such as authentication mechanisms, encryption requirements, and patchable designs, as well as a Software Bill of Materials (SBOM) to monitor vulnerabilities.

Healthcare organizations need to bring their network and procurement strategies in line with FDA cybersecurity advice. This involves confirming compliance by manufacturers, applying suggested network segmentation to medical devices, and developing vulnerability management processes that are compliant with FDA reporting schedules. The guidance also affects hospital IT staff, who have to juggle security patches with FDA-approved change control processes for regulated devices. As threats in cyberspace change, the FDA continues to tighten its strategy, emphasizing cooperation between manufacturers and healthcare providers to ensure device security without disrupting patient care or medical technology innovation (Silvestri et al., 2023).

7. INCIDENT RESPONSE AND RECOVERY

Healthcare organizations need a well-established incident response process for efficiently handling cybersecurity incidents without disrupting patient care. A strong plan includes real-time monitoring, swift containment procedures, and open communication pathways among IT staff, clinical personnel, and management. Special healthcare considerations include ensuring emergency access to important systems during incidents and meeting rigid HIPAA breach notification schedules. Threat response measures should rank threats against potential clinical impact, ranging from ransomware attacks that lock up medical records to hijacked IoT devices impacting patient monitoring systems.

7.1 Data integrity with Response and Recovery

The recovery process is concerned with safely recovering operations and executing mitigation actions. Healthcare networks require expert recovery strategies that authenticate data integrity in the EHR system, ensure medical device performance, and maintain ongoing care provision. Post-incident analysis reveals weaknesses as enhanced security controls eliminate chances of recurrence. Proper recovery also incorporates retraining of personnel and process enhancements to enhance overall cyber resilience within healthcare settings.

7.2 Healthcare-Specific Incident Response Plans

Healthcare organizations need custom incident response plans that take into account the distinct challenges of safeguarding patient information and clinical operations against cyberattacks. In contrast to typical IT environments, healthcare response plans must rank life-critical systems first, maintaining continual access to EHRs, medical devices, and emergency communications. Successful plans integrate clinical workflow into containment plans, with precise escalation paths that involve both technical and medical personnel. They also have to comply with health-care specific laws, such as HIPAA's 60-day breach notification rule and FDA medical device reporting rules, and have detailed audit trails for purposes of verification of compliance.

Effective health care incident response combines specialized considerations like alternative care procedures in the event of system outages and treatment data integrity verification procedures.Periodic tabletop exercises that mimic attacks against hospital systems assist in the identification of gaps in response capacity. In light of data breaches increasingly targeting healthcare, organizations have to constantly revise response plans to react to changing threats while minimizing disruption in the delivery of patient care and sustaining public trust in their security posture (Senevirathna & Kleihorst, 2024).

7.3 Response Protocols

Healthcare companies need customized reaction plans that will counteract attacks that pose risks to data protection and patient care. Actual procedures emphasize isolating affected systems while keeping access to vital medical equipment and EHRs alive via pre-established emergency processes. Quickly, teams have to identify the type, evaluate the encryption extent of data, and analyze effects on clinical activities—all in a manner that maintains forensic value. Healthcare-specific factors involve keeping alternative documentation processes and initiating downtime procedures to continue life-saving treatments during the containment process.

Successful response calls for collaboration among IT security, clinical personnel, and executive management in achieving technical recovery while prioritizing patient safety. Healthcare organizations must set unambiguous decision-making protocols for ransom payment options based on legal guidance and law enforcement advisories. Post-recovery measures involve system validation, vulnerability remediation, and retraining staff to avoid recurrence. Because of the harsh operational and financial impact of health care providers need to test and revise response mechanisms regularly to counter changing threats while complying with regulatory reporting standards for breaches of protected health information.

7.4 Business Continuity Planning

Strong business continuity planning is critical in health care settings to ensure essential operations during cyber-attacks, natural disasters, or system crashes. Good plans put emergency life-saving services first by characterizing critical clinical systems, configuring redundant infrastructure, and providing failover for EHRs, medical devices, and communication networks. Health-specific considerations involve electronic system downtime procedures, emergency documentation protocols, and pre-established escalation routes involving technical and clinical teams. Ongoing risk assessments allow organizations to review possible disruptions to networked systems while maintaining compliance with healthcare regulations that require continuity protection.

Effective business continuity plans include periodic testing via tabletop exercises and mock outages to ensure response capacity. Healthcare organizations need to have current recovery time objectives (RTOs) for key systems and have emergency processes trained to the staff.

7.5 Healthcare Forensic Investigation

Healthcare organizations need advanced forensic investigation expertise to respond effectively to cyber breaches without compromising regulatory compliance and continuity of patient care. Digital forensic activities in healthcare settings have to combine robust evidence collection with the emergency imperative to restore essential clinical systems. Investigators are presented with special challenges when conducting healthcare networks analysis, such as legacy medical devices with minimal logging capabilities, severe chain-of-custody procedures for protected health information (PHI), and balancing preservation of evidence with minimal disruption to treatment. Forensic protocols in healthcare are healthcare-specific, with an emphasis on quick breach scope, attacker methods, and compromised data types identification to accommodate HIPAA's 60-day breach notification requirement.

Practical healthcare forensic investigations utilize specialized tools and techniques that are adapted to medical settings. These involve analysis of medical device logs, EHR audit trail review, and reconstruction of network traffic while preserving data integrity for possible legal actions. Healthcare workflows need to be understood by investigators to differentiate malicious behavior from valid clinical activity. Findings should guide security enhancements, employee training, and revised incident response plans after the investigation (Senevirathna & Kleihorst, 2024).

7.6 Post-Breach Recovery Strategies

Healthcare organizations need to have extensive post-breach recovery strategies in place in order to recover operations securely with continuous patient care. The first step targets system remediation—removing attack vectors, patching vulnerabilities, and ensuring the integrity of EHRs and healthcare devices. Healthcare-specific factors involve recovery prioritization of life-critical systems, treatment data accuracy verification, and instating greater monitoring for areas that have already been compromised. Communication protocols need to resolve regulatory needs, such as HIPAA-recommended patient notification and FDA reportability on impacted medical devices, while still keeping stakeholders informed.

Recovery plans should include lessons learned to enhance network resilience. Security architecture review, revised access controls, and employees' retraining in new procedures fall within that umbrella. Restoration speed must be weighed against rigorous forensic analysis to assure total threat removal prior to full system reintegration. Periodic testing of recovery processes via simulated breach identifies weaknesses and sharpens response capabilities.

8. CASE STUDIES AND LESSONS LEARNT IN HEALTHCARE NETWORK DEFENSE

Examination of actual healthcare cybersecurity breaches is a good source of lessons for enhancing network defense. Such case studies include the 2017 WannaCry attack that paralyzed NHS hospitals, identifying inherent vulnerabilities in legacy systems and patch management procedures. Likewise, the 2020 Universal Health Services attack illustrated the ripple effects of network breaches across multi-facility healthcare systems. All these incidents reinforce common themes: the value of segmenting medical IoT devices from other networks, the necessity of having good backup systems in place, and staff training's role in annulling phishing-driven breaches. Healthcare-centric takeaways teach keeping clinical activities running during breaches while also adhering to strict reporting timeframes mandated by regulatory bodies (Maniraj et al., 2025).

8.1 Healthcare Network Defense

Best practices to emerge from these case studies cite zero trust architectures' efficacy in controlling lateral movement during breaches. Effective healthcare organizations have initiated proactive threat hunting, increased privileged account monitoring, and regular penetration of clinical networks. The lessons are the usefulness of cross-functional incident response groups that involve both clinical and IT leadership and the importance of having offline backup for important patient information.

8.2 Predicting Emerging Threats

The healthcare industry is confronted with a dynamic environment of cyber threats that require proactive recognition and mitigation tactics. Emerging threats include social engineering attacks on healthcare personnel by AI, advanced aimed at interconnected medical devices, and supply chain breaches through third-party providers. Predictive analysis foresees increased risks to cloud-based health data systems and the hacking of 5G-connected medical devices as points of entry into hospital networks. Healthcare-specific weaknesses, including unsecured legacy systems and unpatched IoMT devices, continue to be high priority targets for malicious actors wishing to interfere with the delivery of care or steal coveted patient information. Threat intelligence indicates growing physical and cyber risk convergence, with networked medical devices posing direct threats to patient safety.

To keep pace with these trends, healthcare organizations need to implement predictive security approaches that marry threat intelligence with machine learning-based analytics. Proactive activities such as red team exercises and threat modeling identify vulnerabilities prior to exploitation (Maniraj et al., 2025).

8.3 Security Automation in Healthcare: Strengthening Network Protection

The healthcare sector is increasingly embracing security automation in order to fortify network defense and guard against advanced cyber attacks. Automated solutions facilitate real-time monitoring of electronic health records, medical IoT, and cloud-based systems while minimizing dependence on manual interventions. The major use cases involve AI-powered threat detection analyzing network traffic patterns to flag anomalies, automated patch management of exposed systems, and orchestrated incident response processes that expedite breach containment. Healthcare-specific automation solutions are able to triage alerts by the probable effect on clinical operations so that most critical systems are kept safe without bogging down the security staff. Such technologies also assist in overcoming manpower shortages by executing routine security functions so that staff is free to pursue strategic endeavors while still being compliant with HIPAA and other regulations.

Healthcare security automation must be implemented with careful planning to meet efficiency needs with consideration for patient safety. Solutions need to seamlessly integrate with current clinical workflows and legacy infrastructure and offer audit trails for regulatory purposes. Automated playbooks can automate responses to frequently encountered threats such as unauthorized attempts to access the network, minimizing mean time to remediate. As healthcare networks become more intricate, automation is necessary to continue to ensure strong defenses, monitor distributed environments continuously, and respond quickly to new threats without interrupting critical care delivery services.

8.4 Workforce Training Strategies

Successful cybersecurity training of the healthcare workforce is essential to counteract human-related risks in network defense. Training programs specific to healthcare must extend beyond broad security awareness to cover clinical workflows, vulnerabilities in medical devices, and protected health information (PHI) management. Role-specific training modules must be created for various stakeholders - clinicians require specialized education on secure EHR access and medical device procedures, whereas IT personnel need more advanced training in network monitoring and incident response. Interactive techniques such as phishing simulations and tabletop exercises enhance participation and retention, whereas microlearning strategies provide bite-sized security reminders accommodating hectic healthcare schedules. Training also needs to include regulatory compliance and reporting protocols to support compliance with HIPAA and other regulations.

Reinforcement must be continuous, with periodic refresher courses to compensate for newly emerging threats such as AI-based social engineering attacks on healthcare networks. The efficacy of training has to be monitored using measures like phishing click-through rates, reporting of incidents, and audit findings. Leadership commitment is essential - executives must prioritize and take part in security training to ensure organization-wide adoption. As healthcare is becoming more digital, spending on holistic, role-based cybersecurity training produces a human firewall that reinforces technical controls in safeguarding sensitive networks and patient information.

8.5 Investment Priorities

Healthcare organizations need to strategically invest in fortifying network security while countering emerging cyber threats. Key investment priorities involve the modernization of existing infrastructure, the deployment of zero trust architecture, and the installation of advanced threat detection solutions specific to clinical environments. Key focus areas include shielding Internet of Medical Things (IoMT) devices by segmenting networks, securing clouds for hybrid healthcare systems, and creating strong incident response capabilities. Investments ought to also focus on the automation of compliance tools to make HIPAA and GDPR easier to manage, and security awareness programs to reduce human threats. Ransomware attacks are focusing more on healthcare, so organizations need to strike a balance between preventive controls and detection and response abilities, ensuring that investments are congruent with both today's threats and tomorrow's digital transformation plans.

Long-term investment plans should focus on scalable solutions that evolve along with healthcare's expanding attack surface. These encompass AI-driven security analytics to proactively hunt threats, modular platforms to integrate visibility across far-flung networks, and robust backup systems to enable fast recovery. Training of the workforce continues to be just as important, necessitating constant investment in advanced cybersecurity training for IT staff and clinical workers. With intensified regulatory pressures on the rise, healthcare organizations also need to allocate resources to evidencing security effectiveness through ongoing monitoring and audit readiness. These investments mutually construct a defense-in-depth approach that safeguards patient information and provides uninterrupted delivery of care in an increasingly adversarial cyber environment.

8.6 Roadmap for Resilient Healthcare Networks

Establishing resilient healthcare networks involves an organized roadmap that aligns security efforts with clinical priorities and changing threats. The foundation starts with enterprise-wide risk assessments to define critical assets, vulnerabilities, and possible effects on patient care. Phase one is about the deployment of foundational controls: network segmentation of medical IoT devices, privileged access management, and encrypted communication. Phase two moves to continuous monitoring, threat detection through AI, and automated incident response processes. During the implementation, the roadmap should include regulatory compliance, training programs for staff, and managing third-party risk to develop an integrated defense strategy.

The long-term perspective focuses on adaptive security architectures to be able to handle emerging threats. This entails zero trust deployments, cloud-native security mechanisms for hybrid clouds, and predictive analytics-powered proactive threat hunting. The roadmap should be agile enough to support emerging technologies such as 5G-enabled devices while upholding foundational patient safety goals. Adhering to this graduated pathway allows healthcare organizations to sequentially enhance network resilience without compromising on critical care delivery operations.

9. CONCLUSION

Healthcare network protection has never been more vital as the sector is under mounting cyber threats, facing swift digital evolution. This wide-ranging analysis of security strategies for networks underscores the necessity of a multi-layered security approach that blends innovative technologies such as zero trust architecture and AI-based threat detection with strong policies and ongoing workforce training. The distinctive health environment challenges—such as legacy system security weaknesses, medical IoT threats, and life-critical availability expectations—require unique solutions that reconcile patient care delivery with security. With ongoing ransomware attacks and data breaches targeting the health industry, organizations need to invest in secure infrastructure, proactive threat detection, and incident response measures while ensuring compliance with changing regulations.

Ahead, healthcare network security will need to adapt to evolving threats and facilitate care delivery innovation. Bringing security-by-design methodologies, embracing predictive analytics, and establishing healthcare-dedicated cybersecurity frameworks will be necessary for developing future-proof networks. By executing the strategies outlined—ranging from network segmentation to training personnel—healthcare organizations can develop a security culture that safeguards private patient information, enables continuity of care, and preserves public confidence. The path to cyber-resilient healthcare networks demands sustained effort, effort in collaboration throughout the ecosystem, and acknowledgment that sound network defense is the basis for high-quality patient care in the digital world.

It also retains thematic continuity by correlating security issues to healthcare's fundamental mission—patient safety and continuity of care. Yet, although the content is sound intellectually, flow and logical progression can be enhanced for better readability, coherence, and depth.

The sources cited in this chapter seem to be partly adequate and contextually valid but are not deep, diverse, or recent enough to adequately support an extensive, research-based discussion of healthcare network security. Although the chapter cites some relevant regulatory and technological sources (e.g., HIPAA, GDPR, and NIST), it mostly makes use of generic citations instead of fresh, peer-reviewed, or industry-specific literature representative of the fast-changing nature of healthcare cybersecurity.

REFERENCES

Dzamesi, L., & Elsayed, N. (2025). *A review on the security vulnerabilities of the IoMT against malware attacks and DDoS*. arXiv. https://arxiv.org/abs/2501.07432

Elhoseny, M., Ramírez-González, G., & Abu-Elnasr, O. (2021). Security and privacy issues in Medical Internet of Things: Overview, countermeasures, challenges and future directions. *Sustainability*, *13*(21), 11645. Advance online publication. DOI: 10.3390/su132111645

Erişen, S. (2022). IoT-based real-time updating multi-layered learning system for a special care context during COVID-19. *Cogent Engineering*, *9*(1), 2044588. Advance online publication. DOI: 10.1080/23311916.2022.2044588

European Union Agency for Cybersecurity. (2023). *ENISA threat landscape: Health sector*. https://www.enisa.europa.eu/publications/enisa-threat-landscape-health-sector

Ghubaish, A., Samara, L., Çelik, A., & Al-Ali, A. (2023). *Recent advances in the Internet of Medical Things (IoMT) systems security*. arXiv. https://arxiv.org/abs/2302.04456

IEEE Standards Association. (2024). *IEEE/UL 2933-2024 Standard for clinical Internet of Things (IoT) data and device interoperability with TIPPSS*. https://standards.ieee.org

Kilincer, I. F., Ertam, F., & Sengur, A. (2023). Automated detection of cybersecurity attacks in healthcare systems with recursive feature elimination and multilayer perceptron optimization. *Biocybernetics and Biomedical Engineering*, *43*(1), 30–41. DOI: 10.1016/j.bbe.2022.12.003

Kishor, M., & Chakraborty, C. (2022). Artificial intelligence and Internet of Things based healthcare 4.0 monitoring system. *Wireless Personal Communications*, *127*(2), 1615–1631. DOI: 10.1007/s11277-022-09838-1

Maniraj, S. P., Monisha, J., Amutha, R., Kavitha, R., Shriidhar, P. J., & Srinivasan, C. (2025). Agricultural water conservation through AI-enhanced solar IoT networks. In *Proceedings of the International Conference on Emerging Areas in Research and Studies (ICEARS 2025)*.

Meng, Y., Huang, Z., Shen, G., & Ke, C. (2019). SDN-based security enforcement framework for data sharing systems of smart healthcare. *IEEE Transactions on Network and Service Management*, *17*(1), 308–318. DOI: 10.1109/TNSM.2019.2953489

Mohamadi, A., Ghahramani, H., Asghari, S. A., & Aminian, M. (2024). *Securing healthcare with deep learning: A CNN-based model for medical IoT threat detection*. arXiv. https://arxiv.org/abs/2410.19969

More, S., Singla, J., Verma, S., Ghosh, U., Rodrigues, J. J. P. C., & Hosen, A. S. M. S. (2020). Security assured CNN-based model for reconstruction of medical images on the Internet of healthcare things. *IEEE Access : Practical Innovations, Open Solutions*, *8*, 126333–126346. DOI: 10.1109/ACCESS.2020.3006348

National Institute of Standards and Technology. (2024). *Cybersecurity supply chain risk management practices for systems and organizations* (NIST Special Publication 800-161r1). U.S. Department of Commerce. https://doi.org/DOI: 10.6028/NIST.SP.800-161r1

Nguyen, D. C., Pathirana, P. N., Ding, M., & Seneviratne, A. (2021). BEdgeHealth: A decentralized architecture for edge-based IoMT networks using blockchain. *IEEE Internet of Things Journal*, *8*(14), 11743–11757. DOI: 10.1109/JIOT.2021.3054970

Nguyen, R., Nguyen, H. T., Nguyen, D. C., Pathirana, P. N., & Hossain, M. A. (2021). Secure blockchain enabled cyber–physical systems in healthcare using deep belief network with ResNet model. *Journal of Parallel and Distributed Computing*, *153*, 150–160. DOI: 10.1016/j.jpdc.2021.03.013

Puri, J., & Gochhait, S. (2023). Data security in healthcare: Enhancing the safety of data with cybersecurity. In *Proceedings of the International Conference on Computing and Emerging Sciences (ICCES)* (pp. 1779–1783).

Rachakonda, L., Mohanty, S. P., Kougianos, E., & Sundaravadivel, P. (2021). SaYoPillow: Blockchain-integrated privacy-assured IoMT framework for stress management considering sleeping habits. *IEEE Transactions on Consumer Electronics*, *67*(1), 20–29. DOI: 10.1109/TCE.2021.3054862

Rathore, S., Park, J. H., & Chang, H. (2021). Deep learning and blockchain-empowered security framework for intelligent 5G-enabled IoT. *IEEE Access : Practical Innovations, Open Solutions*, *9*, 90075–90091. DOI: 10.1109/ACCESS.2021.3091540

Ray, P. P., Chowhan, B., Kumar, N., & Almogren, A. (2021). BIoTHR: Electronic health record servicing scheme in IoT-blockchain ecosystem. *IEEE Internet of Things Journal*, *8*(13), 10857–10872. DOI: 10.1109/JIOT.2021.3058794

Senevirathna, N., & Kleihorst, R. (2024). 13 reasons why: Rationale and preliminary statistical approach for classifying electromagnetic disturbances in healthcare environments. In *IEEE Joint International Symposium on EMC Italy/APEMC* (pp. 100–103). IEEE.

Silvestri, S., Islam, S., Papangelou, P., & Sookhak, M. (2023). Cyber threat assessment and management for securing healthcare ecosystems using natural language processing. *International Journal of Information Security*, *22*(6), 1883–1899. DOI: 10.1007/s10207-023-00735-6

Chapter 5
Integrating Blockchain and IoT for Wearable Device Security

Abduvali Sottarov
Termez University of Economics and Service, Uzbekistan

Anorgul Ashirova
Mamun University, Uzbekistan

Temur Eshchanov
Urgench State University, Uzbekistan

Munir Ahmad
https://orcid.org/0000-0003-4836-6151
Survey of Pakistan, Pakistan

ABSTRACT

The integration of blockchain technology with IoT-enabled wearable devices offers a transformative approach to securing sensitive health, fitness, and lifestyle data. Traditional centralized security models are insufficient to address vulnerabilities such as data tampering, unauthorized access, and resource limitations. Blockchain's decentralization, immutability, and smart contract capabilities enable robust authentication, access control, and tamper-proof record-keeping, fostering transparency and trust. While challenges remain, including scalability, energy efficiency, latency, and regulatory compliance, advancements in lightweight architectures, edge computing, and privacy-preserving protocols position blockchain-enabled wearables to create secure, resilient, and user-centric digital ecosystems.

DOI: 10.4018/979-8-3373-4412-6.ch005

INTRODUCTION

The wearable devices have become highly advanced in a short span of time, with mere fitness trackers turning into advanced health monitoring machines, which have the ability to gather, analyze, and relay sensitive physiological and behavioral data. Starting with smartwatches and medical wearables, and moving to augmented reality glasses, they are becoming part of everyday life and are dominant in the areas of health, fitness, and lifestyle uses. Being able to constantly record real-time data, they are invaluable in personal wellness, chronic condition management, and clinical decision-making (Hughes et al., 2023; S. M. A. Iqbal et al., 2021; Poongodi et al., 2020; Sabry et al., 2022).

However, the widespread use of wearables introduces significant security and privacy concerns. Heart rate, blood pressure, location, and even data related to identity are sensitive and are commonly sent via wireless networks or kept in a centralized database, making them vulnerable to unauthorized users, data manipulation, and identity theft (Barbone et al., 2019; Nakayama et al., 2023). Conventional security frameworks that heavily depend on centralized servers and intermediaries are not efficient in securing wearable data because of single points of failure, scaling concerns, and exposure to cyberattacks. These failures substantiate the dire necessity of other methods that guarantee the confidentiality, integrity, and credibility of data produced by the wearables (Boumpa et al., 2022).

A promising remedy to these problems is blockchain technology, which has a decentralized and tamper-resistant ledger and programmable smart contracts. Combining blockchain and Internet of Things (IoT) allows creating secure, open, and verifiable data management systems that are specific to the resource-limited limitations of wearable devices. Such integration may facilitate authentication, user-controlled share of data, and the generation of auditable records of the interactions without the presence of centralized bodies (Adere, 2022; Kamruzzaman et al., 2022; Miaz & Ali, 2020; Nanda et al., 2023).

This chapter discusses how convergence in blockchain-IoT can enhance the security and privacy of a wearable ecosystem. It can examine the challenges inherent in wearable device security, outline the role of blockchain as a trust and resiliency enabler, provide an overview of integration strategies and architectures, and present real-life case studies on the use of blockchain in wearable systems. The chapter also evaluates technical, regulatory, and energy-related challenges that inhibit larger-scale adoption and provides insight into how researchers, developers, and policymakers can create secure, resilient, and privacy-preserving wearable ecosystems.

SECURITY AND PRIVACY CHALLENGES

The accessibility and growing popularity of wearable gadgets have raised concerns about the security and privacy of the data generated by these devices. In contrast to standard computing systems, wearables constantly collect and send highly sensitive data via resource-restricted hardware and wireless networks, usually lacking any well-developed protection measures. This exposes them to cyber threats, especially in the ability to breach personal safety, as well as trust within digital health ecosystems.

Data Sensitivity

The wealth of personal data produced by wearable devices is both intimate and very informative. On a more fundamental level, wearables are used to track vital signs, including heart rate, body temperature, respiration rate, and sleep habits, which give insights into the general health of an individual and their daily activities. Advanced wearables can monitor behavioral patterns, such as physical activity, exercise habits, stress factors, social interactions, and even emotional states based on a physiological response (T. Iqbal et al., 2021; Vijayan et al., 2021).

Medical-grade wearables in the healthcare setting take these features a step further by recording diagnostic-level data, including electrocardiograms (ECG) and blood oxygen saturation levels, continuous glucose levels, and blood pressure levels. This information plays an essential role in patient treatment, the prompt identification of health abnormalities, and chronic disease management. Malicious actors, however, make it an attractive target because of its sensitivity. Wearable data could be used by cybercriminals to commit identity theft, insurance fraud, or black-market trades. Privacy risks are increased by the potential of seemingly harmless data about behavior that, once collected over a long period, can give intimate information about an individual, their lifestyle, habits, place activities, and health weaknesses.

Wearable data breaches have more implications for an individual than for privacy (Zhang et al., 2025). In a healthcare context, breached data may be used to make erroneous clinical decisions, disrupt treatment procedures, and compromise patients' trust in online-based health interventions. In addition, behavioral or location information leaked can put users at risk of physical attacks, stalking, or specifically altering marketing options. This highlights the need to protect wearable information through security solutions beyond the standard methods. Table 1 categorizes examples across different domains.

Table 1. Categories of Wearable Data and Associated Risks

Data Type	Examples	Potential Risks
Basic Physiological	Heart rate, temperature, respiration	Identity theft, profiling, behavioral surveillance
Behavioral	Physical activity, stress indicators	Lifestyle inference, targeted manipulation
Advanced Medical	ECG, SpO_2, glucose, blood pressure	Fraudulent insurance claims, medical identity theft, and misdiagnosis
Location & Routines	GPS tracking, movement patterns	Stalking, exposure to physical threats, and privacy invasion

Vulnerabilities in Communication Channels

Wireless communication protocols used in wearables are mainly Bluetooth Low Energy (BLE), Wi-Fi, Near Field Communication (NFC), and cellular networks to communicate this data to companion devices, gateways, or cloud servers (Dragusin, Bizon, & Bostinaru, 2024; Dragusin, Bizon, Bostinaru, et al., 2024). These protocols facilitate the smooth real-time connection and remote monitoring, but they also pose various points of vulnerability, which are listed below.

- BLE is common because it is power-efficient, but has a high possibility of eavesdropping, man-in-the-middle (MITM) attacks, and impersonation when weak encryption is used or misconfigured. Attackers may steal sensitive information in transit, or they may use pairing mechanisms to gain access.
- Devices based on Wi-Fi are vulnerable to packet sniffing, denial-of-service (DoS) attacks, and network intrusions. Poorly sealed or open networks increase these risks because the attackers may tamper with or intercept the wearable information as it flows.
- A large number of wearables rely on clouds to store and analyze their data as well as to synchronize it. Although cloud-based systems offer scalability and enhanced processing capacity, data is vulnerable to interception during uploading/ downloading, misconfiguration, insider attacks, and attacks against the cloud itself.

These vulnerabilities demonstrate the weakness of wearable IoT systems, in which security lapses in the communication channels may compromise the integrity, accuracy, and confidentiality of essential personal and medical information. The consequences of even small violations of the implementation of protocols can be cascading and threaten the integrity of the whole process. Table 2 summarizes the common communication protocols in wearable IoT ecosystems and the security vulnerabilities associated with each.

Table 2. Communication Protocols and Vulnerabilities in Wearables

Communication Protocol	Advantages (Why Used)	Key Vulnerabilities
Bluetooth (BLE)	Low power, wide adoption	Eavesdropping, MITM attacks, device impersonation
Wi-Fi	High bandwidth, direct cloud	Packet sniffing, DoS attacks, and network intrusion
NFC	Quick, short-range transfers	Skimming, relay attacks, unauthorized access
Cellular	Wide coverage, mobility	SIM cloning, interception, signaling attacks
Cloud Integration	Storage, analytics, sync	Insider threats, misconfigurations, breaches in cloud infra

Threats to Wearable Security

The security threats to wearables are wide-ranging and can be aimed at both the hardware and the network upon which the devices connect. Key threats include:

- Heart rate, GPS, sleep patterns, or behaviour entries can be intercepted in transit by unauthorized parties. Time monitoring enables the attackers to develop comprehensive profiles of users.
- Wearables can be tampered with to send false data to perform inaccurate health analysis, false activity tracking, or a combination of the two, or to provide insurance or research claims. Clinical decisions and user trust can be undermined through such manipulation.
- Malware can use wearable devices or gateways in communication to send erroneous data into the system. This has the potential to interfere with analytics, confuse healthcare providers, or provoke unauthorized reactions.
- Wearable service providers or third-party apps can use personal data without direct user authorization, and this is ethically and legally wrong. There is the possibility of the sale or analysis of aggregated data in ways that the user did not foresee, and this poses privacy and ethical issues.

Such a mixture of threats not only puts in question individual privacy and safety but also undermines the greater confidence in wearable technologies. A user can be reluctant to use new equipment or even join digital health initiatives because they feel that no sufficient protection is implemented to protect their personal information (Barua et al., 2022; Hernández-álvarez et al., 2022; Hora & Kulkarni, 2024). To consolidate the diverse threats facing wearable ecosystems, Table 3 presents key attack vectors, their impacts, and implications for users.

Table 3. Security Threats in Wearable IoT Devices

Threat Type	Description	Implications for Users
Eavesdropping	Interception of sensitive data in transit	Loss of privacy, user profiling, targeted exploitation
Tampering	Manipulation of transmitted or stored data	False health records, misinformed clinical decisions
Spoofing	Impersonation of devices or gateways	Injection of false data, system disruption
Unauthorized Data Use	Data misuse by providers or third parties	Privacy violations, unethical profiling, loss of user trust

Limitations of Centralized Security Models

High-density wearable systems today are created on the basis of centralized security solutions, with the process of authentication, storage, and policy enforcement being delegated to cloud servers or third-party intermediaries (Arif et al., 2020; Li et al., 2023; Tekchandani et al., 2023). Being useful in conventional computing systems, these methods have a few drawbacks in the context of wearables:

- The central servers are points of vulnerability. Power blackouts, malicious operations, or hacking into the server can put the security and availability of the whole wearable network into question.
- As millions of devices produce never-ending flows of data, the extent of centralized systems is limited in processing, authentication, and storage. Latency, service interruptions, or poor performance may result as a result of high traffic.
- Most cryptography protocols and security systems developed to support centralized systems are intensive in computation needs and energy demands. Security-performance trade-offs occur as wearable devices often have short battery life and processing, and thus may not be able to support such operations.
- Users are under the obligation to trust all the service providers or intermediaries to handle and secure their data. This may come into conflict with the

principle of privacy and the law, particularly sensitive health and biometric data, in situations where the providers are not transparent.

Such constraints highlight the importance of decentralized, lightweight, and adaptive security solutions able to address the intrinsic disadvantages of wearable IoT devices. Integration of blockchain, edge-based computing, and privacy-preserving systems is gaining traction as being potential solution to addressing these issues, providing tamper-resistance, resilient, and user-friendly alternatives to centralized security models. Table 4 outlines the weaknesses of centralized security approaches when applied to wearable IoT devices, emphasizing the need for decentralized alternatives.

Table 4. Limitations of Centralized Security Models for Wearables

Limitation	Explanation	Consequences for Wearables
Single Point of Failure	Centralized servers are vulnerable to outages/attacks	System-wide compromise, loss of availability
Scalability Constraints	Difficulty handling millions of continuous data streams	Latency, bottlenecks, degraded performance
High Resource Demands	Complex cryptographic operations exceed wearable device capacities	Battery drain, weakened security-performance balance
Trust Deficits	Reliance on third parties for security and compliance	Lack of transparency, user mistrust, and potential legal conflicts

BLOCKCHAIN AS AN ENABLER OF WEARABLE SECURITY

Weaknesses of the traditional security system to secure the wearable IoT ecosystem have spawned the interest in blockchain as a revolutionary tool of trust, resiliency, and end-user privacy. Using its decentralized, transparent, and immutable infrastructure, the blockchain provides solutions to some of the most significant vulnerabilities of wearable devices, both in terms of data tampering and unauthorized access. The possibility to integrate it into an IoT environment opens opportunities to a secure data exchange, reliable authentication, and autonomous enforcement of privacy-preserving policies.

Blockchain Fundamentals

Blockchain, as a distributed ledger technology (DLT), is a technology that keeps an ever-expanding chain of records, known as blocks, that are cryptographically connected and secured over a peer-to-peer network (Reegu et al., 2023; Tanwar et al., 2020). Its core values are the basis on which it can achieve wearable ecosystems, which are listed below.

- Unlike traditional centralized systems, where a single server or authority governs data, blockchain distributes data across multiple nodes in a peer-to-peer network. This removes any singular points of failure, so that when one compromised server is present, it cannot cause a failure of the system and alter data. Decentralization is also a key property in wearable IoT ecosystems, where resiliency against outages, a cyberattack, or a lost device is improved, and in case a node fails, data can still be available. Decentralized networks also minimize the trust that a user puts into a third-party service provider, since the user has direct control of the data.
- Data cannot be changed or removed once it is added to the blockchain without the decision of the network. This can ensure that there is an auditable history of every interaction and transaction. In the case of wearables, immutability is essential to the integrity of medical, behavioral, and lifestyle data. Biometric data, fitness tracking, and health records are stored in a way that cannot be changed easily, which decreases the chances of fraudulent attempts to change information or unintentional inaccuracies that may interfere with clinical decision-making, insurance claims, or research results.
- Blockchains use consensus algorithms to decide and agree on the validity of transactions. The most popular models are Proof of Work (PoW) (Miraz et al., 2021), Proof of Stake (PoS) (Skh Saad & Raja Mohd Radzi, 2020), Proof of Authority (PoA) (Curran, 2018), and Directed Acyclic Graphs (DAGs) (Byeon & Lee, 2023; Digitale et al., 2022). Wearables, with their limited processing power and energy resources, require lightweight, energy-efficient consensus protocols. As a case in point, PoA enables trusted parties to verify transactions with ease without the need for computation-intensive mining, whereas architectures based on DAGs allow parallel transaction processing, making them capable of supporting large-scale and continuous wearable data sets.

Collectively, the aspects render blockchain naturally competent in overcoming the weaknesses of wearable technologies, such as compromised data, unauthorized access, and malfunction of the centralized system. Blockchain enhances the infrastructure level with security, transparency, and resilience embedded into the wearable systems, which in turn turn wearable ecosystems into trusted digital settings. To clearly highlight the fundamental properties of blockchain and their relevance to wearable IoT ecosystems, Table 5 summarizes the key features and benefits.

Table 5. Blockchain Fundamentals and Relevance to Wearable IoT

Feature	Definition/Mechanism	Relevance for Wearables
Decentralization	Data is distributed across peer-to-peer nodes.	Eliminates a single point of failure, ensures resilience, and provides user data control.
Immutability	Records are tamper-proof once validated	Preserves the integrity of health and behavioral data
Consensus	Network agreement on valid transactions	Enables secure validation with lightweight, energy-efficient protocols

Smart Contracts for Authentication and Access Control

Self-executing programs are coded on the blockchain, which also automatically executes the rules and policies without any intermediaries, known as smart contracts (Hewa et al., 2021; Rahman et al., 2024; Zheng et al., 2020).

- Smart contracts can check the authenticity of wearable devices and related entities and then provide access to the network. This denies attacks of spoofing, and only authorized devices are involved in collecting and communicating data. An example here is a wearable glucose device that may identify itself on the blockchain, and any subsequent effort by a fake device to relay information would be dismissed automatically.
- Smart contracts allow user-controlled and fine-grained access permissions to data sharing. Individuals are in a position to determine who is permitted to access a certain stream of data, its period, and the purpose of doing so. Indicatively, a patient could give a cardiologist access to real-time PDF ECG readings but limit access to insurers or fitness applications to only aggregate summaries. This can provide users with fine control, which is in compliance with the rules and ethics of data privacy.
- Smart contracts can be used to automate regulatory compliance. HIPAA, GDPR, or local privacy legislation requirements can be encoded to dictate the sharing and storage of wearable data at the legal level. The system is instant in flagging or blocking any violation, including unauthorized access or data export, which minimizes the use of post hoc audits and manual enforcement.

Directly implementing these features in the blockchain, wearable ecosystems become less reliant on intermediaries and become more transparent, autonomous, and self-enforcing, improving user trust and system reliability. Table 6 outlines the core applications of smart contracts in wearable IoT ecosystems, illustrating how they enhance authentication, access control, and compliance.

Table 6. Smart Contract Applications in Wearable Security

Application	Mechanism	Benefits for Wearables
Authentication	Verifies device legitimacy before granting access	Prevents spoofing, ensures only trusted devices interact
Access Control	Defines user-specific permissions and sharing rules	Empowers users with granular, privacy-aligned control
Policy Enforcement	Automates compliance with regulatory/legal frameworks	Reduces reliance on audits, ensures GDPR/ HIPAA-aligned data handling

Data Integrity and Tamper-Proof Record-Keeping

Blockchain offers strong systems to maintain the integrity and authenticity of wearable data, such as:-

- All data readings of wearable devices, be it the heart rate, number of steps, or glucose readings, are cryptographically computed as a hash value and are immutable records. This makes sure that the data, when stored, can not be changed without being noticed. This integrity can be used by medical professionals and researchers in clinical decision-making, longitudinal studies, and regulatory filings.
- Blockchain enables stakeholders, such as healthcare providers, insurers, and researchers, to verify the source of data without depending on third parties. Every transaction is time-stamped and traceable, which allows open audit and minimizes the chances of manipulating the data. This can be especially useful in cases where clinical trials or insurance claims are involved and data authenticity is of utmost importance (Hanif et al., 2023).
- Tamper-proof records give users a sense of security that the information stored and transmitted by them is not tampered with or intended to be viewed by others. Blockchain increases the degree of trust in the wearable ecosystem by showing verifiable evidence of data integrity and promoting its adoption.

Furthermore, blockchain allows interoperability when using encryption and anonymization methods, meaning that sensitive information can be safely transmitted to authorized individuals without undermining privacy. This integrity/ auditability/ trust combination makes the blockchain a key building block of secure wearable IoT systems.

Suitability for IoT and Wearables

Even though blockchain was created to be used in financial sectors, its fundamental characteristics can be mapped with the needs of wearable devices powered by IoT. There are certain adaptations:

- Full blockchain clients can be impractically resource-inefficient to run on wearables. Simplified clients, or lightweight nodes, can have a device interact with the blockchain without keeping a full copy of the ledger, reducing memory and energy consumption.
- Edge computing allows processing data at or close to the wearable device before the summaries or hashes are recorded to the blockchain. This minimizes latency, conserves battery power, and optimizes bandwidth usage with no loss of security guarantees.
- Wearable systems can have heterogeneous devices, platforms, and networks. Blockchain is used to securely and standardize data sharing among these multiple systems and can provide uniform authentication, access control, and data integrity across all vendors and protocols.
- Zero-knowledge proofs and homomorphic encryption, as well as off-chain storage, can be used so that sensitive data is kept secret, with blockchain used to perform verification and auditability. Users can prove the validity of information selectively without revealing raw information, which increases privacy and maintains transparency.

These adaptations allow blockchain to be used as a foundation of secure, decentralized wearable ecosystems to support user autonomy, resilient infrastructures, and clear interactions. Blockchain is uniquely positioned to solve the distinct challenges with regard to wearable IoT security by integrating immutable ledger features with smart contracts, privacy-enhancing mechanisms, and resource-conscious architectures to build trust and reliability.

ARCHITECTURES AND INTEGRATION STRATEGIES

Introduction of blockchain into wearable IoT systems needs architectural solutions that are sensitive to security, scale, and resource consumption. Wearable devices are necessarily limited in processing power, storage, and battery capacity, and it is not feasible to use conventional blockchain designs literally. In response, there is a study of hybrid architectures, light consensus mechanisms, and secure data-sharing structures that can make it possible to implement the blockchain without overloading wearable devices.

Blockchain-IoT Architectures for Wearables

The peculiarities of wearable devices require architectural solutions that would be both security- and efficiency-optimized:

On-chain vs. off-chain storage solution solves one of the most important architectural issues of wearable blockchain systems: the amount and rate of data produced by devices. Directly storing all data generated by wearables on the blockchain is not feasible since that would quickly saturate ledger capacity and slow transaction processing, increase costs, and create scalability bottlenecks. As a response, the majority of frameworks implement a hybrid approach, where only necessary metadata, cryptographic hashes, or transaction summaries are stored on-chain, with the rest of the raw data stored off-chain in secure storage, e.g., cloud platforms or edge servers. Such a design can guarantee that the integrity and authenticity of data remain verifiable after blockchain records, so that the stakeholders can verify the provenance without overwhelming the network. Separating critical verification data and high-volume raw datasets enables on-chain/off-chain architectures to be secure and scalable, appropriate to use with ongoing streams of wearable data in healthcare, fitness, and lifestyle applications (Eren et al., 2025).

Edge computing integration is in addition to hybrid storage, where intermediary nodes are deployed between wearables and the blockchain network, where initial data processing, filtering, aggregation, and encryption occur before committing summaries or cryptographic proofs to the ledger (Akkaoui et al., 2020; Yang et al., 2019). This decentralized processing can decrease network congestion, decrease latency, and conserve wearable battery life, which is of primary concern in devices that constantly monitor physiological data. As an illustration, an ECG wearable can process real-time cardiac rhythms at the edge, in order to detect anomalies and transmit only alerts or hash summaries to the blockchain, as opposed to the whole stream of high-frequency data. With prior analytics and cryptographic validation, edge computing can provide guaranteed response time, data confidentiality, and the ability of blockchain networks to scale to massive wearables deployments without performance tradeoffs.

Lightweight nodes allow wearable devices to become actors of the blockchain ecosystem, without the overhead of maintaining the entire ledger or making resource-heavy calculations. These simplified clients may check transaction headers, communicate with smart contracts, and engage with consensus mechanisms, where devices are enabled to authenticate transactions, ensure the integrity of data origins, and preserve trust on the network. The lightweighting nodes enhance memory consumption and computation loads, which translates into the ability of low-power wearables to work to support decentralized data management without compromising the efficiency of the device. This can be used to verify health or fitness metrics in real time, facilitate the sharing of health data securely between multiple stakeholders, and maintain the immutability and transparency that are central to blockchain without affecting the performance of the hardware and software on the device.

Collectively, these hybrid architectural approaches on-chain/off-chain storage, integration of edge computing, and lightweight node participation find a successful compromise between the transparency, immutability, and security of blockchain systems and the feasibility of wearable IoT devices. With these approaches together, wearable systems could provide secure authentication and traceable data management and real-time monitoring, with reduced computational overhead and energy requirements, and strong, user-friendly decentralized networks.

Consensus Mechanisms for Low-Power Devices

The foundation of blockchain networks is consensus algorithms, which make all nodes of the network accept the validity and sequence of transactions (Al-awamy et al., 2025; Upadhyay et al., 2024). Consensus in traditional blockchains is reached in mechanisms such as PoW, which is computationally and energy-intensive, thus not feasible with resource-constrained wearable devices. Wearable systems need lightweight, efficient, and scalable consensus protocols that do not strain device capabilities in order to support continuous data streams but maintain the integrity, security, and trustworthiness of the network.

PoA is a consensus protocol that is very appropriate in wearable IoT networks. Rather than conducting energy-intensive mining, PoA uses a list of already verified trusted emphaticians (such as healthcare institutions, regulatory bodies, or network operators) who can verify transactions. This strategy significantly decreases the computational effort and energy use as well, while realizing a large throughput. In controlled environments where it is possible to verify the identity of a validator, PoA is especially beneficial as it offers both security and efficiency to networks of multiple resource-constrained wearable devices.

Another effective alternative to wearable ecosystems is DPoS. Under DPoS, token holders or participants within the network elect fewer delegates to validate transactions on their behalf. Such a system decreases the amount of energy and computational load on individual devices and preserves network security. DPoS increases the scalability of wearable networks by delegating validation to a set of trusted users, enabling massive amounts of health and fitness data to be processed in near real-time in wearable networks. The strategy facilitates multi-stakeholder multi-moving systems where fast-check is imperative to quick interventions and precise statistics.

DAG-Based Models offer an entirely alternative viewpoint of consensus that can be unique to high-frequency IoT setups. Compared to linear blockchains, DAGs can support parallel processing of transactions without the need to mine. This allows us to verify streams of continuous wearable-generated data (heart rate, glucose levels, activity history, etc.) in real-time with the lowest latency possible. DAG architectures are also able to be scaled by network activity, which facilitates their use in environments where the production of data is necessary to keep up with any real-time monitoring needs.

With considerations of specific limitations of wearable devices in mind, adapting consensus mechanisms can allow balancing security, energy efficiency, scalability, and real-time performance to ensure that decentralized wearable ecosystems operate with high reliability without losing user trust or data integrity.

Secure Data Sharing Frameworks

A wearable ecosystem powered by blockchain can help to securely, transparently, and trustfully share data between multiple stakeholders and ensure that users are in control of their personal data. Verified and tamper-proof data can be accessed directly by healthcare authorities such as hospitals and clinicians through the wearables, thus allowing them to monitor the health of the patient accurately and implement timely interventions. Increasing clinical decision-making capabilities, Blockchain keeps an extensive, auditable history of interactions with patients, improving clinical decisions, and ensuring a clear trail of accountability. The advantage to insurance companies is that wearable data is authenticated in claims processing or by making dynamic premium adjustments to prevent fraud and enable fairness. Confirmed activity records, biometrics, and adherence to health-related policy requirements can be determined without the need to depend on self-reported data, increasing transparency and trust between insurers and policyholders. It also has profound benefits to users and researchers: users can maintain the sovereignty of their data, with smart contract access to third-party applications or research projects selectively, and make informed consent, privacy, and accountability. On their part, researchers receive quality and validated data, and the participants get guaranteed safety of their confidential information. Deterring the use of intermediaries, blockchain creates a clear ecosystem where data integrity, provenance, and access permissions are implemented by protocol means instead of relying on any trust in centralized entities, resulting in a robust and user-friendly wearable data space.

Technical Models

The practicability of blockchain-IoT integration of wearables is evidenced by several practical frameworks:

- MedRec was initially intended to be used in electronic health records and could be modified to integrate wearable data, which would give the patient a single, verifiable record that cannot be changed or removed.
- A blockchain specific to IoT devices, IoTChain is a lightweight, hierarchical blockchain with efficient consensus protocols to use on resource-constrained wearables. Its design balances performance, security, and energy efficiency.
- These models integrate edge computing and blockchain to compute wearable data around the source, crypt summaries on-chain, and to selectively share validated data with trusted parties via smart contracts. This architecture has a low latency, less network load, and saves wearable power.
- A combination of blockchain and advanced cryptographic models, including zero-knowledge proofs or homomorphic encryption, guarantees the privacy of wearable data and retains the transparency, as well. Confirmation of sensitive information can be done without the exposure of raw data and helps with regulatory obligations as well as user privacy.

These models show how blockchain-IoT integration can be theoretically converted to a real-life practice. They cover all of the essential issues of scalability, efficiency, trust, and privacy, proving that wearable ecosystems can be used to manage data securely, decentralize, and be user-friendly. To consolidate the diverse strategies and models discussed in this section, Table 7 provides a comparative overview of blockchain integration approaches for wearable IoT ecosystems.

Table 7. Blockchain Integration Strategies for Wearable IoT Ecosystems

Category	Approach/Model	Key Mechanism	Benefits for Wearables	Challenges/Considerations
Architectures	On-chain/Off-chain Storage	Metadata & hashes stored on-chain; raw data off-chain	Ensures data integrity, reduces ledger overload	Requires secure external storage integration
	Edge Computing Integration	Local preprocessing before blockchain commit	Reduces latency, saves bandwidth & battery	Edge nodes add complexity and must be trusted
	Lightweight Nodes	Simplified clients without a full ledger	Enables wearable participation, conserves resources	Limited capabilities vs. full nodes

continued on following page

Table 7. Continued

Category	Approach/Model	Key Mechanism	Benefits for Wearables	Challenges/Considerations
Consensus Mechanisms	Proof of Authority (PoA)	Validators authenticate transactions	Low energy use, high throughput	Requires trusted validator identities
	Delegated Proof of Stake (DPoS)	Elected delegates validate on behalf of others	Efficient, scalable for real-time health data	Risk of centralization among delegates
	Directed Acyclic Graph (DAG)	Parallel, non-linear transaction validation	Real-time processing, scalable with activity	Less mature than traditional blockchain
Secure Data Sharing	Blockchain-enabled Sharing	Verified, auditable, user-controlled access	Enhances trust for healthcare, insurers, and researchers	Consent & policy enforcement complexity
	Smart Contracts	Automated authentication & permissions	Granular user control, regulatory compliance	Vulnerable to flawed contract coding
Example Frameworks	MedRec	Unified blockchain-based health record system	Immutable, auditable patient histories	Adaptation needed for continuous wearable data
	IoTChain	Lightweight blockchain for IoT	Hierarchical, resource-efficient	Still emerging, limited adoption
	Hybrid Edge-Blockchain Models	Edge processing + blockchain verification	Low latency, scalable, power-efficient	Requires strong edge-cloud synchronization
	Privacy-Preserving Models	Zero-knowledge proofs, encryption	Protects sensitive data, supports compliance	Computational overhead for some cryptographic methods

EXAMPLE APPLICATIONS

The interdependence between blockchain and IoT in wearable devices is not a hypothetical approach; there is a variety of existing applications that can illustrate how this interdependence can improve the level of security, privacy, and trust in fields like healthcare, fitness, and insurance. With the decentralized ledgers and smart contracts, wearables are able to have accurate and tamper-free records and allow users to have control over their personal data.

Healthcare Applications

Wearables in healthcare generate continuous streams of data essential for patient monitoring, chronic disease management, and clinical research. Smart wearables, including smartwatches, ECG, and glucose monitors, measure live health data, including heart rate, oxygen saturation, sleep, and activity. Through the storage of such readings as immutable blockchain records, clinicians can access verified, unmodifiable data to detect and accurately follow the conditions of patients. Smart contracts can automate real-time alerts, including abnormal readings, which shortens response time and enhances patient outcomes. In addition to that, blockchain prevents the malicious or accidental alteration of these records and ensures their integrity between several devices and platforms.

Chronic patients who have diabetes, cardiovascular disease, or even hypertension find secure wearable data-sharing with caring teams to be beneficial. Blockchain allows automatic alert systems through smart contracts when physiological measures fall within or outside predetermined ranges and sends alerts to health practitioners or caregivers. This preventive strategy can allow early interventions, increase the involvement of patients, and decrease hospitalization. Moreover, a granular level of control over access to the health information that the patient needs encourages trust in the patient and adherence to the treatment protocols as well.

It is through blockchain that the integrity and traceability of the wearable-generated data sent into research databases are guaranteed. Patient-reported outcomes are frequently used in clinical trials, and they are likely to be biased and fallacious. Creating a blockchain system to integrate wearable data enables the researcher to verify measurements, keep the participants anonymous, and keep audit trails. This enhances the accuracy of the trial outcomes and minimizes the risk of data manipulation or fraud. The initial testing of blockchain-enabled glucose monitors has shown higher reliability of patient data, reduced the gap between a device and self-reported measurements, and complied with the rules and regulations in research environments.

Fitness and Lifestyle Tracking

Wearable devices used in consumer health and fitness ecosystems constantly gather activity, sleep, and biometric and other measures of behavior, useful information to users and coaches, as well as third-party uses. In this context, blockchain integration is a solution to perhaps the most important issues of trust, privacy, and data authenticity. Increased data accuracy confidence, almost all tamper-proof blockchain records enable users and third-party applications to check the integrity of data gathered by an activity tracker or smartwatch. This guarantees equitable involvement in fitness games, trusted analytics, and trusted metrics of health applications; e.g., confirmed step counts, exercise histories, or heart rate patterns can be shared with confidence with fitness trainers or competitive applications without the threat of being manipulated. Another key advantage is privacy conservation, where users have granular control over the data sharing by smart contracts, namely, which applications or service providers can access which dataset under what conditions and for what duration. This makes it less likely to face risks of unauthorized aggregation, commercial use, or profiling of personal health behavior, and the two elements of blockchain transparency and privacy-preserving mechanisms encourage user confidence in the adoption of wearable devices. Also, gamification and incentive systems are maintained via blockchain, which enables verified wearable data to be used to underpin reward or token-based programs in achieving fitness goals. Activity metrics can be monetized or traded without exposing the users to the risk of losing data because the data is verifiable and cannot be faked; this motivates activity and compliance with wellness programs. Blockchain-enabled wearables, by combining accuracy, privacy, and transparency, build user trust, encourage long-term use, and support new uses in lifestyle, health, and wellness ecosystems.

Insurance and Policy Applications

The use of wearable data to shape personal insurance policies, calculate personal risk, and automate insurance claims is changing the way people have always done insurance. Insurers using blockchain technology can verify that the data utilized in these processes is accurate, untampered, and verifiable, solving critical issues of reliability and trust when it comes to the health and fitness information collected by wearables. Fraud reduction is one of the benefits of blockchain integration. Data collected by wearable devices on immutable blockchains cannot be faked or tampered with, and fraudulent claims of the number of steps, heart rate, or lifestyle records cannot be filed. This can keep the claims processing authentic and can encourage faith between the insurers and policyholders since both groups can be assured that the information presented is genuine.

Another application of blockchain is to support automated claims processing and flexible policy changes with the help of smart contracts. These are self-operating programs that can automatically accept claims or automatically change the premiums when the wearable information is verified. As a case in point, health insurance plans that reward healthy lifestyles can automatically decrease the premiums as exercise routines have been verified or steps taken, as the administrative overhead can be reduced, human error minimised, and the policy can be effectively managed in real time with a direct incentive in relation to healthy behaviour. Other advantages that blockchain-based insurance systems bring are regulatory compliance and auditability.

All information to be used in insurance decisions is kept in a way that can be audited and traced back, compliance requirements are met, and sensitive personal information is secured. Without centralizing raw health data, insurers can preserve verifiable records, contributing to the reduction of liability risks and increasing compliance with privacy, especially in jurisdictions where there are strict data protection laws.

The European market has shown pilot programs that blockchain-enabled wearable data can be used in dynamic insurance programs in practice. These programs demonstrate that confirmed activity counts can be utilized to effectively change premiums and claims in a reliable way, promoting greater engagement with policyholders, building confidence in digital insurance products, and introducing the path towards a wider adoption of blockchain-based wearable insurance products.

Emerging Pilots and Implementations

A handful of pioneering Pilots show how blockchain can be practically implemented in combination with wearable IoT and represent the applications of the technology in practice. MedRec for Wearables builds upon the foundational MedRec blockchain system to include ongoing data streams of wearable data to support secure and auditable health records to supplement existing electronic health records (EHRs). Such integration would provide interoperability across more than one healthcare system and provide traceable, tamper-proof records of patient-generated data, both enhancing clinical decision-making and patient trust.

Another frontier on which startups are experimenting with blockchain-based rewards systems on verified fitness activities is FitnessChain Projects. This is because steps, workouts, and other biometric performances are documented in immutable ledgers, ensuring equity and open-mindedness in awarding incentives. Their decentralized approach to validating activity data also leads to user engagement and healthy behavior within the context of these projects, as well as the way blockchain can strengthen accountability and trust in consumer-focused wearable applications.

Hybrid healthcare platforms integrate wearable devices, edge computing, and blockchain to enable real-time monitoring of chronic disease patients. Such systems are able to work on data on the edge devices locally, provide automated alerts when health metrics rise beyond specified thresholds, and securely exchange verified information between patients, hospitals, and insurers. This kind of integration can lead to responsiveness to health events, increased data security, and build trust among stakeholders, which demonstrates how blockchain-enabled wearables can benefit complex, multi-party healthcare ecosystems.

Privacy-preserving pilots are concerned with safeguarding sensitive wearable information, and they are also verifiable and transparent. Zero-knowledge proofs, selective disclosure of data, and off-chain storage techniques are some of the techniques through which patient and user information can stay secret as important data is stored on blockchain networks. These pilots help to consider regulatory, ethical, and user privacy issues, demonstrating that it is possible to have secure, privacy-based wearable ecosystems without compromising either trust or functionality.

All of these pilots indicate a shift toward the implementation of blockchain-IoT integration in wearable devices beyond the theoretical frameworks, increasing security, privacy, and trust, and expanding the range of business models, dynamic incentive frameworks, and user-centric services. They also show the disruptive power of decentralized technologies in producing robust, open, and ethically accountable wearable ecosystems.

CHALLENGES AND FUTURE DIRECTIONS

Although the idea of integrating blockchain and wearable IoT devices is a potentially successful way to enhance security, privacy, and trust, there are several technical, operational, as well as regulatory concerns to be resolved to achieve the potential. Researchers, developers, and policymakers trying to deploy scalable and resilient wearable ecosystems must understand these challenges.

Scalability and Throughput

One of the biggest challenges to blockchain use in the wearable ecosystem is scalability. Wearables produce large volumes of data (in high frequency and continuity), such as heart rate and blood oxygen saturation, activity history, and sleep cycles. Storing each of the data points on-chain with existing blockchains, particularly those based on energy-intensive consensus algorithms such as Proof of Work (PoW), can rapidly saturate the network.

Even mixed architectures that use off-chain storage or metadata-only approaches are challenged by the need to achieve high levels of transaction throughput. Creating bottlenecks in a large network that consists of thousands or millions of devices transmitting simultaneously can cause delays in the validation of transactions and inconsistencies in data. The integrity, verifiability, and tamper-proof guarantees of blockchain at scale to large wearable data sets must be maintained by innovation in ledger partitioning, sharding, the DAG-based processing of transactions, and lightweight consensus protocols.

In addition, throughput constraints may have a direct effect on the performance of applications. As an example, patient monitoring applications based on the timely transmission of data between devices, healthcare providers, and insurers can be delayed by the update in case of congestion in the network. Scalability solutions should thus be able to trade off speed, security, and decentralization so that large wearable networks can be reliable and responsive.

Energy Efficiency and Resource Limitations

Wearables have a set of inherent resource constraints, such as limited battery capacity, processing power, and memory, and further demands on computational and energy resources by running blockchain clients, even lightweight implementations, may reduce device performance or reduce the time of operation between charges. Energy efficiency can be optimized in several ways: energy-efficient blockchain protocols with streamlined clients, or selective interaction with a blockchain, to save on power consumption and computation overhead without necessarily impacting the integrity of sensitive health or fitness data; efficient cryptography, as classical operations such as asymmetric encryption and digital signatures consume energy, and cryptography such as elliptic curve cryptography (ECC) or hybrid symmetric-asymmetric schemes can substantially lessen the energy consumption; adaptive synchronization schedules, where wearables only transmit their data to blockchain nodes in intervals or thresholds, rather than constantly, reducing the power burden without necessarily affecting the integrity of sensitive information about Trade-offs between energy efficiency and security enforcement are, as such, essential to achieve wearable usability and long-term adoption.

Latency in Real-Time Data Processing

Numerous of the wearable applications, e.g., constant patient information monitoring, emergency medical alerts, or live fitness coaching, demand near-instantaneous data processing, but blockchain itself adds some latency by validating transactions, reaching a consensus, and propagating them across distributed nodes. These delays, even in optimized architectures, can have serious effects on critical applications: real-time healthcare monitoring can be disrupted by delays in alerting of abnormal heart rates or blood glucose levels until blockchain confirmation is provided, in effect compromising patient safety; multi-stakeholder access, where clinicians, insurers, and family members need access to a particular data source simultaneously, can be disrupted by transaction propagation and confirmation delays, hindering timely interventions or decision making; continuous streaming data, such as wearable devices, requires fast aggregation and summarization, but latency in blockchain networks can prevent analytics and predictive modeling, preventing actionable insights. To tackle these issues of latency, it is necessary to incorporate fast consensus mechanisms, off-chain data processing, hierarchies, and edge processing to make sure that important events are given precedence without sacrificing the security and trust guarantees of blockchain.

Legal, Regulatory, and Interoperability Challenges

In addition to the technical problems, there a complicated regulatory, legal, and ethical aspects of the deployment of blockchain-enabled wearable systems. Healthcare regulations that are often stringent against wearable data, such as HIPAA in the United States (Lutkevich, 2019) and GDPR in the European Union (Truong et al., 2020), and decentralized storage, in turn, complicate classic compliance schemes, where robust consent management, data minimization, and privacy enforcement and auditable enforcement are required. There can be clashes in compliance with local laws and regulations governing medical data, personal privacy, and data sovereignty between the host country where the blockchain node is located and the country of origin where the wearable device is sold, so cross-border wearable networks should pay careful attention to regional legal differences. Interoperability is also a major challenge because wearable ecosystems are heterogeneous, including a wide range of devices, communication protocols (e.g., BLE, Wi-Fi, 5G), and different blockchain frameworks; the lack of standardized protocols, APIs, and governance frameworks prevents secure integration, the exchange of data, and the scalable nature of the system. Deployment is also further complicated by ethical concerns, since data ownership, user consent, and transparency should be provided, and individuals should have control over who accesses their data, on what terms, and with what purposes, which is also consistent with both ethical standards and regulatory requirements. It is thus important to find a path through these legal, regulatory, interoperability, and ethical issues to gain wide acceptance and confidence in the use of blockchain-based wearable systems. To provide a structured overview of the issues discussed in this section, Table 8 consolidates the main challenges of integrating blockchain with wearable IoT ecosystems. The table highlights the root causes, real-world impacts, and potential solution pathways, offering a comparative lens across technical, operational, and regulatory dimensions.

Table 8. Key Challenges in Blockchain-Enabled Wearable IoT Ecosystems

Challenge	Root Causes	Impacts on Wearables	Potential Solution Pathways
Scalability & Throughput	High-frequency continuous data streams; resource-heavy consensus (e.g., PoW)	Network congestion, delayed transaction validation, data inconsistencies, and reduced reliability in patient monitoring	Sharding, ledger partitioning, DAG-based processing, lightweight consensus protocols, hybrid on/off-chain storage
Energy Efficiency & Resource Limitations	Limited battery, processing, and memory in wearables; energy-intensive cryptography and consensus	Faster battery drain, degraded device performance, reduced user adoption	Lightweight blockchain clients, optimized cryptography (ECC, hybrid schemes), edge computing offloading, adaptive synchronization schedules
Latency in Real-Time Processing	Consensus delays, distributed propagation, transaction verification	Compromised emergency health alerts, delayed clinician/insurer access, and hindered predictive analytics	Fast consensus mechanisms (PoA, DPoS), off-chain channels, hierarchical structures, edge-based real-time prioritization
Legal, Regulatory & Interoperability	Complex global healthcare regulations (HIPAA, GDPR); cross-border data flows; heterogeneous protocols and blockchains	Compliance conflicts, restricted cross-border data use, integration barriers, and user mistrust	Consent management frameworks, auditable privacy enforcement, standardized APIs/protocols, governance frameworks, emphasis on user data ownership, and transparency

Future Directions

In order to deal with these, research and development are to concentrate on various complementary approaches. Scalable blockchain architectures such as sharding, DAG-based networks, and hierarchical blockchains are being developed to facilitate greater throughput, reduce network congestion, and effectively support the ever-present high-frequency data streams that wearable devices produce. Offloading, including lightweight cryptography algorithms and edge computing integration, and energy-efficient cryptography strategies, helps to lower computational and energy requirements on wearables and maintain security and privacy. Not only privacy-preserving methods such as zero-knowledge proofs, homomorphic encryption, and selective data disclosure allow sensitive data to be kept secret and still enable verification, analytics, and acting on the information. Standardized protocols, APIs, and compliance mechanisms are also being formalized to enable the implementation of wearable blockchain networks across borders securely, with international collaboration needed to develop global ecosystems that are privacy, security, and ethical. Also, adaptive consensus mechanisms are under investigation, where hybrid protocols dynamically adapt the participation and are energy efficient, low latency, and high throughput depending on network conditions and application priorities. With these technical, regulatory, and operational issues resolved, blockchain-powered wearable systems could become resilient, people-focused ecosystems with the potential to enable next-generation healthcare, lifestyle, and insurance applications, as well as security, privacy, and trust for all stakeholders.

CONCLUSION

A new disruptive paradigm in the security of sensitive personal, health, and lifestyle data has emerged with the intersection of blockchain technology and IoT in wearable devices. The classic centralized security models have also been found to be insufficient in the context of the distinct weaknesses of wearables, such as tampering of data, unauthorized access, and the use of devices that may be resource-constrained. With its ability to decentralize, immutable, and automate smart contracts, blockchain can deliver highly reliable authentication, access control, and tamper-proof record-keeping, establishing a less ambiguous and more trustworthy ecosystem for both users and stakeholders.

Although the promise is great, there are a number of challenges. Scalability, energy efficiency, latency, and interoperability should be given due consideration so that they can be implemented practically and seamlessly within large-scale wearable networks. Moreover, compliance with laws and regulations, especially in the area of healthcare and personal data privacy, is a legal obligation; it should be continuously paid attention to to guarantee the compliance of blockchain-based solutions with international standards and expectations of users.

In the future, these limitations can be fixed with the development of lightweight blockchain architectures, edge-computing integration, privacy-preserving cryptography, and standardized protocols. The blockchain-empowered wearables can bring not only facilities of security and privacy but also user control, trust, and transparency in the field of digital health, fitness, and lifestyle management as the research and development process continues. The integration creates the next generation of wearable technologies, opening up the possibility of novel services and applications and protecting the sensitive data on which they depend.

REFERENCES

Adere, E. M. (2022). Blockchain in healthcare and IoT: A systematic literature review. In *Array* (Vol. 14). https://doi.org/DOI: 10.1016/j.array.2022.100139

Akkaoui, R., Hei, X., & Cheng, W. (2020). EdgeMediChain: A Hybrid Edge Blockchain-Based Framework for Health Data Exchange. *IEEE Access : Practical Innovations, Open Solutions, 8*. Advance online publication. DOI: 10.1109/ACCESS.2020.3003575

Al-awamy, A. A., Al-shaibany, N., Sikora, A., & Welte, D. (2025). Hybrid Consensus Mechanisms in Blockchain: A Comprehensive Review. *International Journal of Intelligent Systems, 2025*(1), 5821997. DOI: 10.1155/INT/5821997

Arif, S., Khan, M. A., Rehman, S. U., Kabir, M. A., & Imran, M. (2020). Investigating Smart Home Security: Is Blockchain the Answer? *IEEE Access : Practical Innovations, Open Solutions, 8*. Advance online publication. DOI: 10.1109/ACCESS.2020.3004662

Barbone, A. S., Meftah, M., Markiewicz, K., & Dellimore, K. (2019). Beyond wearables and implantables: A scoping review of insertable medical devices. *Biomedical Physics & Engineering Express, 5*(6), 062002. DOI: 10.1088/2057-1976/AB4B32

Barua, A., Al Alamin, M. A., Hossain, M. S., & Hossain, E. (2022). Security and Privacy Threats for Bluetooth Low Energy in IoT and Wearable Devices: A Comprehensive Survey. *IEEE Open Journal of the Communications Society, 3*, 251–281. DOI: 10.1109/OJCOMS.2022.3149732

Boumpa, E., Tsoukas, V., Gkogkidis, A., Spathoulas, G., & Kakarountas, A. (2022). Security and Privacy Concerns for Healthcare Wearable Devices and Emerging Alternative Approaches. *Lecture Notes of the Institute for Computer Sciences, Social-Informatics and Telecommunications Engineering, LNICST, 440 LNICST*. https://doi.org/DOI: 10.1007/978-3-031-06368-8_2

Byeon, S., & Lee, W. (2023). Directed acyclic graphs for clinical research: A tutorial. *Journal of Minimally Invasive Surgery, 26*(3). Advance online publication. DOI: 10.7602/jmis.2023.26.3.97 PMID: 37712307

Curran, B. (2018). What is Proof of Authority Consensus? (PoA) Staking Your Identity. In *Block Onomi*.

Digitale, J. C., Martin, J. N., & Glymour, M. M. (2022). Tutorial on directed acyclic graphs. *Journal of Clinical Epidemiology, 142*. Advance online publication. DOI: 10.1016/j.jclinepi.2021.08.001 PMID: 34371103

Dragusin, S. A., Bizon, N., & Bostinaru, R. N. (2024). Comprehensive Analysis of Cyber-Attack Techniques and Vulnerabilities in Communication Channels of Embedded Systems. *Proceedings of the 16th International Conference on Electronics, Computers and Artificial Intelligence, ECAI 2024*. https://doi.org/DOI: 10.1109/ECAI61503.2024.10607432

Dragusin, S. A., Bizon, N., Bostinaru, R. N., Enescu, F. M., Teodorescu, R. M., & Savulescu, C. (2024). Analysis of Vulnerabilities in Communication Channels Using An Integrated Approach Based on Machine Learning and Statistical Methods. *Proceedings of the 16th International Conference on Electronics, Computers and Artificial Intelligence, ECAI 2024*. https://doi.org/DOI: 10.1109/ECAI61503.2024.10607483

Eren, H., Karaduman, Ö., & Gençoğlu, M. T. (2025). Security Challenges and Performance Trade-Offs in On-Chain and Off-Chain Blockchain Storage: A Comprehensive Review. *Applied Sciences 2025, Vol. 15, Page 3225, 15*(6), 3225. https://doi.org/DOI: 10.3390/APP15063225

Hanif, F., Waheed, U., Shams, R., & Shareef, A. (2023). GAHBT: Genetic-Based Hashing Algorithm for Managing and Validating Health Data Integrity in Blockchain Technology. *Blockchain in Healthcare Today*, *6*(2). Advance online publication. DOI: 10.30953/bhty.v6.244 PMID: 36798963

Hernández-álvarez, L., Bullón Pérez, J. J., Batista, F. K., & Queiruga-Dios, A. (2022). Security Threats and Cryptographic Protocols for Medical Wearables. *Mathematics*, *10*(6). Advance online publication. DOI: 10.3390/math10060886

Hewa, T., Ylianttila, M., & Liyanage, M. (2021). Survey on blockchain based smart contracts: Applications, opportunities and challenges. In *Journal of Network and Computer Applications* (Vol. 177). https://doi.org/DOI: 10.1016/j.jnca.2020.102857

Hora, A., & Kulkarni, P. (2024). Wearables and Cybersecurity: Navigating the Threat Landscape. *2nd International Conference on Sustainable Computing and Smart Systems, ICSCSS 2024 - Proceedings*, 563–567. https://doi.org/DOI: 10.1109/ICSCSS60660.2024.10625662

Hughes, A., Shandhi, M. M. H., Master, H., Dunn, J., & Brittain, E. (2023). Wearable Devices in Cardiovascular Medicine. *Circulation Research*, *132*(5), 652–670. DOI: 10.1161/CIRCRESAHA.122.322389 PMID: 36862812

Iqbal, S. M. A., Mahgoub, I., Du, E., Leavitt, M. A., & Asghar, W. (2021). Advances in healthcare wearable devices. *Npj Flexible Electronics 2021 5:1, 5*(1), 1–14. https://doi.org/DOI: 10.1038/s41528-021-00107-x

Iqbal, T., Redon-Lurbe, P., Simpkin, A. J., Elahi, A., Ganly, S., Wijns, W., & Shahzad, A. (2021). A Sensitivity Analysis of Biophysiological Responses of Stress for Wearable Sensors in Connected Health. *IEEE Access : Practical Innovations, Open Solutions, 9*. Advance online publication. DOI: 10.1109/ACCESS.2021.3082423

Kamruzzaman, M. M., Yan, B., Sarker, M. N. I., Alruwaili, O., Wu, M., & Alrashdi, I. (2022). Blockchain and Fog Computing in IoT-Driven Healthcare Services for Smart Cities. *Journal of Healthcare Engineering, 2022*. Advance online publication. DOI: 10.1155/2022/9957888 PMID: 35126961

Li, J., Chen, Y., Chen, Y. L., Zhang, W., & Liu, Z. (2023). A smart energy IoT model based on the Itsuku PoW technology. *Results in Engineering, 18*. Advance online publication. DOI: 10.1016/j.rineng.2023.101147

Lutkevich, B. (2019). What is HIPAA (Health Insurance Portability and Accountability Act)? In *WhatIs.com*.

Miaz, M. H., & Ali, M. (2020). Integration of blockchain and IoT: An enhanced security perspective. *Annals of Emerging Technologies in Computing, 4*(4). Advance online publication. DOI: 10.33166/AETiC.2020.04.006

Miraz, M. H., Excell, P. S., & Sobayel, K. (2021). Evaluation of green alternatives for blockchain proof-of-work (Pow) approach. In *Annals of Emerging Technologies in Computing* (Vol. 5, Issue 4). https://doi.org/DOI: 10.33166/AETIC.2021.04.005

Nakayama, A., Ishii, N., Mantani, M., Samukawa, K., Tsuneta, R., Marukawa, M., Ohno, K., Yoshida, A., Hasegawa, E., Sakamoto, J., Hori, K., Takahashi, S., Komuro, K., Hiruma, T., Abe, R., Norimatsu, T., Shimbo, M., Tajima, M., Nagasaki, M., . . . Isobe, M. (2023). Remote Cardiac Rehabilitation With Wearable Devices. In *Korean Circulation Journal* (Vol. 53, Issue 11). https://doi.org/DOI: 10.4070/kcj.2023.0242

Nanda, S. K., Panda, S. K., & Dash, M. (2023). Medical supply chain integrated with blockchain and IoT to track the logistics of medical products. *Multimedia Tools and Applications, 82*(21). Advance online publication. DOI: 10.1007/s11042-023-14846-8 PMID: 37362711

Poongodi, T., Krishnamurthi, R., Indrakumari, R., Suresh, P., & Balusamy, B. (2020). Wearable Devices and IoT. *Intelligent Systems Reference Library, 165*, 245–273. DOI: 10.1007/978-3-030-23983-1_10

Rahman, F., Titouna, C., & Nait-Abdesselam, F. (2024). Fundamentals of Blockchain and Smart Contracts. *Blockchain and Smart-Contract Technologies for Innovative Applications*, 3–37. https://doi.org/DOI: 10.1007/978-3-031-50028-2_1

Reegu, F. A., Abas, H., Gulzar, Y., Xin, Q., Alwan, A. A., Jabbari, A., Sonkamble, R. G., & Dziyauddin, R. A. (2023). Blockchain-Based Framework for Interoperable Electronic Health Records for an Improved Healthcare System. *Sustainability (Switzerland), 15*(8). Advance online publication. DOI: 10.3390/su15086337

Sabry, F., Eltaras, T., Labda, W., Alzoubi, K., & Malluhi, Q. (2022). Machine Learning for Healthcare Wearable Devices: The Big Picture. *Journal of Healthcare Engineering, 2022*(1), 4653923. DOI: 10.1155/2022/4653923 PMID: 35480146

Skh Saad, S. M., & Raja Mohd Radzi, R. Z. (2020). Comparative Review of the Blockchain Consensus Algorithm Between Proof of Stake (POS) and Delegated Proof of Stake (DPOS). *International Journal of Innovative Computing, 10*(2). Advance online publication. DOI: 10.11113/ijic.v10n2.272

Tanwar, S., Parekh, K., & Evans, R. (2020). Blockchain-based electronic healthcare record system for healthcare 4.0 applications. *Journal of Information Security and Applications, 50*. Advance online publication. DOI: 10.1016/j.jisa.2019.102407

Tekchandani, P., Pradhan, I., Das, A. K., Kumar, N., & Park, Y. (2023). Blockchain-Enabled Secure Big Data Analytics for Internet of Things Smart Applications. *IEEE Internet of Things Journal, 10*(7). Advance online publication. DOI: 10.1109/JIOT.2022.3227162

Truong, N. B., Sun, K., Lee, G. M., & Guo, Y. (2020). GDPR-Compliant Personal Data Management: A Blockchain-Based Solution. *IEEE Transactions on Information Forensics and Security, 15*. Advance online publication. DOI: 10.1109/TIFS.2019.2948287

Upadhyay, V., Vaish, A., & Kokila, J. (2024). The need for Lightweight Consensus algorithms in IoT environment: A review. *ACM International Conference Proceeding Series*, 366–376. https://doi.org/DOI: 10.1145/3675888.3676072

Vijayan, V., Connolly, J., Condell, J., McKelvey, N., & Gardiner, P. (2021). Review of wearable devices and data collection considerations for connected health. In *Sensors* (Vol. 21, Issue 16). https://doi.org/DOI: 10.3390/s21165589

Yang, R., Yu, F. R., Si, P., Yang, Z., & Zhang, Y. (2019). Integrated Blockchain and Edge Computing Systems: A Survey, Some Research Issues and Challenges. In *IEEE Communications Surveys and Tutorials* (Vol. 21, Issue 2). https://doi.org/DOI: 10.1109/COMST.2019.2894727

Zhang, B., Chen, C., Lee, I., Lee, K., & Ong, K. L. (2025). A survey on security and privacy issues in wearable health monitoring devices. *Computers & Security, 155*, 104453. DOI: 10.1016/J.COSE.2025.104453

Zheng, Z., Xie, S., Dai, H. N., Chen, W., Chen, X., Weng, J., & Imran, M. (2020). An overview on smart contracts: Challenges, advances and platforms. *Future Generation Computer Systems*, *105*. Advance online publication. DOI: 10.1016/j.future.2019.12.019

Chapter 6
Blockchain-Empowered Data Security and Privacy-Preserving Framework for Wearable Medical Devices

A. Sasikumar
https://orcid.org/0000-0003-1480-4950
SRM Institute of Science and Technology, India

P. Selvakumari
Rajalakshmi Institute of Technology, India

P. Rajasekar
https://orcid.org/0000-0002-1104-9972
SRM Institute of Science and Technology, India

S. Wilson Prakash
SRM Institute of Science and Technology, India

Imran Javeed Settu
Vel Tech Rangarajan Dr. Sagunthala R&D Institute of Science and Technology, India

ABSTRACT

The value of individual lives is anticipated to be enhanced by wearable medical devices. Secure sharing and protecting data privacy are two of the primary technological challenges that smart wearable medical devices must address. A centralized

DOI: 10.4018/979-8-3373-4412-6.ch006

organization that verifies transactions and interaction permissions generally serves as the foundation for medical management devices. Consequently, it is possible to consider this centralized organization a single point of failure. We propose a novel blockchain-empowered wearable device secure system that protects the privacy of medical devices. The proposed framework enhances security and productivity by fusing smart contracts for data processing automation with blockchain technology's decentralized, transparent, and impenetrable features. Smart contracts can quickly identify vulnerable devices that have been compromised or represent a risk to the medical network. Therefore, establishing control over one's own devices protects the data and prevents malicious activity. privacy of the data owner.

1. INTRODUCTION

Wearable medical devices are smart, portable gadgets that utilize sensors and tracking techniques to accumulate, transmit, and visualize personal biological data, including blood pressure, blood sugar levels, and heart rate. By facilitating transmission of data to cloud or hospital records via the Internet or cellular networks, these gadgets allow healthcare practitioners to diagnose and monitor patients remotely in real-time (Iqbal et al., 2021). Medical information is now more accessible and shareable because of the growing use of Internet of Things (IoT) wearable technology. But it has also increased the possibility of privacy violations. Sensitive medical information may be compromised by hostile activity or unauthorized access, which might seriously endanger patients and the related healthcare facilities. It is challenging to address these issues, as traditional centralized data storage techniques are susceptible to abuse and attacks. Thus, it has become increasingly difficult to analyze and share medical data while maintaining data privacy.

The quantity of data required for wearable devices to be useful in healthcare prediction remains a challenge. The real-time data from wearable devices are used for analysis, in that a significant amount of device information are stored, raising security and privacy concerns (Barua et al., 2022). The processing limits of wearable technology create weaknesses and the potential for substantial patient data leaks. The service's dependability and honesty are further concerns. Some components of healthcare may have to be sacrificed to prioritize others. For this area of remote healthcare, which relies on the precision of prediction models and wearable data, service integrity is crucial. The network's flexibility in deploying and providing these predictive healthcare services is another problem. The diversity introduced by wearable devices poses a significant challenge to standardization in IoT networks. Due to this diversity, the medical server must undergo constant repairs and upgrades to remain current with each new wearable device. Finally, concerns related to flexibility prevent the medical system from being entirely financially viable and relevant for extended periods.

A single, widely recognized term for privacy does not exist. For example, Deep et al. (2022) defined privacy in terms of four aspects. The first is the privacy of personal data, which includes the ability to decide how all the information related to medical devices are shared. The right to conceal information about one's actions and decisions is part of the second dimension, which relates to private behaviors and privacy. The third dimension is communication privacy, which includes the individual's freedom to speak without being watched, monitored, or censored. The last component is the individual's right to privacy, which encompasses the authority to manage their own body's integrity, including the use of medical equipment. Although privacy rules primarily cover the confidentiality of personal information, behaviors, and communication, the last dimension is crucial and should be considered in the context of wearable devices. Therefore, rather than attempting to protect privacy at the user's end, medical device control should be enabled.

In typical wearable device administration models, a centralized unit, such as a computing and storage devices, manages the proper validation of each device so that it can connect with other devices. However, due to scale issues and the centralized server ability to act as a computing resource failure, these conventional models are not suitable for wearable devices. To address the problem of device management with centralized solutions, several distributed techniques have been put forth (Sasikumar et al., 2023). As a result, rather than a centralized organization, the medical devices carry out the proper validation. Nevertheless, popular security and privacy methods can sometimes be highly costly to implement on medical devices with limited processing power.

Furthermore, because adversaries can infiltrate medical devices and take control of medical organizations, they can readily compromise user security. Because medical devices have limited resources, such a distributed correct endorsement cannot be reliable. As a result, distributed and reliable proper validation is needed for medical device management. Although the decentralized, secure, and private nature of blockchain technology makes it capable of overcoming these obstacles, its implementation in the medical sector is complicated by the substantial bandwidth cost and latency associated with traditional blockchains. To achieve this, wearable devices can benefit from a lightweight consensus mechanism that removes the computing power required to mine new blocks in conventional blockchain systems.

To address these issues, we propose a safe and private data sharing technique that utilizes blockchain-based device privacy in medical devices. The medical device ciphertext is stored on a blockchain. It ensures data privacy and provides requesters with access to the requested data. Furthermore, without revealing any private information, the blockchain uses a variety of hash algorithms to confirm the legitimacy of the keyword ciphertext. To encourage data owners and data requesters to engage with this system, we create an ideal cost structure.

The following is a summary of the proposed scheme's main contributions.

1. In wearable medical devices, we develop a novel blockchain-based secure architecture that protects privacy and security. Before adding the device to the blockchain, we create a device registration based on multiple hash functions to confirm that the keyword was chosen from a legitimate keyword list. Computational costs are significantly decreased in this method.
2. We provide blockchain-enabled medical devices that use a smart contract and a private decentralized model. Users can only access the requested data if their attribute set matches the access structure provided. While the relevant keyword ciphertext is maintained on the blockchain and validated by a chain code, the original data belonging to the data owners is preserved on the local server. It significantly boosts search effectiveness.
3. To encourage devices to engage with the system actively, we develop a chain code model for medical devices. By a privacy setting derived from a centralized mechanism, the proposed model enables a decentralized verification model. To validate the effectiveness of the proposed system, we have conducted simulation models in comparison with existing techniques.

The chapter structure is as follows. Section 2 deliberates the context of wearable devices and blockchain network for healthcare systems. Section 3 elaborates on related efforts on health data sharing using wearable devices and blockchain-based secure systems. System architecture, workflow, and proposed algorithms are presented in Section 4. In Section 5, the experimental results are presented. We concluded our chapter in Section 6.

2. BACKGROUND

2.1. Wearable Medical Devices

Patients with intermittent or ongoing disability can benefit from long-term support through wearable healthcare devices. Eyeglasses and hearing aids are examples of traditional medical assistance devices; both offer certain health benefits. Data processing features, such as speech recognition, context awareness improvement, alarms, or feedback, are characteristics of more sophisticated systems. These devices include a variety of GPS-based navigation aids for the blind and visually impaired that assist with directions, obstacle avoidance, and navigation. For patients undergoing recovery, wearable therapeutic support devices may include medical help and monitoring features. For patients in high-risk conditions, including following surgery or a heart attack, monitoring equipment may help with rehabilitation by preventing or diagnosing potentially hazardous situations.

The addition of end-to-end intelligence via wearables, audiovisual devices, and other personal IoT equipment successfully improves the reliability, speed, and proactivity of data collection. For instance, they utilize field-programmable gate array (FPGA) encapsulation to offer localized intelligence solutions for end-user devices (Carminati & Scandurra, 2021). As big data and fog computing nodes are developing rapidly, they are being deployed near patients to minimize data transmission loss. While the immediate installation of fog and edge computers delivers computing capacity near the CPU, which can be utilized for model inference, cloud computing primarily focuses on training large datasets (Kavitha et al., 2025; Xu et al., 2019). AI-based medical services may create digital twin representations that precisely represent a patient's unique health features and promptly assess their current physical health condition to help manage chronic illnesses, depending on the patient's health data that has been gathered.

AI-based medical diagnostic techniques primarily comprise deep learning, constraint engines, and large-scale data mining. Big data mining retrieves medical administration models for diagnosing chronic diseases by identifying correlations among vast amounts of data (Thirunavukkarasu & Chinnasamy, 2024). To regulate a user device state, a rule engine applies commercial rules based on ML training and testing. Machine learning builds a multi-layer complicated framework or multiple layers of processing made of numerous nonlinear changes for processing various types of data to integrate basic characteristics to create a more intangible, organized, high-level visualization of a user's device recording information for analysis, given the growing amount of available medical care data and the rapid growth of ML. With the use of ML-based wearable technology, chronic illness health data can be autonomously processed quickly and efficiently, leading to supplemental diagnoses with fewer medical resources.

2.1.1 Trend analysis on wearable medical devices

Rapid market expansion: There has been some discrepancy in the reported estimates of the wearable medical device market's rapid expansion. The market is expected to reach around USD 42.7 billion in 2024, according to pessimistic professional estimates. By 2025, it is forecast to reach nearly USD 54.0 billion, with a high multi-year CAGR continuing until the late 2020s. Other market studies indicate a bigger starting point (about USD 91.2 billion in 2024) and consistent, robust growth over several years. This difference shows how different the segments are defined (consumer wearables vs. clinical wearables), as well as how strong the need is for continual and remote surveillance. The increased volume of sensitive personal health data acquired at the edge due to a bigger installed base and higher clinical usage raises the stakes for strong privacy, authenticity, and integrity measures.

Growing relevance of privacy-preserving computation: The use of privacy-preserving methods, such as federated learning (FL), homomorphic encryption (HE), and access control, is on the rise in healthcare machine learning and analytics, according to research and review articles. HE and DP are transitioning from conceptual proofs-of-concept to realistic pilots that incorporate performance design for actual workloads; FL has grown quickly for cooperative model development that does not need centralizing raw patient data. To strike a compromise between practicality and legal/compliance requirements (GDPR/HIPAA), it has grown more practicable to combine FL with HE or DP, or to deploy computing inside hardware secure buffers.

Blockchain as an integrity & access-control layer: Market estimates indicate growing enthusiasm and economic predictions for blockchain and distributed-ledger technologies in healthcare, with an increasing number of pilot EHR exchanges, consent registries, and clinical study audit trails. However, the exact market statistics for these technologies vary somewhat between these publications. Authenticity and consent tracking might benefit from blockchain's irreversible audit trail and decentralised control of keys, but there are still practical obstacles to overcome, such as scaling, confidentiality of on-chain data, and legal compliance. Instead of replacing efficient secure storage or privacy-preserving computing, blockchain is most useful for wearables as an additional layer (audit trails, consent/meta-records, key database) (Hellsten et al., 2021).

Ecosystem & regulatory drivers: Cybersecurity and equipment management throughout their lifecycle are becoming more important as the Medical-IoT (MIoT) ecosystem grows at a rapid pace (connected implants, remote monitoring devices, etc.). The certification of devices, the reporting of incidents, and data management are becoming more important to healthcare organizations and regulators. A combination of device-level safety, secure firmware/TEE, insights that preserve privacy, and transparent authorization and permission levels is what integrated systems that address these constraints favour.

Consolidation of design pattern: The current trend in wearable healthcare architecture is towards hybrid solutions. This means that we should (a) avoid storing protected health information (PHI) on public chains; (b) encrypt data locally or on the device itself; (c) conduct analytics using privacy-preserving algorithms (FL, HE, DP); and (d) record relevant metadata, consent, and audit logs on a trusted blockchain to ensure distributed access control and counterfeit-proof authenticity.

Figure 1. illustrate the wearable medical devices market-size projection from 2024 to 2032. In this case we have considered two scenarios in which curves are plotted in the figure 1.

Using projection/CAGR data, a conservative scenario was developed using data from Grand View Research, with a base of around USD 42.7B in 2024. Fortune Business Insights has projected an optimistic scenario with a base value of around USD 91.2B in 2024 and an alternative CAGR. There will be massive amounts of sensitive clinical data created at the network's periphery even if we assume conservatively that the market will continue to grow far into the 2030s.

Figure 1. Wearable Medical Devices: Market-size trend analysis.

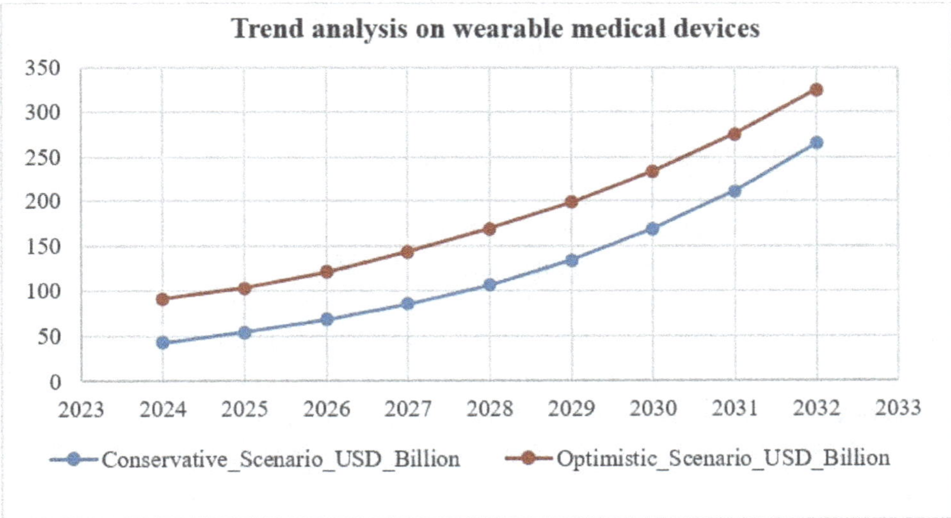

For the management of chronic illnesses, the technology and procedures for gathering most healthcare data, including heart rate, pulse, fasting glucose, and blood pressure, are comparatively advanced. Pose assessment is currently a substantial area of research that is linked to the recognition of long-term conditions, comprising heart and lung disorders. The complete value of the perspective and identification data is excellent. Wearable visual position markers, computer vision-based bone key localization techniques, and electromyogram and skin electronics wearable sensor devices are now the primary ways used to capture attitude data.

2.2 Blockchain and AI integrated Wearable Medical Devices

Improved services for patients will be provided by investigating AI techniques in conjunction with wearable technologies. However, gathering and analyzing patient physiological information in a timely way though maintaining device privacy is a serious challenge in the management of medical devices (Sivakumar et al., 2024). Restrictions related to device safety and privacy often prevent the exchange of personal health information between medical facilities. Furthermore, several replicas and available machine learning schemes lack thorough testing, verification, and accountability. Blockchain network may be a viable resolution to this issue, offering provenance and transparency of health data by serving as a common record for organizing information in a distributed, safe, and reliable style.

To safeguard patient privacy, the distributed ledger system uses smart contracts to manage wearable device co-chain data. It also uses an integrated consensus plugin to facilitate exchange of value and cross-chain data exchange across various blockchain platforms (Griggs et al., 2018). The quality of managing chronic illnesses will be enhanced by the grouping of AI, wearable devices, and blockchain network, which will also facilitate increased efficiency, automation, data security, and privacy (Baucas et al., 2023; Rajathi et al., 2024). To continually enhance the relevant algorithm model, a hypothetical technological procedure with blockchain and AI can learn data from medical wearable devices and share it to a specific data management structure unit or a cloud platform. Currently, the primary focus of study is on the key issues and difficulties associated with the anticipation and treatment of chronic sicknesses. With the use of blockchain for privacy protection and trustworthy data tracking, patient data can be gathered via wearable technology and securely shared with healthcare organizations (Khan & Abaoud, 2023). AI technology can help medical organizations manage vast amounts of data related to chronic diseases. By ensuring the internet-based synchronized estimation speed for several wearable sensors, completing the multifaceted estimation of blood glucose, pressure, pulse, oxygenated blood content, humidity, breathing, and posture via an adaptive procedure, and successfully resolving the overall estimation problem of multi-point identification health, wearable technology can offer crucial assistance for digital twins.

2.3 Security Challenges of Using Wearable Medical Devices in Healthcare

The following issues are raised by wearable IoT devices, despite their potential to improve healthcare services.

1) Privacy of information and network security: By using wearable technology to gather patient data, the healthcare service's server gains more endpoints. These remote services make it easy to collect and monitor data. But when more devices are added, the network becomes more vulnerable. There are more potential

points of vulnerability for unscrupulous individuals to exploit and steal data when there are more endpoints. Better security is therefore more in need as the network expands. Additionally, the user data communicated from wearable devices to computing devices raises privacy apprehensions; thus, as the system rises with more medical devices, apprehensions about user privacy and network security also increase.

2) Data Security and Accuracy: Real-time diagnostics and early identification of a patient's disease and medical abnormalities are aids of employing wearable devices in healthcare. The sensor's reliability and its analysis plan, however, may have an impact on this. If the sensor or the assessment technique is subpar, there is a significant chance of misdiagnosis. The way the data is gathered and kept on the server may also be a source of errors. The integrity of the physiological information collected by the wearable devices must be maintained during its transfer from the device to the server. It guarantees that the information is up to date and accurate, given the source's current state. Additionally, careful data processing during aggregation is necessary to provide a precise patient assessment. Inaccurate results will be produced by a service that is unable to effectively and adequately gather, transmit, and process the data. For a medical service that leverages wearable IoT devices to be efficient, the reliability and precision of data must be addressed.
3) Networking Design Versatility and Responding: Wearable gadgets bring in various sensors and data-gathering and processing technologies. Healthcare services should incorporate them into their systems due to their numerous benefits. However, because changes occur often, advances and enhancements are iterative. It determines the rate at which existing infrastructures must keep up, even if it is an indication of technical progress and improvements in the healthcare industry. Because IoT networks require constant standardization, device variety has long been a challenge. Services that utilize this new technology should be able to monitor the expansion process, as it is still in its early stages. The same applies to wearable medical equipment. Since new viruses and illnesses frequently emerge, there is a great demand for technology that can identify each one. But every new technology meant that the service had to change. Reduced flexibility in networks leads to resource loss. Some even lose their entire infrastructure and services. Due to the constantly changing nature of wearable IoT devices, healthcare networks must be flexible and adaptive in their design (Guk et al., 2019).

3. RELATED WORK

Access control, privacy, and authenticity are only a few of the safety features that blockchain technology offers, and it has recently become an exciting technology (Asaithambi et al., 2022; Xie et al., 2021). Blockchain technology is attracting an increasing number of cybersecurity experts from various industries, including healthcare, due to its intrinsic qualities, which include transparency, immutability, and permanence. In (2020), Sun et al. presented architecture for tracking and monitoring changes to the setup of IoT devices. They utilized a private blockchain to store the device's configuration information, as well as any potential updates. The administrators have access to and are responsible for the preservation of the adjustment history. Thus, by monitoring and auditing the setup of IoT devices, this paradigm promotes security.

A private Ethereum blockchain was utilized by Griggs et al. (2018). Sensors engage with a smart device (such as a tablet or smartphone) in the system's architecture, which then connects to smart contracts immediately. After analyzing the supplied data, the latter notifies patients and medical professionals. Keep in mind that only transactions of events that have happened are stored in the ledger; gathered data is not. Thus, Blockchain properties are used to provide a secure remote patient monitoring solution. However, a significant drawback of the suggested approach is the time required for data to be transmitted from the smart device to the blockchain node.

Blockchain has emerged as a novel approach to conventional wearable healthcare device data exchange due to its distributed and secure nature. Chain codes were implemented on the blockchain by Rahman et al. (2021) to guarantee the safe completion of transactions. Jin et al. (2019) proposed a dependable and cooperative strategy for encrypting data stored in the cloud and securely exchanging it via blockchain as the volume of medical data increases. However, blockchain encounters performance issues due to the massive storage of information, which is exacerbated by the increasing number of data transfers between various medical institutions. To reduce storage and processing demands, Dwivedi et al. (2021) integrated IPFS with blockchain, storing data hashes within blockchain transactions. To reduce storage overhead and time costs, Ali Zouaghi et al. (2025) proposed a personal data confidentiality protection strategy that encrypts raw data stored on IPFS using an enhanced homomorphic encryption algorithm.

Meanwhile, user access control is required in decentralized data exchange due to the sensitive nature of wearable devices. To guarantee that only approved devices can access the data, each medical entity should have clearly defined access permissions. A distributed architecture for safe electronic health record sharing was proposed by Wang et al. (2019), who utilized blockchain smart contracts to provide a reliable platform and an attribute-based constant-size encryption technique to ensure restricted access. A hash-based anonymized authentication system was subsequently created by Li et al. (2015) to safeguard the personal security and access rights of data requesters. But using the blockchain to store data in plaintext might result in privacy violations. To achieve scalable access control, Jiang et al. (2022) proposed a medical data-sharing approach that utilizes attribute-based encryption techniques.

This plan, however, cannot guarantee the accuracy of user data, which could be detrimental to the interests of data demanders. The blockchain-based medical record safeguarding privacy exchange strategy proposed by Liu et al. (2018) combines content-extraction authentication techniques with CP-ABE-based access control methods in a collaborative manner. To decrease the danger of patient information leaks, the index is stored on a consortium blockchain that is impenetrable, while the actual medical data is maintained in the cloud. However, storing a large amount of encrypted medical data may decrease system efficiency due to the blockchain's computational performance limitations. Researchers have utilized sketch data structures to enhance search performance, thereby addressing challenges in medical data storage and effective searching. A medical data-sharing architecture that uses blockchain smart contracts for authorization control was proposed by Chen et al. (2021). By implementing a bidirectional conversion that synchronizes the entire dataset with these sections, this design enhances search performance by dividing the data into fine-grained parts and sharing them with various nodes.

MedAccess HBPF Duggegowda & Ramamoorthy (2024) adopted a distributed integration of information, as well as access control for health information across different divisions and levels, aiming to address the traits that include significant difficulty in managing health information, complex information subjects, and incomplete security of privacy. They achieved this by utilizing innovative contract technology to implement accessibility control of healthcare data on the blockchain. There are three contract tiers at MedAccess. Patient information regarding identity is managed through registration agreements, and data permission administration is accomplished through authorization contracts. Individual patient data and related role rights are bound by linked contractual SCs. The hybrid blockchain-edge design was proposed by Boumezbeur & Zarour (2022). This architecture uses edge intelligence and blockchain technologies to implement smart contracts for managing access controls of electronic health records. Sasikumar et al. (2024) used smart contracts to develop an attribute-based access management system for Industrial IoT.

The dynamic, dispersed, and dependable access control issues in an open Internet of Things setting were resolved by this plan. A data exchange and access control system was presented by Tanveer et al. (2022) and is utilized for communication between smart wearable devices. Through access control contracts, registration contracts, and judgment contracts, the system offers efficient access control administration and enables data sharing and authentication. Smart contract-based authentication and access control provide concepts for safeguarding the privacy of medical data; however, the issue of establishing the identity and authority of patients and physicians in smart contracts remains unresolved, particularly in the context of diagnosis facilitated by medical wearables.

In contrast to all previous research projects, our approach transfers security and privacy from medical devices to an externally controlled blockchain network using smart contracts. To (i) enforce an umbrella contract among multiple unknown users without the assistance of a reliable third party, (ii) confirm the security settings for permissions established by the confidentiality choices of the medical device owner before permitting any medical device to interact with additional devices, and (iii) prevent any dreadful attempts by analyzing the behaviors of medical devices to detect any virus attempt and quickly block the identified devices, smart contracts are being used.

4. THE PROPOSED BLOCKCHAIN-BASED PRIVACY PRESERVING WEARABLES MEDICAL DEVICE

In this section, we introduce revolutionary blockchain-based architecture for securing wearable medical devices. To assess the viability of the proposed strategy, a system will be implemented based on the proposed design, and chain code will be examined. To gauge the efficacy and efficiency of the proposed framework, the performance of the established scheme will also be presented.

4.1. A proposed four-layer framework overview

The four levels that make up the framework of the developed system are shown in Figure.2. The first layer is the physical layer of wearable devices, which includes wearable medical equipment such as weight scales, glucometers, and blood pressure monitors. Their job is to record vital signs, including blood pressure, and breathing rate, in real-time.

- A network gateway and internal storage unit, like a server and memory management unit, comprise the second layer, which is known as the gateway and storage layer. The gateway sends the vital signs data it has collected to healthcare computing devices. The storage and server then communicate with the decentralized database and the blockchain network. Additionally, the incoming data is encrypted by the server before being stored in a decentralized, off-chain database. To get real-time vital sign data, device information, and device state, the healthcare server also sends client-generated tasks.

- We proposed the decentralized blockchain as the third layer to perform secure device data transactions. It uses peer-to-peer databases for decentralized devices. Decentralized storage, on the other hand, is a peer-to-peer interactive program standard that uniquely identifies each file using resource addressing. The hash of the information saved in the decentralized database is created by IPFS and sent to the blockchain network. The Blockchain network layer, which is the third layer, utilizes a permissioned blockchain to guarantee that only authorized individuals can access the system. As a result, the Hyperledger Fabric architecture is used to oversee the execution of access control policies, wearable medical device registration, network gateway, and device enrollment.

Figure 2. The proposed blockchain integrated Privacy-Preserving Framework for Wearable Medical Devices.

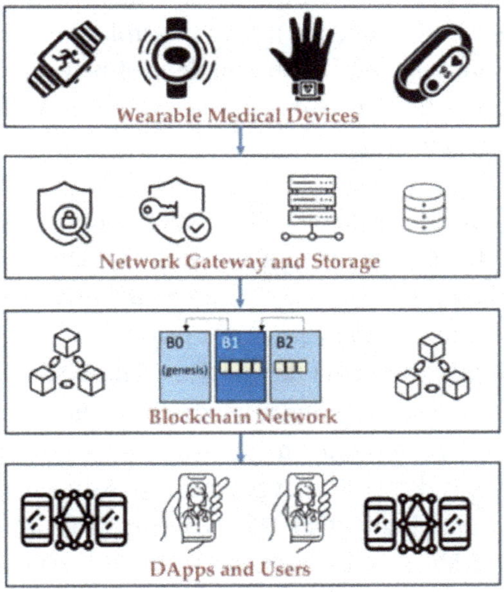

- The fourth layer, the Dapp layer, suggests a decentralized remote device monitoring application. This application uses APIs to connect to deployed smart contracts and operates on a peer-to-peer network. Users can utilize features such as access control description, device health record administration, and supervising provided by this decentralized application. This layer also includes the user's layer, comprising lab workers, doctors, nurses, and patients who utilize the DApp and benefit from its features. Furthermore, a blockchain network administrator is enrolled. The admin user can add, update, and remove peers in addition to creating, joining, and deploying chain code. As an administrator, we suggest a certain Ministry of Health organization. In the blockchain network, each user is represented as a node, and each node must have a specific role, such as administrator, peer, orderer, member, or client.

4.2. Privacy-Preserving Wearable Device Management

To ensure privacy preservation, we suggest defining a blockchain-based wearable device management context using chain codes. This framework would enforce the data owner's authority over wearable devices by identifying any potential misbehavior and turning off the devices that are detected. This section outlines the primary capabilities of the framework as well as our suggested smart contracts.

We have developed three smart contracts to automate device functions (i), Privacy permission setting, Ownership, and device Control. These are suggested to give the data owner the ability to specify and implement privacy permission settings. These agreements impose the data owner's privacy choices on the behavior of smart devices based on each data output.

(i) Privacy Permission Setting chain code: Each wearable device that is aware of this chain code address can utilize it by calling its specified functionalities. It is generated by the data owner and housed on the private BC. The purpose of the privacy permission setting chain code is to allow smart devices to request consent before interacting with other devices. This chain code defines the following functions: (i) The local Store, which allows the smart device to save its data gathered privately and confirm approval; (ii) External Store, which checks whether the medical device has approval to transmit the information it has gathered to be saved on an outside storage; (iii) Read, which checks whether the medical device has authorization to obtain data obtained medical devices with in the network after confirming permissions; (iv) Write, which allows a medical device to add and/or alter the required information gathered by other medical devices in the network if it is allowed; and (v) monitor, which allows the smart device to confirm authorization to receive periodic information from a different device.

(ii) The data owner creates the smart property contract to store the addresses of its own wearable devices. A privacy permission chain code is associated with a collection of data outputs for each medical Device. The Ownership smart contract also enforces the data device control over the medical devices and their outputs. The 'Add New Wearable Device' function allows you to add a new medical device by providing its address, output, and the address of the related privacy permission setting chain code. It specifies several functions, including: (ii) replace medical Device function, which allows an existing medical device to be removed, (iii) change medical Device function, which allows an existing medical device to have its description changed aside from the set of its outputs, By describing the new output, the (iv) add medical device output function allows an existing medical device to have a new output added. Modifying the summary of an established medical device output is possible with the (v) medical device output function. Removing an established medical device from an existing IoT device is possible with the (vi) medical device output action.

(iii) The data owner creates the device control chain code, which allows the data owner to specify the privacy settings for every smart Device output, check authorizations before granting any device accessibility to other devices and prevent a smart device from using a resource if it sends numerous requests in a short period. By examining the behavior of smart devices, the device control chain code is designed to identify any malicious activity quickly. The privacy setting add function, which allows a smart device to have a new privacy setting based on its data output through setting the action to be performed on the data, its authorization, and its permitted recurrence threshold, is one of the functions it specifies. (ii) The privacy setting update feature allows you to change the permissions linked to an action on a single smart device's output. The (iii) settings for privacy remove function allows you to remove authorization from a previous smart device; (iv) misbehavior penalty function allows you to keep track of all the IoT device misbehaviors and calculate how long a smart device penalty will last when any misbehavior is found; and (v) verify permission function allows you to examine the behavior of the smart Device before granting the communication the transmitter accessibility to the data that was requested output.

4.3. Framework's Main Functions

Our privacy-preserving wearable device organization, which is based on the suggested chain code, has the following features.

(i) Adding privacy permission settings to each medical device.
(ii) Enrolling a new medical device to the network system.
(iii) Imposing the privacy permission settings.

The following describes the dynamic component of the context that depends on these functions.

1. Adding a new medical device to the registry. An owner can register new wearable devices using the following procedures to make managing their own smart devices easier:
   - Step 1: Write and assemble a chain code for privacy permission setting.
   - Step 2: Organize the generated chain code onto the private blockchain by sending a transaction.
   - Step 3: Write and assemble a chain code for ownership.
   - Step 4: Install the generated chain code onto the private blockchain by sending a deal.
   - Step 5: Guide a transaction to invoke the add wearable device function specified in the Ownership chain code. This adds a new medical device by providing the address of the related Privacy Permission Setting smart contract, an medical device address, and a medical device output.
2. Setting Up Privacy Permissions on Every Medical Device. The owner can use the following procedures to provide the privacy permission settings for each medical device to specify the privacy preferences for how each one should operate:
   - Step 1: Develop a device that controls the chain code by writing and assembling it.
   - Step 2: To invoke the privacy setting function, send a transaction. By specifying the action to be performed on the information, its authorization, and the permitted occurrence threshold—the maximum number of requests that may be made within a short period—a new privacy permission option can be added to the device control smart contract.

The blockchain address of the Privacy Permission Setting smart contract was sent to the newly installed smart device.

3. The Privacy Permission Settings are being enforced. The following procedures may be used by the smart device to interact with its related Privacy Permission Setting smart contract and get permission to carry out the required action:
   - Step 1: By specifying the required target (such as the output of a medical device) and the action that is to be performed on the target, a transaction is sent to contact any function specified in the Privacy Permission Setting smart contract to get authorization to carry out the necessary operation.

- Step 2: Use the function called Step 1 to internally call the verify Permission function specified in the device control chain code.
- Step 3: After confirming the smart device's authorization and behavior, send out the Return Request Result event with the relevant choice.
- Step 4: Acquire the relevant ruling.

As previously stated, the activity of every medical device is monitored to ensure the desired activity or identify any potential misconduct. To achieve this, we present the algorithms for misbehavior penalty and permission function verification, as specified in the device Control smart contract. These algorithms are explained in detail in Algorithms 1 and 2.

When any misbehavior is discovered, Algorithm 2 Privacy Preserving seeks to calculate the length of activity and place the received misbehavior into a dynamic array that holds the smart device's detected device records. The privacy-preserving algorithm returns the calculated penalty after receiving as input the subject, the desired medical device output, the requested action, the type of misactivity, and the time at which the activity occurred. Punishment is essentially the block duration compared to the subject, measured in minutes, during which the subject is unable to perform any action using its smart contract.

Table 1. Algorithm 1: Wearable Medical Device Registration

Input: The device information (m_d); Device ID v_{id}, Device public key pk_d
Output: Valid or invalid device
Computing the device sign $v'_{id} = sign(h(m_d), pk_d$
if $v'_{id} = v_{id}$ then
$addr_d = GetBlockAddr(pk_d)$
if IsExist($addr_d$)=false then
select $seckey_{id} \in d_p$
Compute $pk_d = seckey_{id} \cdot g$
Compute Device ID = $h((seckey_{id}, pk_d), h(m_{id}))$
Calculate cyphertext = $enc(seckey_{id}, pk_d)$
Store {$addr_d$, cyphertext, v_{id}
end if
else
exist
else
return invalid device
end if

Table 2. Algorithm 2: Privacy Preserving Scheme Design

```
if Wearable Device is not registered, then
Register Device address
Assign device role and generate a random ID key K
else
if device role is not mentioned exist then
Retrieve user role
end if
end if
Wearable Device Data list = []
for device data in database do
Wearable Device Data List.append(Data)
end for
for device data in wearable device data list do
Keyword Index= Extract Keyword Index (Device Data)
Allow Access= False
for role assign in permission to device role do
if role assign= Ture
Break
end if
end for
if allow access and access request== Keyword Index then
Display Device Data
end if
end for
```

This is calculated by storing a record array of misbehaviour, known as the Misbehaviour List, for each subject. The penalty is then calculated based on the variety of subject records of misbehaviour and the frequency threshold at which a particular action is triggered on a single device output. Ensure the user has been previously registered. If not, the system will randomly select a key and assign the associated user role, also recording the user's address. The software will allocate a role to the user if they have been added and haven't been allocated one before. The list of medical data should then be obtained from the data source and saved in a list named "Wearable Device Data List." Next, extract each data's keyword index by iterating over the medical data list. Next, determine if the user's position has the authority to access the current medical information. The system sets the "Allow Access" variable to True if authorization is granted. The system displays the relevant medical data to the user when the request for entry matches the phrase in the index and the user has sufficient access privileges.

5. EXPERIMENTAL SETUP AND PERFORMANCE INVESTIGATION

To verify the effectiveness of the suggested wearable framework in terms of average transaction throughput and read throughput, we run several experiments in this section. We have employed Hyperledger blockchain tool developed by the open-source foundation, which enables system users to assess the functionality of blockchain applications. In addition to a single orderer node, we consider several established network factors for experimental analysis, such as five medical devices representing the members. The amount of time required to execute a chain code to access device data stored in decentralized storage is used to measure latency in the suggested system. We calculate throughput as the quantity of verified transactions per second. Read throughput and transaction throughput are the two subcategories of throughput.

Figure 3. The read transaction throughput analysis of proposed system.

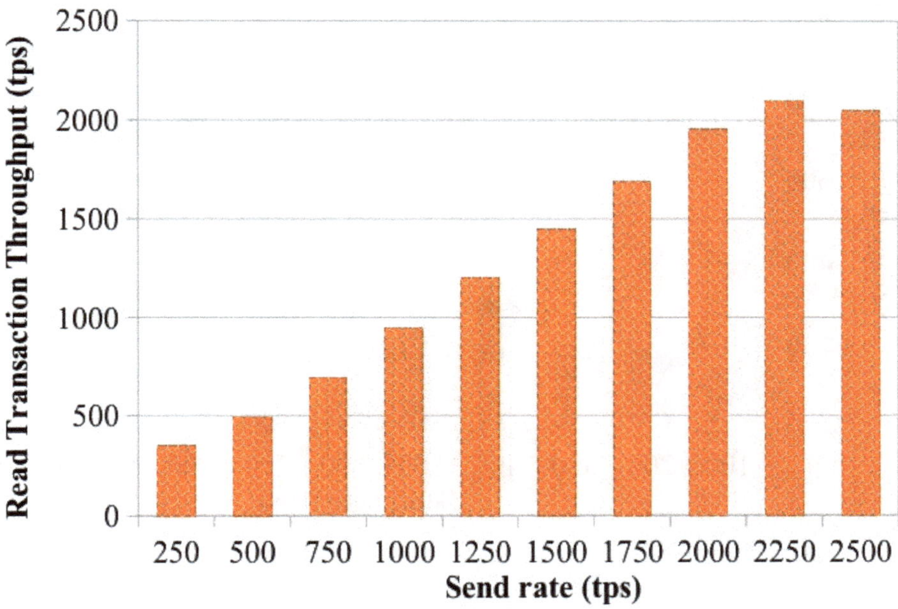

The read throughput is defined as the number of transactions carried out throughout the blockchain system within the specified period. Similarly, the transaction's throughput is the total number of successful transactions completed on the distributed ledger system within the specified period. We subtract the total number of incorrect transactions from the total number of operations to obtain successful ones. By varying the transmission rate from 250 to 2500 operations per send, as illustrated in Fig. 3 with an alternative machine utilization arrangement, the reading throughput of the developed system is evaluated. The graph shows that in the ideal situation, read transaction throughput rises sharply to its maximum and then slightly declines after transmit rate 2000, which is regarded as the perfect case.

Similarly, as shown in Fig. 4, the transaction throughput is assessed by changing the transmit rate between 100 and 1000 transactions per second. The graph indicates that when the send rate reaches its maximum of 1,010 transactions per send, the average transaction throughput also increases. Furthermore, 850 transactions per second is the ideal rate for transactional throughput; when the send rate increases, the throughput begins to decline.

Figure 4. The Average throughput analysis of proposed system.

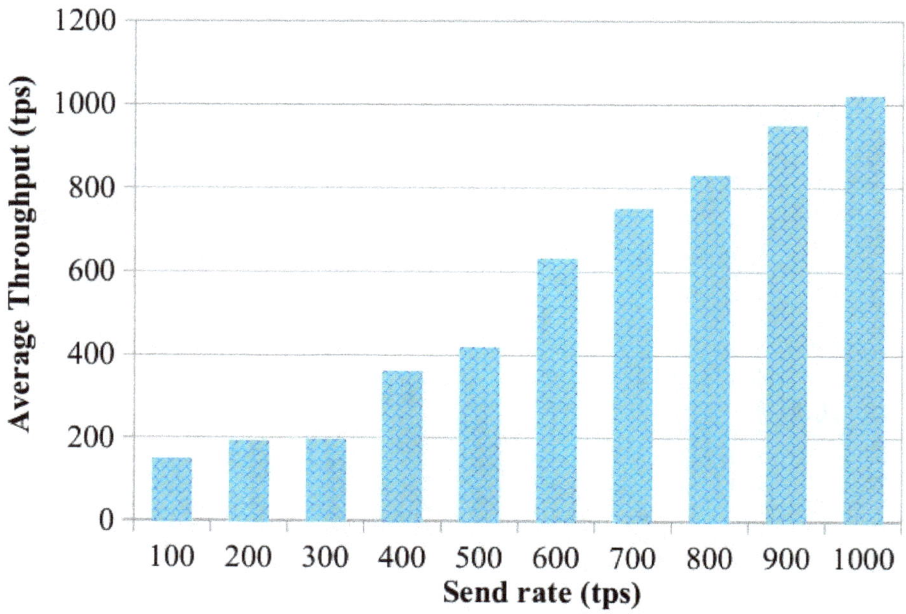

This section assesses the effectiveness of the proposed framework in terms of computational time cost. We experimented to determine how long it would take one miner node to confirm a privacy authorization establishing a description transaction that called the privacy setting add operation and a Privacy Authorization Transaction Request that called the verify authorization function defined on the device control smart contract to assess the performance of our solution. Initially, we ran a test to see how long it took to invoke the privacy setting add and check permission methods. The computing cost of the two operations for a single smart device is shown in Figure 5. To add a new privacy authorization setting or check the behavior of a single medical device, just 130 ms is required.

Additionally, using the settings for privacy add function takes longer to complete than using the verify permission method. This is explained by the fact that when using the Privacy Setting Add function, a new state on the chain code must be initialized with numerous details, including the data output, the action to be performed on the data, its authorization, and its permitted frequency threshold. We then repeated the experimentation with more smart devices under the control of a single miner node. The computational expense of the two procedures is shown in Figure 5 as the number of smart devices increases from 1 to 5. The range of processing times is between 150 and 750 ms. We find that the number of smart devices multiplied by the processing time for each smart device equals the total processing time. Therefore, the miner's computer power is needed to reduce the time required for processing as the number of smart devices increases.

Figure 5. The processing time analysis of different medical devices in the blockchain network

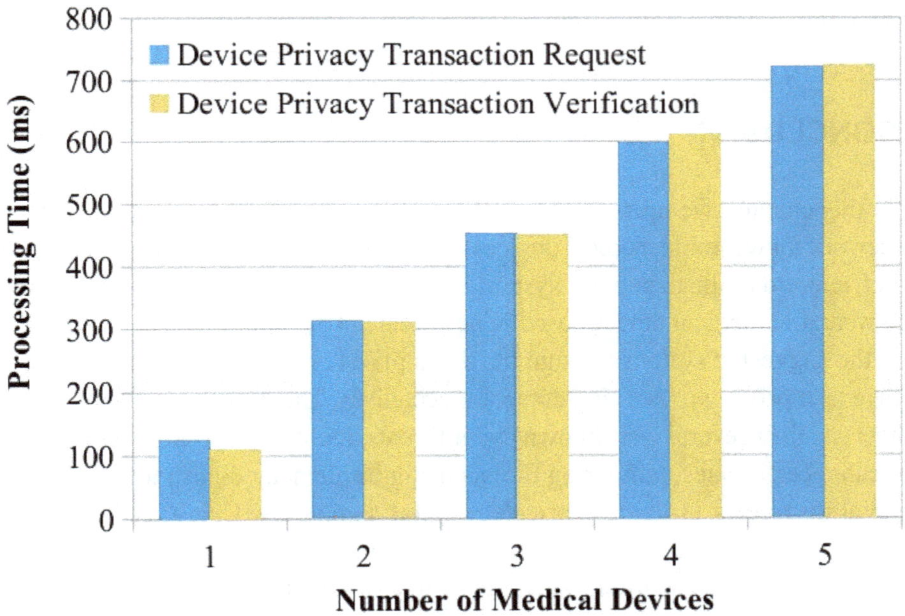

The performance assessment of current blockchain technologies in terms of latency and throughput is presented in Table 3, following an examination of the security and privacy aspects of the proposed system, as well as its essential features, and other blockchain-based medical devices that were evaluated. This helps determine whether the suggested system performs better than other comparable systems. It is clear from the numbers displayed that the suggested blockchain system offers the best throughput and the lowest latency for both reading queries and executing transactions.

Table 3. The overall performance comparison of proposed system with existing blockchain based system for healthcare application.

Reference	Transaction Throughput (Read)	Average Throughput	Read Latency (Average)	Transaction Latency (Average)
Jamil et al., 2020	2310 tps	58 tps	452 ms	2989 ms
Jamil et al., 2021	2382 tps	65 tps	452 ms	2950 ms
Proposed	2450 tps	1210 tps	210 ms	2450 ms

The proposed blockchain-based wearable medical system outperforms other researched blockchain-based healthcare systems in terms of operational metrics, according to the comparison results shown in Table 3. Thus, proposed blockchain helps to provide safe and effective remote device monitoring and exchange of medical data.

6. CONCLUSION

In this chapter, we present a blockchain-based, distributed, privacy-preserving framework for wearable medical devices. The proposed solution establishes a secure and efficient data management system by participating in blockchain technology with wearable medical devices used in healthcare. To monitor the user's vital signs data, the suggested system's design utilizes a private blockchain and decentralized storage as a privacy preserving control mechanism. The proposed system's design protects against several well-known cyber threats, including spoofing attacks using fabricated certificates, tampering threats using implemented hash techniques, and repudiation threats utilizing fabricated digital signatures. Using chain code, the suggested architecture utilizes blockchain not only to store transactions but also to manage access to the information saved in a distributed, off-chain database. To overcome centralized security concerns, the decentralization design included a de-centralized blockchain network, a decentralized off-chain database, and a distributed medical device monitoring application. As a result, the chosen strategy provides secure access to patient medical information, along with additional benefits for data confidentiality and privacy. Additionally, we conducted several tests to demonstrate the efficiency of the suggested remedy. Next, the cost of calculation time and the overhead of scalability are examined. Lastly, we contrast our suggestion with the current methods. It's also important to keep in mind that using blockchain results in storage overhead costs. To address this issue, we aim to save only the most recent blocks in our next work. Miners don't need to keep the entire blockchain on file for an extended period. To maintain the blockchain's immutability, they can only preserve the hash of the blocks that came before it, not the complete blocks.

REFERENCES

Ali Zouaghi, Y., Mahamdioua, M., Lahoulou, A., & Chettibi, S. (2025). Privacy preserving biometric authentication based on fully homomorphic encryption, blockchain, and IPFS data storage. *Multimedia Tools and Applications*. Advance online publication. DOI: 10.1007/s11042-024-19234-5

Asaithambi, S., Ravi, L., Kotb, H., Milyani, A. H., Azhari, A. A., Nallusamy, S., & Vairavasundaram, S. (2022). An energy-efficient and blockchain-integrated software defined network for the industrial Internet of Things. *Sensors (Basel)*, *22*(20), 7917. Advance online publication. DOI: 10.3390/s2220791 PMID: 36298266

Barua, A., Al Alamin, M. A., Hossain, M. S., & Hossain, E. (2022). Security and privacy threats for Bluetooth Low Energy in IoT and wearable devices: A comprehensive survey. *IEEE Open Journal of the Communications Society*, *3*, 251–281. DOI: 10.1109/OJCOMS.2022.3141912

Baucas, M. J., Spachos, P., & Plataniotis, K. N. (2023). Federated learning and blockchain-enabled fog-IoT platform for wearables in predictive healthcare. *IEEE Transactions on Computational Social Systems*, *10*(4), 1732–1741. DOI: 10.1109/TCSS.2022.3193138

Boumezbeur, I., & Zarour, K. (2022). Privacy-preserving and access control for sharing electronic health record using blockchain technology. *Acta Informatica Pragensia*, *11*(1), 105–122. DOI: 10.18267/j.aip.185

Carminati, M., & Scandurra, G. (2021). Impact and trends in embedding field programmable gate arrays and microcontrollers in scientific instrumentation. *The Review of Scientific Instruments*, *92*(9), 091101. Advance online publication. DOI: 10.1063/5.0056719 PMID: 34598486

Chen, Y., Meng, L., Zhou, H., & Xue, G. (2021). A blockchain-based medical data sharing mechanism with attribute-based access control and privacy protection. *Wireless Communications and Mobile Computing*, *2021*, 6685762. Advance online publication. DOI: 10.1155/2021/6685762

Deep, S., Zheng, X., Jolfaei, A., Yu, D., Ostovari, P., & Bashir, A. K. (2022). A survey of security and privacy issues in the Internet of Things from the layered context. *Transactions on Emerging Telecommunications Technologies*, *33*(6), e3935. Advance online publication. DOI: 10.1002/ett.3935

Duggegowda, D., & Ramamoorthy, U. (2024). MedAccess HBPF: A privacy-preserving hybrid-blockchain framework for secure and efficient cloud-based electronic health record sharing. *SN Computer Science*, *5*(8), 1018. Advance online publication. DOI: 10.1007/s42979-024-03245-8

Dwivedi, S. K., Amin, R., & Vollala, S. (2021). Blockchain-based secured IPFS-enable event storage technique with authentication protocol in VANET. *IEEE/CAA Journal of Automatica Sinica, 8*(12), 1913–1922. https://doi.org/DOI: 10.1109/JAS.2021.1004209

Griggs, K. N., Ossipova, O., Kohlios, C. P., Baccarini, A. N., Howson, E. A., & Hayajneh, T. (2018). Healthcare blockchain system using smart contracts for secure automated remote patient monitoring. *Journal of Medical Systems*, *42*(12), 248. Advance online publication. DOI: 10.1007/s10916-018-0993-x PMID: 29876661

Griggs, K. N., Ossipova, O., Kohlios, C. P., Baccarini, A. N., Howson, E. A., & Hayajneh, T. (2018). Healthcare blockchain system using smart contracts for secure automated remote patient monitoring. *Journal of Medical Systems*, *42*(12), 248. Advance online publication. DOI: 10.1007/s10916-018-0993-x PMID: 29876661

Guk, K., Han, G., Lim, J., Jeong, K., Kang, T., Lim, E.-K., & Jung, J. (2019). Evolution of wearable devices with real-time disease monitoring for personalized healthcare. *Nanomaterials (Basel, Switzerland)*, *9*(6), 813. Advance online publication. DOI: 10.3390/nano9060813 PMID: 31146479

Hellsten, T., Karlsson, J., Shamsuzzaman, M., & Pulkkis, G. (2021). The potential of computer vision-based marker-less human motion analysis for rehabilitation. *Rehabilitation Process and Outcome*, *10*, 11795727211022330. Advance online publication. DOI: 10.1177/11795727211022330 PMID: 34987303

Iqbal, S. M. A., Mahgoub, I., Du, E., Leavitt, M. A., & Asghar, W. (2021). Advances in healthcare wearable devices. *NPJ Flexible Electronics*, *5*(1), 9. Advance online publication. DOI: 10.1038/s41528-021-00107-x

Jamil, F., Ahmad, S., Iqbal, N., & Kim, D. H. (2020). Towards a remote monitoring of patient vital signs based on IoT-based blockchain integrity management platforms in smart hospitals. *Sensors (Basel)*, *20*(8), 2195. Advance online publication. DOI: 10.3390/s20082195 PMID: 32294989

Jamil, F., Kahng, H. K., Kim, S., & Kim, D. H. (2021). Towards secure fitness framework based on IoT-enabled blockchain network integrated with machine learning algorithms. *Sensors (Basel)*, *21*(5), 1640. Advance online publication. DOI: 10.3390/s21051640 PMID: 33652773

Jiang, Y., Xu, X., & Xiao, F. (2022). Attribute-based encryption with blockchain protection scheme for electronic health records. *IEEE Transactions on Network and Service Management, 19*(4), 3884–3895. DOI: 10.1109/TNSM.2022.3193664

Jin, H., Luo, Y., Li, P., & Mathew, J. (2019). A review of secure and privacy-preserving medical data sharing. *IEEE Access : Practical Innovations, Open Solutions, 7*, 61656–61669. DOI: 10.1109/ACCESS.2019.2915024

Kavitha, D., Chinnasamy, A., & Selvakumari, P. (2025). Intelligent decision-making framework for big data using enhanced honey badger-based adaptive hybrid deep learning network. *International Journal of Data Mining and Bioinformatics, 29*(1-2), 193–222. DOI: 10.1504/IJDMB.2025.10060345

Khan, M. F., & Abaoud, M. (2023). Blockchain-integrated security for real-time patient monitoring in the Internet of Medical Things using federated learning. *IEEE Access : Practical Innovations, Open Solutions, 11*, 117826–117850. DOI: 10.1109/ACCESS.2023.3326145

Li, C. T., Weng, C. Y., Lee, C. C., & Wang, C. C. (2015). A hash based remote user authentication and authenticated key agreement scheme for the integrated EPR information system. *Journal of Medical Systems, 39*(11), 144. Advance online publication. DOI: 10.1007/s10916-015-0371-8 PMID: 26349803

Liu, J., Li, X., Ye, L., Zhang, H., Du, X., & Guizani, M. (2018). BPDS: A blockchain based privacy-preserving data sharing for electronic medical records. In *2018 IEEE Global Communications Conference (GLOBECOM)* (pp. 1–6). IEEE. https://doi .org/DOI: 10.1109/GLOCOM.2018.8647939

Rahman, M. Z. U., Surekha, S., Satamraju, K. P., Mirza, S. S., & Lay-Ekuakille, A. (2021). A collateral sensor data sharing framework for decentralized healthcare systems. *IEEE Sensors Journal, 21*(24), 27848–27857. DOI: 10.1109/JSEN.2021.3123456

Rajathi, V., Chinnasamy, A., & Selvakumari, P. (2024). DUTC Net: A novel deep ulcer tissue classification network with stage prediction and treatment plan recommendation. *Biomedical Signal Processing and Control, 90*, 105855. Advance online publication. DOI: 10.1016/j.bspc.2024.105855

Sasikumar, A., Ravi, L., Devarajan, M., Selvalakshmi, A., Almaktoom, A. T., Almazyad, A. S., & Mohamed, A. W. (2024). Blockchain-assisted hierarchical attribute-based encryption scheme for secure information sharing in industrial Internet of Things. *IEEE Access : Practical Innovations, Open Solutions, 12*, 12586–12601. DOI: 10.1109/ACCESS.2024.3356789

Sasikumar, A., Ravi, L., Devarajan, M., Vairavasundaram, S., Selvalakshmi, A., Kotecha, K., & Abraham, A. (2023). A decentralized resource allocation in edge computing for secure IoT environments. *IEEE Access: Practical Innovations, Open Solutions*, *11*, 117177–117189. DOI: 10.1109/ACCESS.2023.3324732

Sivakumar, C. L. V., Mone, V., & Abdumukhtor, R. (2024). Addressing privacy concerns with wearable health monitoring technology. *Wiley Interdisciplinary Reviews: Data Mining and Knowledge Discovery, 14*(3), Article e1535. https://doi.org/DOI: 10.1002/widm.1535

Sun, S., Folarin, A. A., Ranjan, Y., Rashid, Z., Conde, P., & Stewart, C.RADAR-CNS Consortium. (2020). Using smartphones and wearable devices to monitor behavioral changes during COVID-19. *Journal of Medical Internet Research*, *22*(9), e19992. Advance online publication. DOI: 10.2196/19992 PMID: 32877352

Tanveer, M., Ahmad, M., Nguyen, T. N., & Abd El-Latif, A. A. (2022). Resource-efficient authenticated data sharing mechanism for smart wearable systems. *IEEE Transactions on Network Science and Engineering*, *10*(5), 2525–2536. DOI: 10.1109/TNSE.2022.3216837

Thirunavukkarasu, J., & Chinnasamy, A. (2024). Enhancing the preciseness of prediction in heart disease diagnosis by utilizing machine learning. In 2024 *International Conference on Advances in Computing, Communication and Applied Informatics (ACCAI)* (pp. 1–9). IEEE. https://doi.org/DOI: 10.1109/ACCAI61015.2024.10587654

Wang, Y., Zhang, A., Zhang, P., & Wang, H. (2019). Cloud-assisted EHR sharing with security and privacy preservation via consortium blockchain. *IEEE Access : Practical Innovations, Open Solutions*, *7*, 136704–136719. DOI: 10.1109/ACCESS.2019.2943154

Xie, Y., Lu, L., Gao, F., He, S. J., Zhao, H. J., Fang, Y., & Dong, Z. (2021). Integration of artificial intelligence, blockchain, and wearable technology for chronic disease management: A new paradigm in smart healthcare. *Current Medical Science*, *41*(6), 1123–1133. DOI: 10.1007/s11596-021-2487-8 PMID: 34950987

Xu, S. S.-D., Chen, C.-H., & Chang, T.-C. (2019). Design of oneM2M-based fog computing architecture. *IEEE Internet of Things Journal*, *6*(6), 9464–9474. DOI: 10.1109/JIOT.2019.2932248

Chapter 7
Strengthening Data Integrity in Healthcare Through Blockchain Technology for Enhanced Patient Privacy in the Digital Age

N. Nasurudeen Ahamed
https://orcid.org/0000-0002-2777-8870
United Arab Emirates University, UAE

Thangavel Murugan
https://orcid.org/0000-0002-2510-8857
United Arab Emirates University, UAE

ABSTRACT

Health consciousness is increasingly becoming a priority among urban populations, leading many to embrace digital healthcare services, such as wearable devices. These innovations have become integral to daily life, significantly improving diagnostic and treatment processes as healthcare professionals and patients adopt medical wearables. However, concerns regarding the protection of sensitive medical data and information integrity remain prevalent. To address these critical privacy issues, we propose a blockchain-based data integrity solution that utilizes the InterPlanetary File System (IPFS) for decentralized data storage. This innovative platform offers a secure, censorship-resistant environment for managing health-related documents, ensuring both accessibility and authenticity. By storing patient information on

DOI: 10.4018/979-8-3373-4412-6.ch007

IPFS, we can decentralize data management and permit access only to authorized users, effectively safeguarding sensitive information against breaches. We explore the implications of health consciousness in urban populations, focusing on digital healthcare adoption.

1. INTRODUCTION

1.1 Overview of Health Consciousness in Urban Populations

In high-population countries like India and China, individuals' engagement in health activities is significantly influenced by their level of health consciousness. Several variables affect the health consciousness of Chinese inhabitants. Older persons tend to have lower levels of health consciousness than younger individuals, influenced by socio-demographic and economic factors. Males tend to be less health-conscious than females. Residents with partners tend to be more health-conscious than those without partners. Individuals with higher levels of education tend to be more health-minded. Middle-income individuals are more aware of their health compared to those with lower incomes. Residents with higher family economic status and prior medical experiences tend to be more health-conscious (Shi et al., 2025). Obesity is a nutritional disease, one of the most serious of the twenty-first century, that has spread on a global scale. Overweight and obesity, which were once thought to be problems in high-income countries, are now affecting low- and middle-income countries, particularly in cities. Overweight and obesity rates among children and adolescents are steadily increasing. Obesity and overweight are caused mainly by an imbalance of calories consumed and expended. Obesity in children is connected with an increased risk of noncommunicable diseases, but it also generates poor psychosocial impacts (Lewandowska et al., 2025). As more people migrate from rural to urban areas in China (Su et al., 2024), they encounter distinct challenges in accessing healthcare services. Population movement optimises labour allocation, thereby promoting a country's social and economic progress. Migrants often experience lifestyle changes and obstacles in their jobs, healthcare, housing, and insurance (Song et al., 2025).

1.2 Importance of Digital Healthcare Services

Digitalization is playing an increasingly significant role in nearly every aspect of society. Healthcare has only lately begun to digitalize procedures and services on a larger scale. The researchers use the term “digital health” to encompass a broad range of concepts, including eHealth, mobile health (mHealth), telehealth, and telemedicine. Digital health is "an advancement in the way healthcare provision is conceived and delivered by healthcare providers through the use of technological tools to track and enhance the well-being and health of patients and to empower patients in the management of their own and their families' health." Furthermore, digital health services are available at all times and from any location, promoting patient empowerment and facilitating collaborative decision-making (Maier et al., 2021).

Digital health presents many opportunities and the prospect of improving the quality of patient care. Machine learning, mobile apps, sensors, wearables, and telehealth have the potential to enhance traditional clinical history, assessment, differential diagnoses, and treatment paradigms. The most recent pandemic has accelerated our progress toward this future, but there are still significant challenges ahead, including: ensuring proper evaluation and intelligent implementation of new technologies; integrating data into care records; and, perhaps most importantly, appropriate clinical support for digital tools. Patients should benefit from this technology without placing an additional burden on their physician/provider. Older obstacles may be tackled, but new challenges will develop, particularly in ensuring the benefits of better care are realized for those without access, all the way to using a smartphone or accessing the web. Clinicians must continue to be advocates for patients and each other as we counsel one another regarding digital health (Butcher & Hussain, 2022).

1.3 Rise of Medical Wearables for Diagnosis and Treatment

The use of consumer wearable technology has grown in popularity. These have routinely included wrist wearables such as watches and activity bands, gloves, insoles, headgear, and rings. Wearables use implanted sensors to collect physiological information (mostly passively) and then relay the data to the device or to a smartphone app when paired. This has provided clinicians with more data than has ever been available for assessment, much of which is not captured in traditional electronic health records; it is often presented as reports across multiple apps. Many of the technologies were designed with goal-oriented measures of exercise, physical fitness, or rehabilitation; however, there has been an increased focus on identifying, monitoring, and delivering interventions for early-onset disease. The large technology companies have made a hefty investment, suggesting they identify a possible revenue opportunity. Year-on-year growth for these devices has remained strong; the smartwatch market saw a 24% increase in 2021 and shipped over 40 million units in the last quarter of 2021 (Butcher & Hussain, 2022).

Technological disruptions and innovations have caused a more dramatic shift in the health care environment and other industries/parts of the global economy. In academic literature, this change in phenomena charge is known as the Fourth

Industrial Revolution (4R). New technologies, including: blockchain; big data; the Internet of Things (IO); artificial intelligence (AI); self-driving vehicles; remote sensing, which includes satellite imagery and drones; wearables, which are simply a noun identifying that the device is worn, not the user; robots; genome editing; augmented reality; 3D printing; and biotechnologies, provide plenty of evidence for health care organization chaos and the concept of 4R. An example of a wearable device, also known as a fitness band or smartwatch (Sharma et al., 2020), is a fitness band or smartwatch.

1.4 Objectives of the Chapter

The purpose of this chapter is to analyze the implications of health consciousness in urban societies, with a particular focus on the utilization of digital healthcare services. It seeks to demonstrate the benefits of wearable devices in improving diagnostic and treatment processes, while recognizing the serious issues surrounding data privacy and integrity. The implementation of a blockchain-based solution focuses on data integrity through the InterPlanetary File System (IPFS).

2. HEALTH CONSCIOUSNESS AND THE ADOPTION OF DIGITAL HEALTHCARE

2.1 Trends in Health Awareness Among Urban Dwellers

Human health is a significant concern among global policymakers and scholars from various academic fields. Healthcare is an assumed right, irrespective of one's socio-economic status, and has very real consequences for people's health outcomes, life experiences, and overall well-being. Specifically, healthcare is the most essential urban service because its regular functioning affects the breadth of other choices. Importantly, healthcare is often output-constrained, particularly in developing countries, and it costs more than other services (Su et al., 2024).

The rapid growth of urban populations and transportation-related greenhouse gas emissions continues to challenge the smart city agenda for sustainable development, enhancing public health, environmental quality, and urban liveability. Smart healthcare wearable devices and applications have no precedent for utilization in urban transportation networks. The integration of smart wearable healthcare devices (SWH) with new mobile applications can counteract the adverse effects of transportation modes, encourage and support healthy lives, and contribute to thoughtful urban planning and design. Although SWH devices and applications can benefit physical and mental health in smart cities, their uptake in urban transportation networks remains limited as cities continue to grow. SWH devices can be used to monitor work-life balance, physical activity, and allow access to real-time health data (Kazmi et al., 2024)

Cardiovascular disorders (CVD) represent one of the major worldwide health issues, causing high morbidity and mortality across communities. In recent years, wearable technology has advanced, evolving from simple fitness monitors to advanced health-monitoring devices central to the delivery of cardiovascular care. Early fitness trackers were predominantly focused on step counting, calorie consumption, and overall physical activity levels, providing limited indicators of cardiovascular health (C-SYS). Newer developments in wearable technology, driven by advances in sensor technology and miniaturization, have included performance-monitoring wearables for photoplethysmography (PPG), electrocardiography (ECG), and blood pressure monitoring (Sultana et al., 2025).

2.2 Impact of Digital Healthcare Services on Patient Engagement

Digital healthcare services, including telemedicine, mobile health (mHealth) applications, wearable devices, and electronic health records (EHRs), have entirely changed patient engagement with clinicians. This advancement has notably increased patient engagement and allowed patients to take a more active role in their health journey.

Wearables are mobile, multi-use, small, flexible devices that can be worn on the head, limbs, or torso, such as helmets, bands, and belts. Such devices combine sensors or utilize standard sensors including three-dimensional accelerometers, gyroscopes, photoplethysmography, external skin temperature, and electrodermal activity to calculate metrics related to gait, energy expenditure, physical activity, brain activity, oxygen saturation, heart rate and its derivatives, blood pressure, or biomarkers in biofluids, such as saliva, blood, or tears. Wearables are typically linked with novel applications that make it easy to communicate user measurements and findings. Wearables use algorithms to produce outputs related to user biometrics and behaviours, providing feedback to users and motivating regulated lifestyle changes (Menassa et al., 2025).

Sleep is the most potent form of rehabilitation for athletes and supports optimal performance. However, athletes often suffer from sleep challenges. Typically, sleep duration in athletes is recorded over periods of no more than 2 weeks, and often only 1 month, during long-term sleep assessments. Short-term sleep duration does not account for transient events, will not accurately capture an individual's sleep trends and patterns, and hinders thorough evaluations of sleep quality. Therefore, an athlete's sleep should be monitored over time. Wearable smart devices that offer a better user experience, ease of use, and immediate sleep feedback are being implemented for everyday monitoring among athletes as science and technology advance (Dai et al., 2025).

Figure 1. Types of Digital Healthcare Services

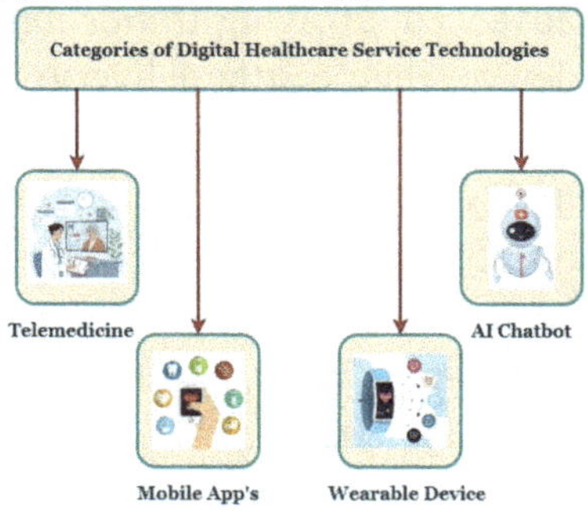

Figure 1 depicts the taxonomy of digital healthcare services. In the present era, digital healthcare services make it easier for patients to diagnose themselves. However, in this chapter, we discuss wearable gadgets for monitoring patient data and protecting sensitive information.

2.3 Role of Medical Wearables in Preventive Healthcare

Wearable health technology is predicated on the integration of digital technologies and healthcare systems, a trend that has advanced rapidly over the past few decades. Initially developed for fitness and wellness tracking, including heart rate and physical activity capabilities, wearables today represent advanced medicine, providing continuous health monitoring and personalized care. Wearables span all types of devices, including smartwatches, fitness trackers, and even medical-grade wearables that track and monitor vital signs such as heart rate, oxygen saturation, and blood glucose levels. The proliferation of wearable technology is driven by advances in biosensors, compact electronics, and wireless communications, enabling real-time monitoring and analysis of health data. Wearable health technology has proven valuable for personal health and clinical use by enabling timely assessment of healthcare concerns and chronic conditions, supporting early detection, management, and patient outcomes. Wearable technology has progressed from simple fitness trackers that improved activity tracking to sophisticated medical devices that provide continuous health monitoring, real-time data analysis, and predictive health information. Wearable health technology has altered the course of healthcare, as continuous monitoring of vital signs and access to real-time health data have enabled more accurate assessment of patient status and improved ultimate patient outcomes. The emergence of gadgets featuring countless sensors across various types of wearable technologies helps manage health concerns for both patients and healthcare professionals. Wearables not only provide helpful diagnostic information but may also enable predictive assessment, indicating the probability of a health concern and helping prevent life-altering disorders before they occur (Obianyo et al., 2024).

Proactive healthcare aims to minimize the likelihood of chronic diseases through early detection, continuous monitoring, and lifestyle management. Medical wearables, or smart devices that track physiological and biometric measures such as oxygen levels, heart rate, steps, and sleep quality, are critical for real-time health monitoring and behaviour change. Several healthcare devices are presented in Table 1. The illustrations (Figure 2) below show the various wearable devices, and Table 1 describes their performance.

Figure 2. Types of Healthcare Wearable Gadgets.

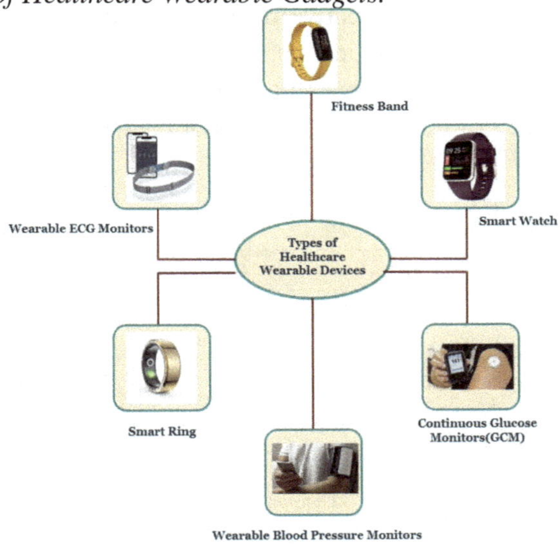

Table 1. Performance of Healthcare Gadgets.

S.No	Classification of Wearable Gadgets	Performance
1	Smart Watch	Track your heart rate, ECG, steps, sleep, and oxygen saturation.
2	Continuous Glucose Monitors (CGM)	Monitor blood sugar levels in real-time for people with diabetes.
3	Wearable ECG Monitors	Identify abnormalities and abnormal heartbeat.
4	Smart Rings	Track your sleep, temperature, and stress levels.
5	Fitness Bands	Track your daily activity and calorie consumption.
6	Wearable Blood Pressure Monitors	Constant monitoring of blood pressure

2.4 Case Studies of Successful Wearable Implementations

In this section, we addressed preventive medicine and chronic illness management, organized by disease area and application. Many countries use medical wearable devices. The following is a list of several countries and their wearable devices for healthcare uses. Table 2 discusses the use cases of medical wearable devices.

Table 2. Healthcare Gadgets Case Studies

S.No	Country	Gadgets	Goal	Results
1	USA	Apple Watch (Smart Watch)	To Detect Irregular Heart Rhythms	Early Detection
2	USA/Asia /Europe	Oura Ring (Smart Ring)	To Detect Sleep and Illness	Early Detection of Illness (Including Fever)
3	USA	Breathing Monitor	To identify the Stress	To Reduce the Stress
4	Netherlands	Chest Patch	Constant tracking of vital signs to detect illness early.	Detecting signs of disease early allows for suitable action.
5	UAE	Fitness Trackers	Physical Fitness	Increased community knowledge of preventive fitness.
6	Overseas	Continuous Glucose Monitors (CGMs)	Management of diabetes	Enhanced control of glucose

3. CHALLENGES IN DATA PRIVACY AND INTEGRITY

3.1 Overview of Sensitive Medical Data

The clinical context is an important factor in identifying and treating patients in healthcare. The notion of "clinical" encompasses both "laboratory" (where the patient's physical samples are tested to assess injuries or problems) and "data" (data recorded in other facilities during laboratory procedures). This environment is an important source of data for healthcare. However, in recent years, the value of this environment has increased, as this data is considerably more sensitive than other areas of patient data, particularly with respect to ethical concerns related to linking it to individuals. Hackers, fuelled by financial gain or other motives, are more likely to target and steal this "medical data". An example of this data would include patient information that is more sensitive than other patient data. The clinical context is an important area of focus in the data collection of sensitive patient data in healthcare. Cybercriminals are always looking for opportunities to exploit their victims for personal or financial gain. Therefore, securing sensitive data is a vital concern (Martínez et al., 2023).

Personal and sensitive data are commonly handled in both research and industry. Even with various methodological improvements in protecting sensitive data, the practice often lacks an overview and guidance on how to use the available data protection methods and instruments. A health insurance firm wishes to share individual-level data with colleges and hospitals for analytical purposes. To accomplish this purpose, it generates scientific-use files. For instance, we examined the degree of geographical heterogeneity and the influence of health insurance-related characteristics using anonymized patient claim data from Switzerland's largest insurance provider (Templ et al., 2022). In today's world, there is an abundance of data relating to patients' healthcare records. With the emergence of vast amounts of healthcare data, the confidentiality and security of this data are critical. Computer scientists, engineers, medical physicians, and attorneys are all worried about the security and privacy of patients' healthcare information. Our purpose is to address the various acts and statutes related to patient healthcare data. The authors also provide an overview of how modern internet-connected healthcare devices, such as BANs (including IoT wristbands for pulse, temperature, and skin condition monitoring), pacemakers, EEG and ECG devices, and ICU medical gadgets, contribute to the massive volume of healthcare information (Vyas et al., 2021).

Health information (commonly referred to as personal health information, PHI, or medical data or health information) is data or information about an individual's mental or physical health, diagnosis, care, and historical conditions. In general, health information is any information that could be utilized to identify an individual. Wearable and IoT data, such as heart rate, sleep, and glucose levels, are used to represent health information.

3.2 Common Threats to Data Privacy and Security

The healthcare facility is a key source of sensitive patient data. Cybercriminals seek to steal this data for their benefit. Therefore, securing sensitive data is a vital concern (Martinez et al., 2023). EHR systems face challenges in interoperability, user interface complexity, and data security, hindering seamless patient care and healthcare delivery. The electronic health record (EHR) has transformed healthcare by improving the availability, accessibility, and analytics of patient data and enhancing care quality. However, EHRs confront issues in interoperability, flexibility, security, privacy, and standardization (Rathore et al., 2025). The rise of innovative healthcare systems has led to substantial online data sharing between doctors and patients. However, this open communication channel makes it vulnerable to attacks. The healthcare sector prioritizes privacy and security. Security measures are in place to prevent unauthorized access to patient data. Authors highlight and explore security and privacy issues in edge-based competent healthcare (Alzu'Bi et al., 2024).

- Device authorization.
- Confidentiality.
- Data manipulation.
- A compromise between hardware and software.
- Privacy and safety risks.
- Common edge computing attacks.
    - Eavesdropping.
    - Denial-of-Service (DoS) Attacks.
    - Distributed Denial-of-Service (DoS) Attacks.
    - Data Tampering Attacks.
- Safety of data Outsourcing.

Data used in the provision of health care is subject to both internal and external threats, including the potential for data leaks during information sharing between various parties. A breach of data integrity occurs when an inadvertent change occurs during data storage, retrieval, or processing, which may result from: a compromise of data integrity motivated by malicious intent, an equipment failure (e.g., a power outage), or human error. Changes resulting from unauthorized access to a system may also be classified as unauthorized data access events. If access to keys is unauthorized, this may ultimately compromise data confidentiality (Alzu'Bi et al., 2024).

3.3 Impacts of Data Breaches on Patients and Providers

In the healthcare industry, data breaches are extremely costly not only to healthcare organizations, such as hospitals and insurance providers, but also to patients and society. In contrast to user IDs and passwords, which can be quickly changed after a data breach occurs, a patient's health status remains. Health information can also be used for months or years for a variety of purposes, including medical fraud and bogus insurance claims (Park et al., 2025).

A consequence of increased digitalization is that cybersecurity has become an essential part of the technology landscape. We see health service providers beginning to integrate electronic health records (EHRs) into the Internet of Medical Things (IoMT), signalling a move toward more digitally connected systems, with data increasingly significant in the healthcare response. This change provides a major opportunity to improve the quality of care for patients and the effectiveness of service delivery; however, it also introduces significant cybersecurity risks into the health service system. Personal health information is sensitive and, therefore, fascinating to cybercriminals. In healthcare, a breach of this personal health information could threaten patient safety or privacy. The landscape of cybersecurity vulnerabilities in the healthcare system means there are multiple pathways for a breach (In Figure 3) to occur, including the two most likely pathways: hacking or deliberate attacks, and accidental disclosures. The litany of human factors that influence data breaches in healthcare often serves as the primary pathway for them. The most likely risks identified by ENISA in the healthcare sphere include ransomware, data-related threats, intrusion, DDoS/DoS/RDDoS attacks, supply chain breaches, malware, and others. During the COVID-19 pandemic, there were many reports of data breaches involving various healthcare organizations worldwide, driven mainly by insider threats or improper system configurations (Nemec Zlatolas et al., 2024).

Figure 3. Effects of a Data Breach

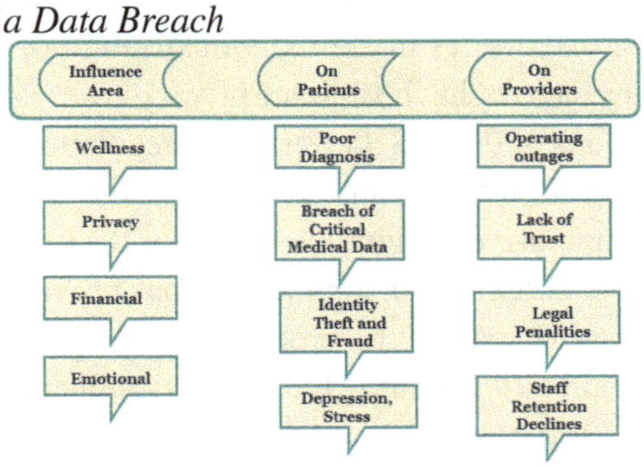

In healthcare, a data breach occurs when unauthorized individuals or organizations access patients' protected health information. These events can be pretty serious for healthcare organizations. Healthcare data breaches are the most expensive in the United States across all sectors. Healthcare organizations that are frequently breached incur approximately $8 million in lost revenue, litigation costs, and public relations costs (e.g., patients lost after a breach). The Office of Civil Rights within the U.S. Department of Health and Human Services oversees organizations that have experienced a data breach involving more than 500 patients. Healthcare is particularly vulnerable to data breaches, accounting for more than half of all breaches in the United States. The incident is much worse if it is severe, such as a breach conducted by malicious actors or involving a larger number of patients. In contrast, the impact is alleviated mainly if hospital visits are halted, as this may, in fact, cause harm to patients, particularly those who require follow-up questions for their chronic illnesses (Chen et al., 2025).

3.4 Regulatory Framework and Compliance Issues

In 1996, the United States passed the Health Insurance Portability and Accountability Act (HIPAA). The Health Insurance Portability and Accountability Act (In Figure 4) is a healthcare law created by the United States (US) that lays out universal standards for regulatory oversight of patient information (including sensitive information) throughout its lifecycle (Khan & Rudman, 2025).

The significance and application of the aforementioned rules/standards had to adjust to the evolving health systems across our world. Over time, consistent methods for recognizing and deterring violations of these rules had to be adjusted as well. Even though patients are becoming increasingly aware and protective of their information, the entity type has a moral and ethical obligation not to put patients at risk, which is a disadvantage to them and may result from information breaches. As a product of artificial intelligence in cancer research, its use continues to increase, as does the number of discoveries in the individualization of patient care. As the United States, like many nations, has health care privacy laws regarding patients' data. The primary clarifications of the U.S. Government regulations for safeguarding as a component of the protection of patients' protected health information (PHI) often but not always remain inclusive of multiple facets, of these, the Privacy Rule sets out provisions of patient consent and communications provision, and the Security Rule outlines general provisions of the process of protecting or safeguarding. In addition, the Breach Notification Standards impose an obligation on a covered entity to notify not only those involved but also appropriate entities of a breach of secure information within a reasonable time. Moreover, from an ethical perspective, the precondition requiring a patient's consent to the confidentiality of sensitive medical information is an essential construct of medical ethics (Maguluri et al., 2024).

Figure 4. HIPAA Regulations and Accreditation.

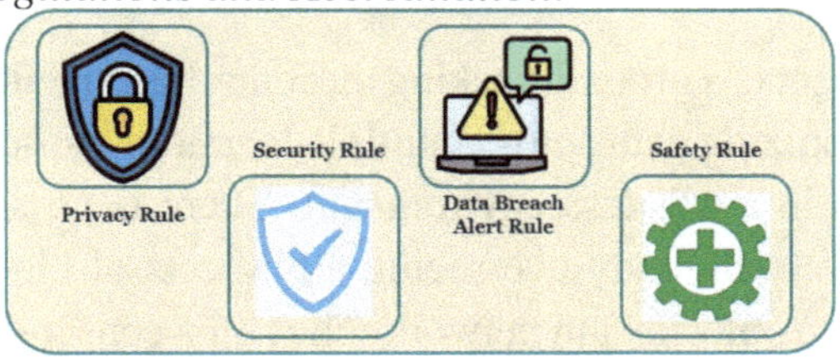

To summarize, patients have privacy rights and protections afforded by HIPAA. Healthcare providers, health plans, and healthcare clearinghouses must comply with these federal standards to perform certain electronic transactions and implement system adjustments to implement the physician accountability system for transactions to protect personal health information. Privacy standards encompass patients' rights to their health and medical care information. Practically speaking, any health care provider that is expected to comply with these federal privacy rules for transactions (and therefore implement privacy safeguards), as well as health care providers that are not required to comply with the administrative simplification rules (and therefore may not implement electronic data interchange privacy safeguards), and perhaps practitioners that are the smallest, who, reports suggest, never get onto a computer, will be expected to implement the privacy rules, through hard copy records. If a provider strays from the customary use and disclosure rules, the practitioner is responsible for offering the sender the option to consent, assent, or object to certain disclosures. The stakes for using improvised health care data daily are high. In addition to legal and financial ramifications, privacy violations can erode the community's confidence, goodwill, and capital. Therefore, ensuring that health care providers understand the privacy rules, have resources in place to comply, are updated on the rules and any updates, and receive technical assistance in following them are significant parts of a safeguarding privacy approach (Maguluri et al., 2024).

4. BLOCKCHAIN TECHNOLOGY AND ITS APPLICATION IN HEALTHCARE

4.1 Introduction to Blockchain Technology

Blockchain represents a groundbreaking, decentralized method for sharing, replicating, and synchronizing data across multiple locations worldwide. It guarantees a secure transaction in a trustless environment. There is no singular, centralized administrator or governing body overseeing all aspects of blockchain technology concerned with data. A blockchain network relies on a consensus model among all participating organizations to complete a new transaction. Blockchain technology is also built on DLT, but, by its very nature, it is immutable. Once a user in a blockchain network decides to perform a transaction, the request is recorded in the ledger, and a copy of the ledger is made publicly available to all other users of the network. All users validate the transaction on a node, and once everyone agrees to confirm the node's authenticity, it is added to the network. To alter or manipulate the transaction, you would have to compromise more than 51% of the network's nodes, which is virtually impossible. The consensus algorithm is at the core of every blockchain network. It is how a consensus is reached amongst multiple nodes to add a block to the blockchain network. Most attributes of any blockchain network are determined by the consensus algorithm, including, but not limited to, the accessibility, scalability, degree of decentralization, latency, throughput, security, network overhead, computational overhead, and storage overhead. Therefore, each consensus algorithm is likely to serve the needs of its respective application. The consensus algorithm for Bitcoin is PoW. Several consensus methods are being created for various uses (Namasudra & Akkaya, 2023). Figure 5 represents the types of consensus algorithms.

Figure 5. Taxonomy of Consensus Algorithms

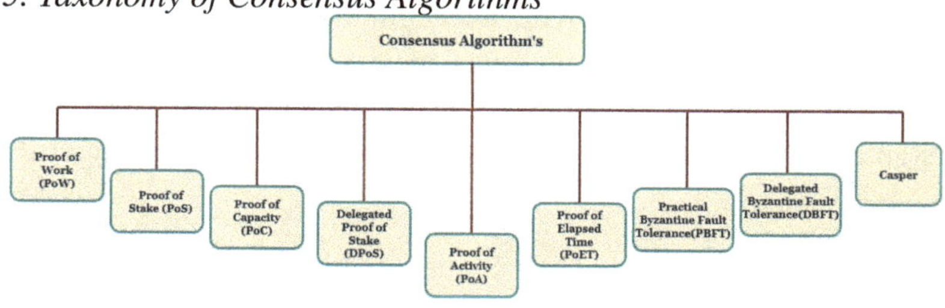

- **Varieties of Blockchain:** A blockchain network can include a few or millions of nodes distributed worldwide. Blockchain is classified into three types: (i)

public, (ii) private, and (iii) consortium, which are determined by the network layer architecture.

- **Characteristics of Blockchain**: Due to its unique qualities, blockchain is now used in a wide range of sectors and use cases. Some of the key properties of blockchain are discussed as follows:
  - Stronger security.
  - A decentralized network.
  - Unalterable.
  - Transparent.
  - Distributed ledger.
  - Consensus.
  - Quick settlement.
  - Chronological data.
  - Intelligent agreement.
- **Benefits of Blockchain**: Blockchain technology is one of many digital technologies that can help organizations achieve their goals. The primary benefits of blockchain technology are outlined below:
  - Data security.
  - Verifiability.
  - Decentralization.
  - Traceability.
  - Privacy.
  - Faster processing.
  - There is no third-party intervention.
  - Provenance.
  - Automation.
- **Applications of Blockchain in Industry**: The following are some examples of blockchain technology uses in industry:
  - Supply Chain Management.
  - Healthcare.
  - Real Estate.
  - Media.
  - Energy.

4.2 Key Features of Blockchain: Security, Transparency, and Immutability

The blockchain technology is rapidly changing the paradigm of data security. Blockchain is a secure, tamper-proof alternative to centralized data storage. The digitization of information and the rapid proliferation of data have created a growing need for more secure technology. Increased vulnerability to data breaches, unauthorized infiltration, and cyberattacks is driving the development of sophisticated security procedures and practices for centralized systems. While blockchain technology was initially proposed in 2008 with the introduction of Bitcoin, the concept of a decentralized system for data storage and security is evolving rapidly and may address the inadequacies of many of today's centralized systems. Blockchain involves a decentralized ledger that contains secure, transparent, and tamper-proof transactions. Each block contains a list of transactions, all linked cryptographically to the preceding block to form a chain of blocks. Decentralization in blockchain is the basis for preventing a single party from controlling the entire network. This promotes trust and protects the overall safety of the data storage. (Verma et al., 2024).

- **Security Characteristics of Blockchain**: The implementation of a cryptographic hash serves as an example of a security feature. Every block in the blockchain contains a cryptographic hash of the previous block, a timestamp, and transaction data. The hash function maintains the integrity of the data in the block and generates a unique output (hash) for every input. Therefore, if the data were to change in any way, a different hash would be generated, revealing possible fraud.
- **Applications of Blockchain in Information Safety**: It ensures secure data storage, and the Blockchain secures data stored across a distributed network. This decentralised model protects data from being stored in a single location, thereby limiting an engaged party's ability to steal or access it.
- **Secure Transfers**: Blockchain technology ensures transparent and immutable record-keeping for accurate and verified financial and non-financial transactions, benefiting a wide range of applications.
    Digital currencies are secure digital currencies (such as Bitcoin and Ethereum) that employ blockchain for transaction validation. Healthcare.
    Supply chain: Monitoring and verifying the movement of items across the supply chain to assure legitimacy and prevent theft.
- **Healthcare Data Security:** Healthcare institutions have the capacity to utilize blockchain or similar technology as a means of appropriately storing patient records and relatively granting access to confidential material to authorized individuals only in a secure manner. The act of doing this not only enhances trustworthy privacy and information governance but also organizes and coordinates health care.

Blockchain is a decentralized ledger system that enables secure, transparent, and tamper-proof record-keeping. Each block comprises a list of transactions that are cryptographically linked to the previous block, forming a chain of records.

Blockchain's decentralised nature means no single party controls the entire network, improving safety and confidence (Verma et al., 2024). The Fundamental Elements are listed below:

- **Transparency:** Each interaction on a blockchain is visible to all participants, ensuring transparency and accountability. *Example:* Healthcare Applications. As wearable technology evolves and plays an increasingly important role in healthcare, addressing these ethical and legal challenges will be crucial to maintaining public trust and ensuring its responsible use. Stronger legislation, user-centred policies, and greater openness in data collection and use can help protect individuals' rights while enabling wearable technology to realize its full potential to revolutionize healthcare (Obianyo et al., 2024).
- **Immutability:** Once assigned to a blockchain, information cannot be changed or deleted. This permanence is enabled by cryptographic hashing within the consensus mechanism. Example: Healthcare Applications. Blockchain offers a distributed ledger with decentralized management. A feature of blockchain is that cryptocurrency transactions cannot be reversed, thereby eliminating the possibility of tampering with private and secure information. As shown in the Supply Chain, key participants include manufacturers, distributors, vendors, consumers, retailers, and healthcare providers such as hospitals. Blockchain technology increases trust through transparency. The event request-response architecture supports the movement of each product in the chain among authenticated entities. Smart contracts on the blockchain record all transactions among organisations (Singla et al., 2024).

4.3 How Blockchain Addresses Data Privacy Concerns

In recent years, the storage of Electronic Health Records (EHRs) in mobile cloud environments has undergone tremendous transformation, as the use of mobile devices and cloud computing enables the exchange of medical data between patients and health authorities. This state-of-the-art paradigm offers low operational costs, flexibility, and use of electronic health records (EHRs). However, concerns about data privacy and network security are raised in the new paradigm for e-health systems. It is challenging to safely share EHRs among mobile users while maintaining high security levels in the mobile cloud. This study introduces a new blockchain system for safely storing health data on the cloud to support the authentication and certification of health data. The blockchain employs strong encryption and authentication, including an upgraded version of Blowfish (Verma Garima, 2024).

Blockchain technology represents a significant advance in addressing security issues in healthcare data management. Blockchain's primary advantage is that it ensures data integrity using cryptographic hashing. Each block has a unique hash derived from its data and the previous block's hash. Because of this cryptographic connection, the blocks form a chain that is tamper-proof or tamper-resistant. Any attempt to change the data in a block once it is recorded in the blockchain would require changing every subsequent block in the chain, thereby compromising data integrity (Adeghe et al., 2024).

Healthcare analytics has revolutionized how authors analyze large, complex health datasets. Safeguarding the privacy of sensitive healthcare data should be factored into this process. It proposes an architecture for privacy-preserving healthcare analytics using zk-SNARKs, blockchain, and a multi-tenant cloud environment. Traditional cryptographic methods can secure data at rest, but may fall short of safeguarding data during analytical queries. Authors employ zk-SNARKs in our method to ensure privacy-preserving analytics while verifying the accuracy of computations, without requiring the release of raw data. In multi-tenant cloud-based systems, secure data sharing and processing must be considered in the development of healthcare innovations, telemedicine, and policy decisions (Babu & Jothi, 2024).

In recent years, the health informatics academic community has shown considerable interest in developing a safe, practical solution for storing large volumes of medical data, primarily through cloud-based storage using centralized architectures. However, using a cloud-based storage architecture creates several issues, including data ownership, interoperability with other platforms, fault tolerance, and security and privacy concerns. Thus, there is a need to create a resilient architecture that can validate and overcome the constraints and limitations posed by these issues. The study describes a patient-centric system, HealthRec-Chain, for storing and sharing sensitive medical reports and photographs. The HealthReChain framework uses the Interplanetary File System (IPFS) to enable automated, secure storage of health data. Security is assured through Java-enabled GPG encryption, which provides state-of-the-art privacy and security (Kumari et al., 2024).

Capable health care, also known as IoT-based health care, applies IoT technology to the health care industry. IoT devices enable health care professionals to monitor patients remotely, support in-home care, and notify them when there is a deviation in the patient's condition, leading to improved outcomes and more effective monitoring of chronic health conditions. Health care using an IoT approach, however, must adhere to strict safety standards to protect patient information. An approach may involve using blockchain technology to protect health information while it is stored, along with associated permissions to share data with health care providers. The decentralized structure of the blockchain and its use of advanced encryption techniques reduce hackers' ability to alter or compromise medical information. IPFS, or the Interplanetary File System, meets regulatory requirements for storing and sharing data efficiently with approved medical professionals. The smart contract's functionality automates permission assignment and removal, providing additional layers of security for the applicant's health information. This study describes the design and anticipated outcomes of a blockchain-based remote monitoring system for patients with life-changing chronic medical conditions. The system uses distributed blockchain for data security, IPFS for data storage and sharing, DApps for data collection and access to the blockchain, and encrypted data for additional anonymity (Rani et al., 2024).

Blockchain in healthcare safeguards the confidentiality of information through:

- Providing Patients Direct Access.
- Keeping Only Reliability Proofs On-Chain.
- Using Encryption and Strong Cryptographic Techniques.
- Maintaining a Permanent, Verifiable Record of Data Access.
- Preventing Critical Points Where Data Can Be Compromised.

4.4 Case Studies of Blockchain in Healthcare Applications

The introduction of blockchain technology positively impacts data security, privacy, and interoperability, making it a possible technological solution for EHR management. The nature of its decentralized system makes it resistant to data breaches and enables secure, patient-directed health data sharing. Blockchain can improve data integrity and interoperability, as demonstrated by two case studies—one from Estonia and the other, the MedRec project by Canada's Massachusetts Institute of Technology.

- **MedRec by MIT:** MedRec is an electronic health records blockchain-based application developed by the MIT Digital Currency Initiative to enhance interoperability, privacy, and control of patients' medical data while having a permanent record accessible to multiple physicians. MedRec encompasses "smart" contracts that document interactions between patients and providers, allowing patients to govern access to their medical information, while addressing privacy issues and enabling an accessible health care journey across different institutions. The testing of MedRec provides a glimpse into the possibilities of blockchain for improving data integrity, enhancing privacy, and reducing duplicate testing - all of which contribute to better health care record management overall. (Raju et al., 2024).
- **Estonia's eHealth System**: In 2016, Estonia was the first country to implement a project for managing the electronic health records (EHRs) of its 1.3 million residents using blockchain technology. The project guarantees that patient data is tamper-proof, increasing transparency in patient-centred care

delivery and enabling health care providers to access patient information securely. Estonia's EHR system uses a blockchain-based application with cryptographic hashing to verify data validity, reduce data breaches, increase trust, and support healthcare interoperability. This seamless, interoperable healthcare solution is scalable and secure, and serves as a model for other countries (Raju et al., 2024).

Blockchain can revolutionize global healthcare standards by promoting a secure, interoperable, and patient-centred ecosystem with the proper support and development.

5. INTERPLANETARY FILE SYSTEM (IPFS) FOR DECENTRALIZED DATA STORAGE

5.1 Overview of IPFS and Its Functionality

The InterPlanetary File System (IPFS) is classified as a Peer-to-Peer distributed file system. IPFS is an off-chain storage solution. IPFS uses SHA-256 (Secure Hash Algorithm) to create a data hash that serves as a content identifier (CID). CID protects data integrity. A minor change in the data causes a significant change in the CID. IPFS uses content addresses rather than location addresses. A centralized system operates on location addressing. To obtain a file, the client asks the server for its full location, and the server then transfers the file. An example of that is content addressing. Users will request a file from peer nodes based on its content. Patients generate the data using the Sensor and DApp. The data is encrypted using AES. IPFS is an off-chain solution for storing generated data and generating a CID for the data. The CID is entered as a key in the blockchain. The doctor may want to initiate a request to access the patients' data. The smart contract validates their authority to access and sends them the relevant CIDs for the encrypted data. Finally, using symmetric and private keys, the data and keys are decrypted (Rani et al., 2024).

Blockchain integration improves the security, privacy, and sustainability of the healthcare industry. Blockchain solutions, such as IPFS, are helping improve and manage patient care by addressing security and access issues associated with wearable devices and remote monitoring. While blockchain technology can help improve security, typical advantages of using blockchain and the IPFS protocol for content distribution include decentralization, immutability, transparency, accountability, and security. Scalability is also an important advantage of this framework. The blockchain's limited block size prevents the storage of files of any size directly on its general ledger, requiring a decentralized network to maintain. This system architecture is not without limitations. This problem is being solved using IPFS and blockchain. These improvement frameworks enable decentralized scaling. Essentially, these two systems enable the secure management and storage of large amounts of data while preserving the essential properties of decentralization, immutability, and security. The integration of IPFS to blockchain will also support patient records in the healthcare domain and help offer justified accessibility (Tiwari et al., 2025).

The combination of blockchain technology and IPFS creates a decentralized framework for managing healthcare data. This combination provides a secure, traceable, and immutable storage mechanism for medical images and diagnostic results. The following Figures 6 and 7 shows the process of storing and retrieving data on IPFS.

Figure 6. Patient Data Stored into IPFS.

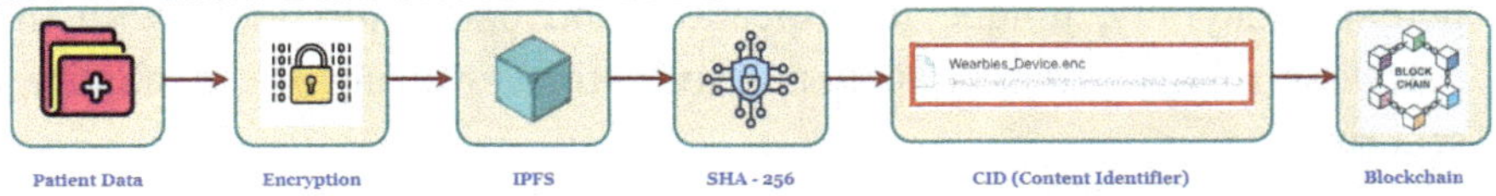

Figure 7. Patient Data Access from IPFS.

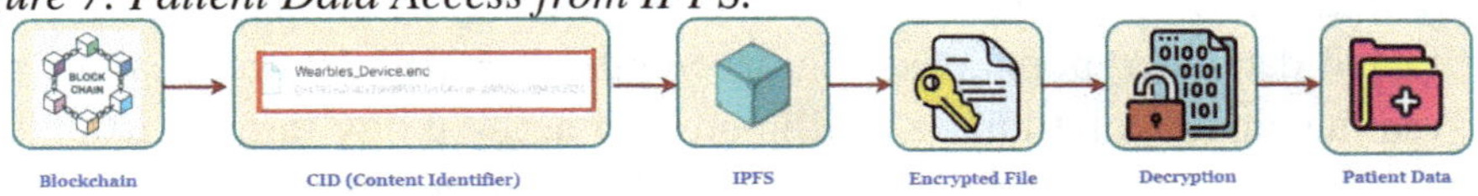

IPFS provides a scalable storage mechanism. IPFS enables distributed storage by distributing files across several heterogeneous nodes. Files are disseminated and replicated across multiple nodes, eliminating the need for a centralized server or storage location. The advantages of using a distributed file storage model include scalability, as storage capacity increases as more nodes access and use it. The distributed model allows multiple nodes to download and deliver files, improving scalability by enabling simultaneous retrieval of files across nodes. With more users and nodes, requests can run concurrently, with a node retrieving information from the storage system of a peer. The distribution of nodes increases the number of peers storing the files and increases storage capacity, enabling scalability in the storage model (Rani et al., 2024).

IPFS Provides:

- Decentralized File Sharing.
- Deduplication.
- Immutable and Verifiable Data.

5.2 Advantages of Using IPFS in Healthcare Data Management

Researchers have introduced a healthcare system for managing chronic illnesses that utilizes IoT, Blockchain, and IPFS technologies. This technology provides a variety of benefits for remote patient monitoring. It enables the collection, sharing, and safety of everyday data (Azbeg et al., 2022).

- **Security:** The privacy of patient data is protected in our system through the use of smart contracts that regulate access to this data. Thus, medical data is protected and cannot be accessed by unauthorized persons.
- **Privacy:** The privacy of patients is protected through the blockchain's inherent anonymity, unique identification, and data encryption, with third-party control over access to patient information, ensuring confidentiality and security.
- **Integrity**: Blockchain technology enhances data integrity by storing hash data with mutability features, regulating access through smart contracts, and enabling traceability by recording all data alterations and operations, thereby preventing tampering and ensuring secure storage.
- **Availability:** Blockchain enhances system security by combining IoT devices and data encryption, ensuring decentralization and data replication, preventing single-point failure, and improving accessibility through healthcare equipment, mobile devices, and decentralized applications (DApps).

5.3 Integration of IPFS with Blockchain Technology

Protecting healthcare data using IPFS and Blockchain requires significant effort, and researchers still have a long way to go. Blockchain provides content integrity, immutability, and dependability. IPFS stores data in a distributed and secure environment. Researchers use a variety of technologies in a variety of scenarios, such as IoT wearables and connections to Wi-Fi access points for real-time data storage and security. Consortium Blockchain can enhance the robustness of these efforts and enable telesurgery in conjunction with 5G, virtual reality, and robotics. (Kumar et al., 2021).

Blockchain technology represents a paradigm shift, offering an innovative, secure, and decentralized platform that facilitates the safe storage, sharing, and retrieval of Electronic Health Records (EHRs), addressing the limitations of traditional healthcare infrastructure. This paper proposes a blockchain-enabled framework for EHR in health care because it can potentially allow health care organizations to manage fail-safe and tamper-proof (auditable) health care ledgers in a decentralized system. Hospitals and physicians will serve as lightweight nodes in this approach; patients will be either full nodes or lightweight nodes. A blockchain-enabled framework with an InterPlanetary File System (IPFS) for off-chain storage is proposed to allow optimal EHR management in the health care network. This integrated framework enables patient health data to be stored in a decentralized, distributed architecture with fine-grained access controls. A patient-centric paradigm protects health data privacy by appropriately granting ownership of health data to the patient. The design of the blockchain provides native security and anonymity, all based on the proper application of cryptographic algorithms—data encryption and IPFS storage further benchmark security (Jayabalan & Jeyanthi, 2022).

Benefits of Combined:

- Ensures that data cannot be manipulated without notice.
- Secure communication, verified history, and automatic authorization.
- Data management is both fast and ethical.

5.4 Use Cases Demonstrating IPFS in Healthcare

The decentralized architecture and cryptographic protocols of blockchain make medical data less susceptible to unauthorized access or alteration by hackers. The InterPlanetary File System (IPFS) is an effective solution for storing and sharing data, allowing authorized medical professionals access to that information. Automating the granting or revocation of access to patient data via smart contract functionality is another way to streamline the process (Rani et al., 2024).

Use Case 1: Safe Preservation and Sharing of Medical Images - Massive files, such as MRIs, CT scans, and X-rays, can be securely uploaded to IPFS for safe preservation and sharing.IPFS securely stores and shares medical images, ensuring data integrity and preventing duplicates. It reduces storage costs, enhances accessibility, and prevents picture tampering.

Use Case 2: Patients' health information (lab results, medications, and diagnoses) is secured and kept on IPFS. Patient-Centered Health Records securely store patients' health information on IPFS, with smart contracts managing access permissions to enhance data ownership, privacy, and cross-institutional sharing.

Use Case 3: The process of tracking medical device and drug supply chains involves storing certificates, manufacturing records, and shipping data in IPFS.IPFS stores data on medical device and drug supply chains, utilizing blockchain technology for real-time verification, counterfeit protection, and enhanced traceability.

6. PROPOSED BLOCKCHAIN-BASED DATA INTEGRITY SOLUTION

To ensure the safety and privacy of patient-sensitive data on wearable devices, this chapter discusses integrating IPFFS with Blockchain Technology.

6.1 Architecture of the Proposed Solution

The suggested system suggests collecting sensitive patient data via wearable devices. Once you have collected this sensitive information, save it as a CSV file. We encrypt the data before storing it directly on IPFS (using AES). The encrypted file is stored in IPFS, where its CID is retrieved, and then stored in the Blockchain. Share the password securely with approved recipients. Figure 7 illustrates the proposed framework for storing patients' records on a blockchain.

Initially, we encrypted patient critical information before uploading it to IPFS. The figures below show the uploaded IPFS file and the encrypted file.

We created a smart contract in Solidity (using the Remix IDE) to hold a CID containing patient-sensitive information. Once you have verified the integrity of patient-sensitive details, you can access the CID utilizing the patient's contract address, if it is the same, to retrieve the correct CID. If somebody attempts to modify their user address, we will be unable to retrieve the correct CID of the patient's sensitive information. The results of our proposed strategy are presented in the Figure 8 below.

Figure 8. Proposed framework for a Patient-Sensitive Data Store on IPFS.

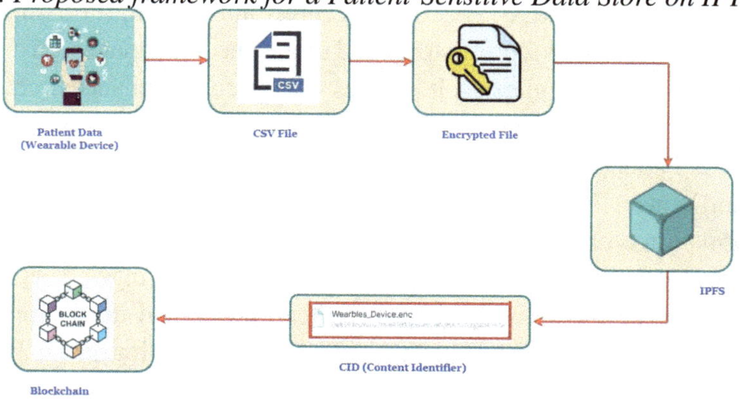

Figure 9. To Upload a Patient's Encrypted File into IPFS.

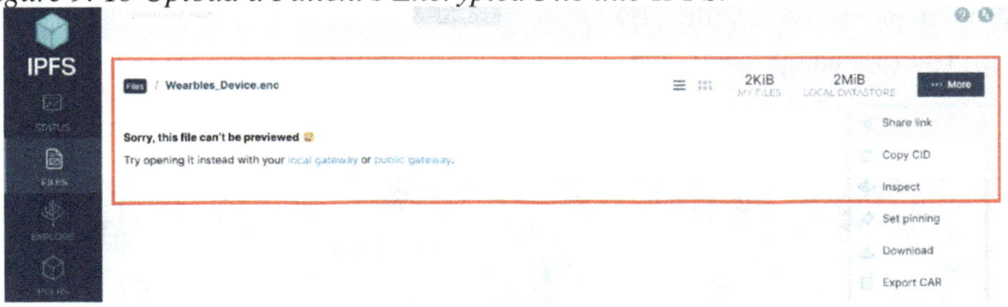

Figure 9 illustrates how to upload a patient's encrypted file to IPFS and retrieve the CID of the specific data. The unique CID (Figure 10) of a patient's wearable gadget is an encrypted file.

Figure 10. CID of Wearable Devices of Patient Data.

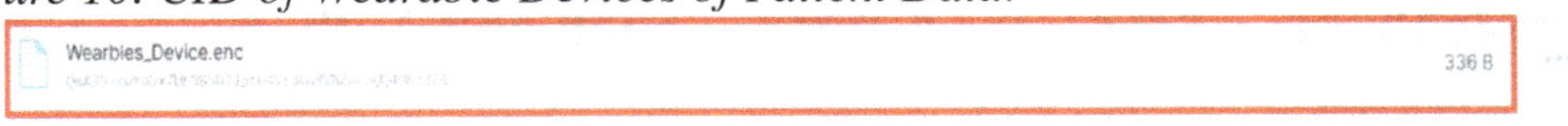

Figure 11. To Store / Retrieve CID.

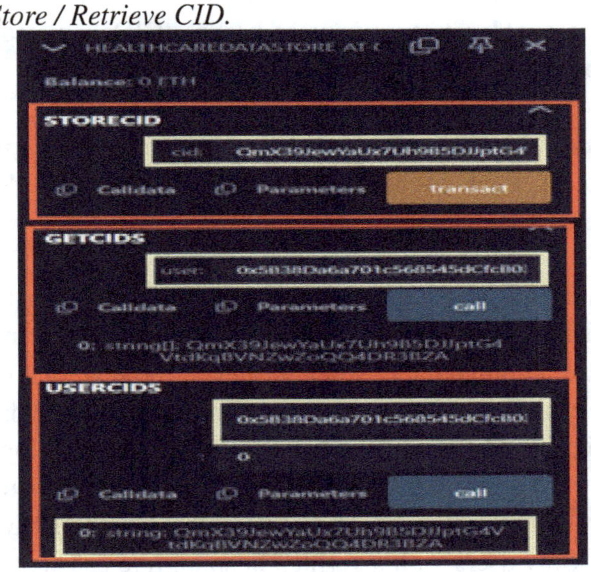

Figure 11 discusses how to store and retrieve the CID of sensitive patient information using wearable medical equipment and the Remix Ethereum smart contract.

Figure 12 indicates that if anyone attempts to edit the patient's contract address, they will be unable to access the CID of the patient's sensitive information, indicating an error in the manipulated data.

Figure 12. Manipulated Address

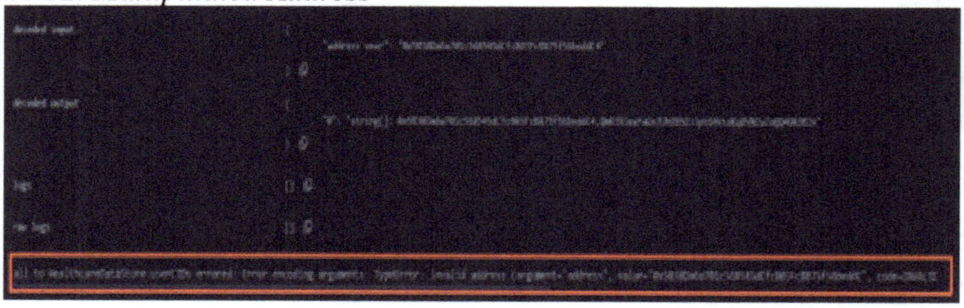

6.2 Mechanisms for User Authentication and Authorization

The Methods for user identification and permission in healthcare applications that use IPFS and blockchain.

- IPFS can store huge files, including medical photos, EHRs, and lab data.
- Blockchain technology saves content hashes (CIDs), metadata, and smart contracts for access control purposes.

We must ensure that only authorized users (doctors, nurses, patients, and researchers) can upload, view, or share data. Users can verify their identities without relying on a centralized database.

The authentication of patients' sensitive information describes blockchain-based verifiable credentials. In IPFS, patient-sensitive information is stored and generates a unique CID. Nobody can change anything; only authorized individuals can view it; however, no one tampered with the data.
The authorization to access the patient's sensitive information through wearable devices and to create a smart contract between the patient and the wearable device. Only the patient and their designated doctor have access to the file's CID. "Only users with a verified hospital role can write new records." Blockchain-based enforcement ensures transparency and accountability.

Benefits of Decentralized Data Management

- **Enhanced Data Accessibility and Integrity**: Patient records, medical scans, and lab results are dispersed across multiple nodes, ensuring that even if a hospital server fails, data remains accessible.
- **Data Security and Tamper-Proofing**: IPFS stores data using a cryptographic hash (CID), and any modification to a file generates a new CID, making tampering readily identifiable.
- **Patient-Focused Data Management**: Patients can easily share their health information by providing their CID. Encourages systems that give the patients discretion over who can access or use their data, through data privacy requirements such as HIPAA.
- **Transparent and auditable access**: When combined with blockchain technology, record-keeping and data sources become unchangeable. Assists hospitals in adhering to audit requirements while also building confidence with their patients.

6.3 Future Implications for Healthcare Providers and Patients

Healthcare Providers:

- **Auditing:** Immutable blockchain records and IPFS content hashes facilitate confidentiality and traceability. Helps meet regulatory requirements (GDPR, HIPAA) without requiring extensive manual audits.
- **Data Sharing:** Hospitals, clinics, laboratories, and research institutes can securely exchange patient data, medical images, and clinical trial results in real-time. It is easier to enable cross-border care and telemedicine.

Patients:

- **Confidentiality and Safety**: Decentralized systems, along with encryption, safeguard data against centralized breaches. Patients do not have to trust a single company with all of their sensitive information.
- **Greater confidence and honesty:** Patients can see when, why, and who obtained their personal information. Increases confidence in digital health systems.

7. CONCLUSION

7.1 Summary of Key Points

This chapter recommends safeguarding sensitive patient information by applying medical wearable devices in urban society. Urban populations are becoming increasingly aware of their health and fitness levels; however, the modern urbanization of the world has heightened the sensitivity of patient data to the point where it is no longer as secure as it was in the past—especially if it leaks. In this way, we preserve patient information that is publicly available while ensuring that sensitive patient information is no longer exposed through modern medical devices and that it is permanently protected. Blockchain is a new technology that enables transparency and trust in the handling of personal information for patients and service providers. Likewise, the interplanetary file system (IPFS) provides enhanced security and privacy. In this, we propose moving patient information to IPFS. The IPFS file creates a unique tag, called a content identifier (CID). The IPFS CID list is referenced and stored in a blockchain. Regarding the respective data integrity protocols, we also write smart contracts to enhance data integrity. Essentially, we verify and ensure that the CID is linked to specific patient data. Should the CID be altered or amended, errors will be received by all parties involved. In this way, we maintained patient safety and security.

7.2 Future Directions for Research and Development

We will use this notion in the future across a variety of techniques, such as federated learning to improve privacy and XAI (Explainable Artificial Intelligence) to increase usability.

7.3 Final Thoughts on the Role of Technology in Enhancing Healthcare Data Integrity

The use of contemporary technologies (blockchain, IPFS, encryption, and smart contracts) restores trust, accuracy, and robustness to healthcare data, enabling transparent, patient-centered, tamper-proof management of health data. Medical wearable technologies provide providers with real-time information and continuous monitoring in healthcare. However, the value of medical wearable technologies depends upon the integrity, privacy, and openness of the data. The ability to use blockchain and similar technologies promotes trusted, patient-centered, and data-driven approaches to healthcare.

8. REFERENCES

Adeghe, E. P., Okolo, C. A., & Ojeyinka, O. T. (2024). Evaluating the impact of blockchain technology in healthcare data management: A review of security, privacy, and patient outcomes. *Open Access Research Journal of Science and Technology, 10*(2), 013–020. https://doi.org/DOI: 10.53022/oarjst.2024.10.2.0038

Alzu'bi, A., Alomar, A. A., Alkhaza'leh, S., Abuarqoub, A., & Hammoudeh, M. (2024). A review of privacy and security of edge computing in smart healthcare systems: Issues, challenges, and research directions. *Tsinghua Science and Technology*, *29*(4), 1152–1180. DOI: 10.26599/TST.2023.9010090

Azbeg, K., Ouchetto, O., & Jai Andaloussi, S. (2022). BlockMedCare: A healthcare system based on IoT, blockchain, and IPFS for data management security. *Egyptian Informatics Journal*, *23*(2), 329–343. DOI: 10.1016/j.eij.2022.03.001

Babu, S. B., & Jothi, K. R. (2024). A secure framework for privacy-preserving analytics in healthcare records using zero-knowledge proofs and blockchain in multitenant cloud environments. *IEEE Access : Practical Innovations, Open Solutions*, *12*, 109846–109864. DOI: 10.1109/ACCESS.2024.3433571

Butcher, C. J. T., & Hussain, W. (2022). Digital healthcare: The future. *Future Healthcare Journal*, *9*(2), 113–117. DOI: 10.7861/futurehosp.9-2-113

Chen, D., Chou, S.-Y., & Peng, X. (2025). Impacts of hospital data breach on healthcare quality. *Health Services Research.* Advance online publication. DOI: 10.1111/1475-6773.14439

Dai, J., Xu, X., Chen, G., Lv, J., & Xiao, Y. (2025). Sleep-wake patterns of fencing athletes: A long-term wearable device study. *PeerJ*, *13*, e18812. Advance online publication. DOI: 10.7717/peerj.18812

Jayabalan, J., & Jeyanthi, N. (2022). Scalable blockchain model using off-chain IPFS storage for healthcare data security and privacy. *Journal of Parallel and Distributed Computing*, *164*, 152–167. DOI: 10.1016/j.jpdc.2022.02.005

Kazmi, S. M. A., Khan, Z., Khan, A., Mazzara, M., & Khattak, A. M. (2024). Leveraging deep reinforcement learning and healthcare devices for active travelling in smart cities. *IEEE Transactions on Consumer Electronics*. Advance online publication. DOI: 10.1109/TCE.2024.3389668

Khan, N., & Rudman, R. J. (2025). IoT medical device risks: Data security, privacy, confidentiality, and compliance with HIPAA and COBIT 2019. *South African Journal of Business Management, 56*(1), 4796. Advance online publication. DOI: 10.4102/sajbm.v56i1.4796

Kumar, S., Bharti, A. K., & Amin, R. (2021). Decentralized secure storage of medical records using blockchain and IPFS: A comparative analysis with future directions. *Security and Privacy, 4*(5), e162. Advance online publication. DOI: 10.1002/spy2.162

Kumari, D., Parmar, A. S., Goyal, H. S., Mishra, K., & Panda, S. (2024). HealthRec-Chain: Patient-centric blockchain enabled IPFS for privacy-preserving, scalable health data. *Computer Networks, 241*, 110223. Advance online publication. DOI: 10.1016/j.comnet.2024.110223

Lewandowska, A., Rudzki, G., Lewandowski, T., Bartosiewicz, A., Próchnicki, M., Stryjkowska-Góra, A., Laskowska, B., Sierpińska, M., Rudzki, S., & Pavlov, S. (2025). Overweight and obesity among adolescents: Health-conscious behaviours, acceptance, and the health behaviours of their parents. *BMC Public Health, 25*, 418. Advance online publication. DOI: 10.1186/s12889-025-18045-5

. Maguluri, K. K., Ganti, V. K. A. T., & Subhash, T. N. (2024). Advancing patient privacy in the era of artificial intelligence: A deep learning approach to ensuring compliance with HIPAA and addressing ethical challenges in healthcare data security. *International Journal of Medical Toxicology & Legal Medicine, 27*(5). (Advance online publication expected)

Maier, E., Reimer, U., & Wickramasinghe, N. (2021). Digital healthcare services. *Electronic Markets, 31*(4), 743–746. DOI: 10.1007/s12525-021-00502-y

Martínez, A. L., Gil Pérez, M., & Ruiz-Martínez, A. (2023). A comprehensive model for securing sensitive patient data in a clinical scenario. *IEEE Access : Practical Innovations, Open Solutions, 11*, 137083–137098. DOI: 10.1109/ACCESS.2023.3335122

Menassa, M., Wilmont, I., Beigrezaei, S., Knobbe, A., Artola Arita, V., Bridge, L., Verschuren, W. M. M., Rennie, K. L., Franco, O. H., & van der Ouderaa, F. (2025). The future of healthy ageing: Wearables in public health, disease prevention and healthcare. *Maturitas. Article, 108254*. Advance online publication. DOI: 10.1016/j.maturitas.2025.108254

Namasudra, S., & Akkaya, K. (2023). Introduction to blockchain technology. In Namasudra, S. (Ed.), *Blockchain and its applications in Industry 4.0* (pp. 1–28). Springer Nature Singapore., DOI: 10.1007/978-981-99-2174-8_1

Nemec Zlatolas, L., Welzer, T., & Lhotska, L. (2024). Data breaches in healthcare: Security mechanisms for attack mitigation. *Cluster Computing*, *27*(7), 8639–8654. DOI: 10.1007/s10586-024-04401-8

Obianyo, C., Ezeamii, V. C., Idoko, B., Adeyinka, T., Ejembi, V. E., Idoko, J. E., Obioma, L. O., & Ugwu, O. J. (2024). The future of wearable health technology: From monitoring to preventive healthcare. *World Journal of Biology Pharmacy and Health Sciences*, *20*, 36–55.

Park, E., & Lim, J. H. (2025). The impact of healthcare data breaches on patient hospital visit behavior. *International Journal of Research in Marketing*. Advance online publication. DOI: 10.1016/j.ijresmar.2025.01.003

Raju, N., & Quazi, F. (2024). Blockchain applications in electronic health records (EHRs) [Preprint]. *SSRN*. https://doi.org/DOI: 10.2139/ssrn.5026829

Rani, D., Kumar, R., & Chauhan, N. (2024). A secure framework for IoT-based healthcare using blockchain and IPFS. *Security and Privacy*, *7*(2), e348. Advance online publication. DOI: 10.1002/spy2.348

Rathore, N., Kumari, A., Patel, M., Chudasama, A., Bhalani, D., Tanwar, S., & Alabdulatif, A. (2025). Synergy of AI and blockchain to secure electronic healthcare records. *Security and Privacy*, *8*(1), e463. Advance online publication. DOI: 10.1002/spy2.463

Sharma, R., & Kshetri, N. (2020). Digital healthcare: Historical development, applications, and future research directions. *International Journal of Information Management*, *53*, 102105. Advance online publication. DOI: 10.1016/j.ijinfomgt.2020.102105

Shi, Z., Du, X., Wang, D., Paek, S. C., Kitcharoen, P., Li, J., & Marohabutr, T. (2025). Social capital and health consciousness based on regional differences in China: A cross-sectional study. *Frontiers in Public Health*, *13*, 1598121. Advance online publication. DOI: 10.3389/fpubh.2025.1598121

Singla, D., Kumar, S., Gulzar, Y., Mir, M. S., Gupta, D., Jaziri, W., Sassi, N., & Arora, S. (2024). Designing and implementing a resilient immutability mechanism for enhanced supply chain management in e-healthcare systems. *Frontiers in Sustainable Cities*, *6*, 1403809. Advance online publication. DOI: 10.3389/frsc.2024.1403809

Song, Y., Liu, J., Yan, S., Ma, M., Silver Tarimo, C., Chen, Y., Lai, Y., Guo, X., Wu, J., & Ye, B. (2025). Factors influencing health service utilization among 19,869 China's migrant population: An empirical study based on the Andersen behavioral model. *Frontiers in Public Health, 13*, 1456839. Advance online publication. DOI: 10.3389/fpubh.2025.1456839

Su, R., Huang, X., Chen, R., & Guo, X. (2024). Spatial and social inequality of hierarchical healthcare accessibility in urban system: A case study in Shanghai, China. *Sustainable Cities and Society, 109*, 105540. Advance online publication. DOI: 10.1016/j.scs.2024.105540

Sultana, S., Hriday, M. S. H., Haque, R., & Das, M. (2025). (in press). Health monitoring through wearables: A systematic review of innovations in cardiovascular disease detection and prevention. *Strategic Data Management & Innovation.*

Templ, M., & Sariyar, M. (2022). A systematic overview of methods to protect sensitive data provided for various analyses. *International Journal of Information Security, 21*(6), 1233–1246. DOI: 10.1007/s10207-022-00887-5

Tiwari, K., & Kumar, S. (2025). Accelerating healthcare data access: A blockchain and decentralized indexing approach. *Concurrency and Computation, 37*(15–17), e70172. Advance online publication. DOI: 10.1002/cpe.70172

Verma, G. (2024). Blockchain-based privacy preservation framework for healthcare data in cloud environment. *Journal of Experimental & Theoretical Artificial Intelligence, 36*(1), 147–160. DOI: 10.1080/0952813X.2023.2270649

Verma, P., & Ram, B. (2024). Application of blockchain technology in data security. *IP Indian Journal of Library Science and Information Technology, 9*(1), 51–55. DOI: 10.18231/j.ijlsit.2024.009

Vyas, A., Abimannan, S., & Hwang, R.-H. (2021). Sensitive healthcare data: Privacy and security issues and proposed solutions. In Kanagachidambaresan, G. R., Maheswar, R., Manikandan, V., & Ramakrishnan, K. (Eds.), *Emerging technologies for healthcare: Internet of Things and deep learning models* (pp. 93–127). Wiley., DOI: 10.1002/9781119792338.ch5

KEY TERMS AND DEFINITIONS

Blockchain: A decentralized digital ledger that records transactions across multiple computers in such a way that the registered transactions cannot be altered retroactively, ensuring data integrity and security.

Decentralized Storage: A system that distributes data across multiple locations or nodes rather than relying on a central server, enhancing data availability and redundancy.

Digital Health: The use of technology to improve health and healthcare delivery, encompassing various forms of health-related data, applications, and services available through digital means.

eHealth: The range of health services and information delivered or enhanced through the internet and related technologies, aimed at improving health outcomes and promoting patient engagement.

InterPlanetary File System (IPFS): A peer-to-peer hypermedia protocol designed to make the web faster, safer, and more open, allowing users to share and store files in a decentralized manner.

Machine Learning: A subset of artificial intelligence that enables computer systems to learn from data patterns and improve their performance on specific tasks without explicit programming.

Medical Wearables: Devices that can be worn on the body and that monitor, collect, and transmit health-related data, enabling continuous health tracking and personalized healthcare solutions.

Patient Empowerment: The process by which patients gain control over their health care decisions, increasing their involvement in managing their health conditions and treatment options.

Telehealth: The delivery of healthcare services through digital communication technologies, allowing patients to receive care remotely and improving accessibility to medical professionals.

Wearable Devices: Electronic devices worn on the body that track and gather data on various health metrics, such as heart rate, physical activity, and sleep patterns, thereby contributing to health monitoring.

Chapter 8

Hardware Security and Challenges in Wearable and Implantable Medical Devices

S. Nithiya
Department of Computing Technologies, SRM Institute of Science and Technology, Kattankulathur, India

K. Suresh
Department of Information Technology, Sri Venkateswara College of Engineering, Sriperumbudur, India

S. Pandikumar
https://orcid.org/0000-0002-2535-3780
Acharya Institute of Technology, India

S. Srividhya
https://orcid.org/0000-0002-7827-6045
Department of Data Science and Business Systems, SRM Institute of Science and Technology, Kattankulathur, India

K. Jawahar Jonathan
https://orcid.org/0009-0000-4941-6937
Acharya Institute of Technology, India

R. Soniya
https://orcid.org/0009-0005-8124-0288
Acharya Institute of Technology, India

ABSTRACT

The growth of health information technology, especially through wearable and implantable medical devices, has transformed patient care by facilitating continuous health monitoring. Devices such as fitness trackers and pacemakers play a pivotal role in tracking vital signs and supporting proactive health management. Despite the substantial benefits of these technologies, they also pose significant security and privacy risks. Unauthorized access, data breaches, and device malfunctions are critical concerns, as these vulnerabilities can jeopardize patient safety. This chapter delves into the security challenges associated with wearable and implantable

DOI: 10.4018/979-8-3373-4412-6.ch008

devices, focusing on threats like remote attacks, signal interference, and potential device compromise. The chapter concludes by exploring future directions for secure, reliable, and user-friendly medical devices to ensure patient safety in an increasingly interconnected healthcare landscape.

1. INTRODUCTION TO WEARABLE AND IMPLANTABLE MEDICAL DEVICES

Non-invasive wearable medical technology offers innovative solutions for accurately collecting health data. Biosensors play a vital role in preventing diseases, enabling early diagnosis, and supporting personalized treatment plans. Applications include pain management, psychological monitoring, and tracking vital health states such as glucose levels, sleep patterns, and brain activity. Emerging technologies like electronic skin patches, which adhere directly to the body, emulate human skin and connect to smartphones, enabling data transfer to cloud-based systems for comprehensive health monitoring. Traditionally, patient monitoring was centered within hospitals, but it has now evolved into a remote, patient-centric approach. This shift allows for more comprehensive data collection on a patient's health, supporting deeper analysis, early diagnosis, and the development of precision medicine. Implantable medical devices play a crucial role in healthcare by monitoring critical functions, such as heart performance, providing medical professionals with timely and precise data to inform diagnoses and treatment plans (Salunkhe et al., 2024). These devices often feature external accessibility and may include storage capabilities for comprehensive data management.

1.1 Types of Wearable Gadgets

Wearables comprise four main categories: smart glasses and headgear, smart watches, wearable medical devices and fitness trackers. All of these have three enabling technologies that make them smart:

✓ Sense and translate data;

Wearables are equipped with various sensors that detect and measure physical parameters such as heart rate, movement, temperature, and environmental factors like air quality. These sensors translate the gathered data into digital signals, which can then be processed and analyzed.

✓ Collect and prepare data for transmission

Once the data is captured, wearables clean, filter, and organize it to ensure it is accurate, reliable, and formatted properly. This step often involves integrating data from multiple sensors to provide a comprehensive view of the user's health or activity.

- ✓ Transmit data to off-site storage for processing and reporting.
- ✓ devices for further processing, analysis, and reporting. This enables real-time monitoring, remote access, and the ability to track long-term trends, which are crucial for both personal and clinical use.

Table 1. Types of wearbles its examples

Smart glasses and headgear	**Fitness trackers**	**Smart watches**	**Wearable medical devices**	**Smart clothing and accessories**
e.g.Google glasses and Samsung's Gear VR;	e.g.Fitbit, Nike FuelBand, and Microsoft Band;	e.g. Apple and Android watches and ;	e.g.Medtronic Continuous Glucose monitoring system and the ZIO Wireless Patch;	e.g.Visijax products, Levi's Smart Jacket

Cyberattacks on IoT devices pose significant risks, especially when managing sensitive health data, as they can result in physical harm and jeopardize lives. Such vulnerabilities affect not only the functionality of the devices but also the well-being of individuals. Wearable devices have created another attack vector and, if not appropriately controlled or governed, they can facilitate the compromise of data confidentiality, availability and integrity for users and organizations (Sandhiya et al., 2022). These attacks can lead to unauthorized access to personal health data, manipulation of device functions, and disruption of critical healthcare services, threatening patient safety and privacy. As the number of connected devices grows, the risk of security breaches increases, demanding more stringent protection measures, figure1 shows the wearable and implantable devices.

Figure 1. Wearable and implantable devices (Referred from Microsystem Technologies)

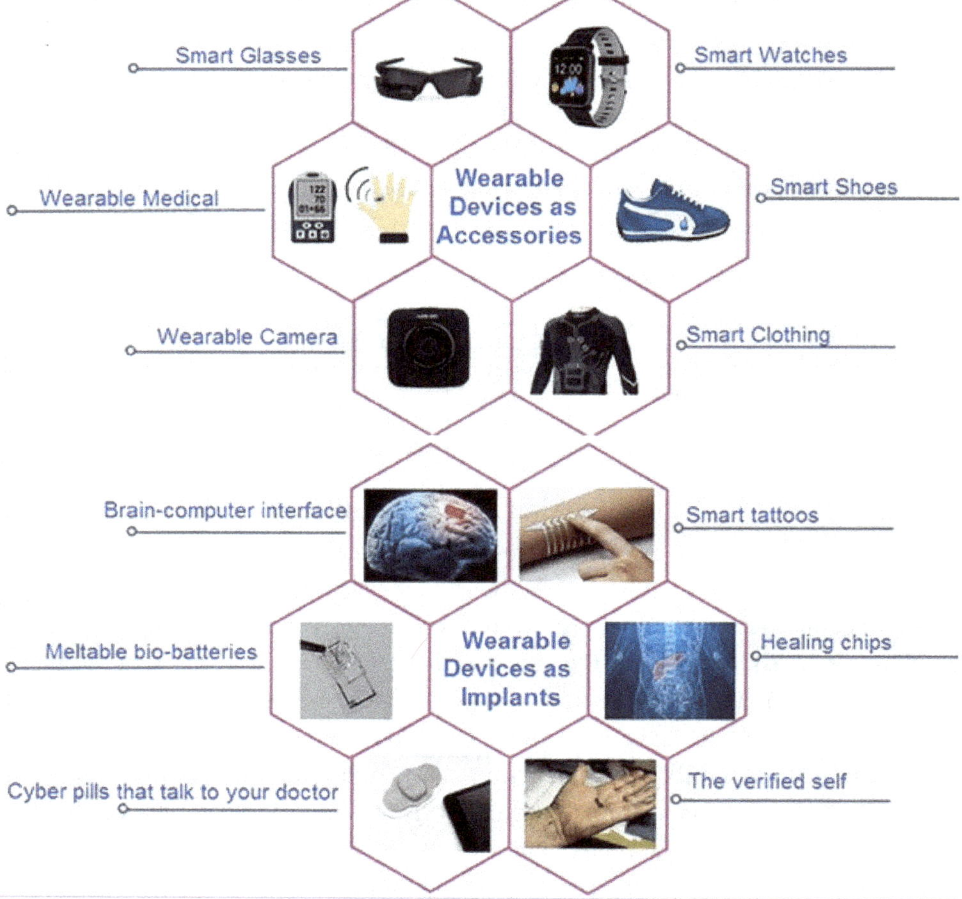

With the growing population, affordable healthcare devices are becoming increasingly essential to help individuals access timely medical intervention and prevent emergencies. However, the wearable device market and manufacturers face significant challenges in delivering reliable products that ensure the security of medical data and seamless communication with clinicians, caregivers, and doctors and figure2 shows the market strategy of wearable devices use. Additionally, the rapid advancement of technology and the integration of new features create further complexities in maintaining device performance and meeting regulatory standards.

Figure 2. Wearable usage market scenario

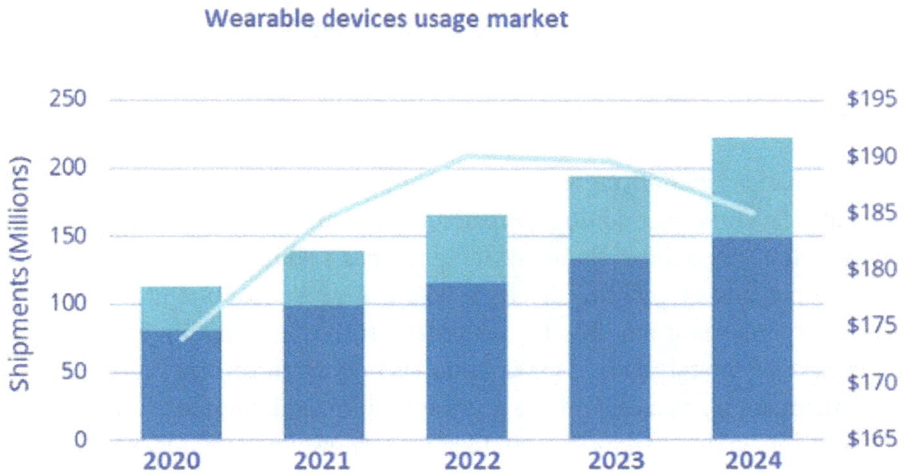

1.2 Key Objectives of wearable and implantable devices

a. *Early Detection of Health Issues:*

This helps in the early detection and prediction of diseases, so that potential emergencies can be prevented before they happen. Through sensors that monitor heart rate, blood pressure, and other indicators, wearables can identify subtle changes in health patterns that may indicate the onset of a serious condition. This proactive approach allows for timely intervention, which improves the chances of successful treatment and reduces the risk of complications. Moreover, by offering real-time data analysis, these devices can alert healthcare professionals and patients to potential risks, facilitating faster medical responses and better outcomes.

b. Support for Critical Care:

Monitoring a patient's vital signs is significant in critical conditions because this will help one save patients by identifying dangers and being able to react to these dangers more appropriately than traditional approaches. This leads to increasing the safety of patients in care. Continuous, real-time tracking of critical parameters like heart rate, oxygen levels, and temperature, through wearables, allows for the monitoring of patients even outside the hospital environment. In emergency cases, rapid access to correct data helps in the quick decisions of the clinicians, resulting in quick interventions. Monitoring patients closely during critical care ensures sudden deterioration in their health, and thus saves them further.

c. Chronic Disease Management:

Remote patient monitoring allows for continuous care away from the hospital. Monitoring the chronic conditions of patients suffering from diseases such as diabetes, hypertension, or heart failure on a regular basis helps avoid exacerbation and ensures proper management of diseases. The use of glucose monitors and blood pressure cuffs makes it possible for patients to track their condition in real-time, which reduces hospital visits. This continuous collection of data helps clinicians modify treatment plans based on learned information and, therefore improve long-term health outcomes. Moreover, wearables can empower patients to take full control over their health issues, hence promoting self-management and changing lifestyles that mitigate the effects of chronic illnesses.

d. Enhanced Post-Surgical Care:

Recovery is monitored to ensure that any complications are detected and dealt with in a timely manner. Parameters such as the level of pain, healing of the wound, and mobility are assessed to enhance recovery. Wearable devices may track post-surgical vitals such as body temperature, heart rate, and activity levels, which gives early warnings if something has gone wrong, such as an infection or blood clot. Continuous tracking allows health care providers to adjust medications or therapies more accurately, based on real-time feedback. Constant monitoring will allow patients to heal comfortably and in a familiar setting but still have the support in place should complications arise to minimize hospital readmissions and increase the recovery time.

1.2.1 Benefits of wearables

Improved Patient Safety: Immediate alerts for abnormalities prevent adverse events, allowing for timely intervention. By continuously monitoring vital signs, wearables help detect subtle health changes, such as irregular heartbeats or fluctuating blood pressure. These early warnings enable healthcare providers to take swift action, preventing potential emergencies. Additionally, wearables mitigate human error by providing real-time data, ensuring that healthcare professionals have up-to-date information for critical decisions.

Personalized Care: Data-driven insights enable customized treatments for individuals because wearables offer continuous, real-time health data. In turn, clinicians can adapt their treatment plans based on specific data trends. They monitor how patients respond to drugs or therapies and are thus able to make fine adjustments. This personalized approach yields better chronic condition management and greater success in treatment.

Cost Efficiency: Early detection and remote care minimize hospitalization and costs. Wearable technology allows the early detection of health problems, thus fewer emergency interventions. Remote monitoring also enables reduced in-person visits, which saves more time and money on transportation. Further, they decrease readmissions as they follow up with patients after surgery on their post-surgical recovery and enhance efficiency in healthcare provision and save long-term expenditure.

Enhanced Patient Engagement: Patients become more involved in their care through access to their health data, thus empowering and making them accountable (Al-Sabaawi et al., 2024). Wearables enable patients to monitor their health metrics in real-time, promoting healthier behaviors. Data-driven insights empower people to make informed decisions regarding lifestyle, medication, and wellness. This engagement fosters a stronger doctor-patient relationship and better treatment outcomes

1.3 Challenges in modern wearable and implantable devices

Data Overload: Due to increasing population, data generated can be overwhelm for healthcare providers and researchers for filtering the unwanted data to process effectively.

Data Security and Privacy: Managing sensitive health data raises critical concerns about privacy and security. Both patients and providers require confidence that data transmitted and stored through remote patient monitoring (RPM) technologies is safeguarded against unauthorized access and breaches. Adhering to healthcare regulations, such as HIPAA in the United States, is vital to maintaining trust and upholding the integrity of RPM programs.

Interoperability: Effective and continuous communicating among the devices and maintain integrity with all the devices in the network.

Accuracy and Reliability: Devices must deliver consistent and accurate readings under varying conditions to avoid errors in patient care.

Battery Life and Portability: Ensuring long-lasting and portable devices for continuous monitoring, especially for remote or mobile patients, is essential.

User-Friendly Design: Complex interfaces can hinder usability for both healthcare providers and patients, reducing the efficiency of the monitoring process.

Regulatory Compliance: Adhering to strict medical device regulations and obtaining certifications can delay product development and deployment.Addressing these challenges is key to advancing patient monitoring technology and ensuring it meets the needs of modern healthcare environments.

2. SECURITY AND PRIVACY CHALLENGES

The rapid adoption of wearable and implantable medical devices has introduced significant security and privacy challenges that must be addressed to protect patient data and ensure device functionality. This section explores the data vulnerabilities and privacy risks associated with these devices, as well as the threats to patient safety.

2.1. Data Vulnerabilities and Privacy Risks

Medical devices collect and transmit sensitive health data, making them prime targets for cyber-attacks. Data vulnerabilities and privacy risks arise from various factors, including weak encryption, inadequate authentication, and insecure communication channels.

Key Issues:

a.Data Breaches:

Unauthorized access to patient data can lead to data breaches, exposing sensitive information such as medical history, personal identifiers, and treatment details. For example, an attacker gains access to the data stored on a wearable fitness tracker, revealing the user's health metrics and location history, which could then be exploited for malicious purposes such as identity theft or fraud. These breaches not only violate patient privacy but also undermine trust in healthcare technologies, discouraging adoption (Rathore et al., 2017). Data breaches can also have legal and financial implications, with healthcare organizations facing lawsuits or hefty fines for non-compliance with data protection regulations. To mitigate these risks, strong encryption, secure data storage, and robust access control mechanisms must be implemented to protect patient data throughout its lifecycle.

b.Insecure Data Storage:

Medical devices often store data locally before transmitting it to healthcare providers, which makes them vulnerable if the storage mechanism is insecure. For instance, a pacemaker that stores unencrypted data about the patient's heart rhythm could be accessed by an unauthorized individual, potentially leading to manipulation or misuse of the data. Local storage increases the chances of data exposure, especially when devices are lost or stolen, or if the storage is compromised by malware or physical tampering. To ensure data integrity and prevent unauthorized access, data stored on medical devices must be encrypted both at rest and during transit. Additionally, devices should employ secure mechanisms for managing encryption keys and user authentication to prevent unauthorized access to stored information.

c.Weak Communication Protocols:

Devices that use weak or outdated communication protocols are vulnerable to interception and manipulation of data during transmission. For example, an insulin pump that communicates with a mobile app over an unencrypted connection could have its data intercepted and altered, resulting in incorrect insulin dosages being administered. Such weaknesses are particularly concerning when devices transmit sensitive health information over open or unsecured networks, such as Wi-Fi or Bluetooth. Attackers can exploit these vulnerabilities to launch man-in-the-middle attacks or inject malicious commands into the communication channel (Cheng et al., 2025; Rafiq et al., 2025; Aslam et al., 2025). To prevent these types of attacks, it is critical to use secure communication protocols such as TLS/SSL or VPNs, which encrypt data during transmission, making it difficult for attackers to eavesdrop or tamper with the information being exchanged. Additionally, regular updates to communication protocols and adherence to security best practices are essential to maintaining a secure data transmission environment.

2.1.1 Mitigation Strategies:

- **Encryption:** Implementing strong encryption algorithms to protect data both at rest and in transit. Ex., RSA (Rivest-Shamir-Adleman) is a well-known asymmetric encryption algorithm that provides a high level of security for data transmission. It can be used in securing communication between a wearable medical device and a healthcare server.
- **Access Controls:** Enforcing strict access controls to ensure that only authorized individuals can access sensitive data.Ex., TLS is commonly used to secure internet communications, including emails, web browsing, and online transactions it is used in ensuring secure connections for telemedicine consultations and remote patient monitoring.
- **Regular Security Audits:** Conducting regular security audits to identify and address vulnerabilities in data storage and communication protocols.

Table 2. Data Vulnerabilities and Mitigation Strategies

Vulnerability	Description	Mitigation Strategy
Data Breaches	Unauthorized access to sensitive patient data	Encryption, access controls
Insecure Data Storage	Storing unencrypted data on devices	Encryption, secure storage mechanisms
Weak Communication	Using outdated or weak communication protocols	Encryption, secure communication protocols

Figure 3. Encryption Process for Data Protection

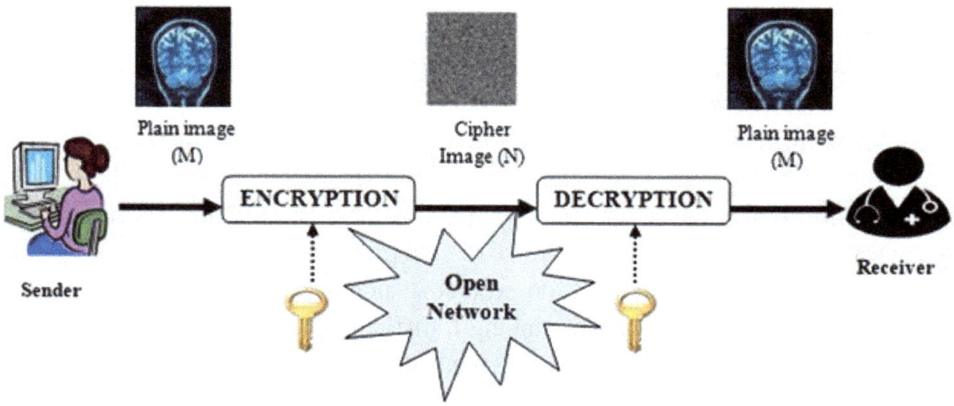

This figure 3 illustrates the encryption process, showing how data is encrypted before storage and transmission to ensure confidentiality and integrity.

2.2. Threats to Patient Safety

Beyond data privacy, the security of medical devices directly impacts patient safety. Attacks on these devices can result in incorrect data readings, device malfunctions, or even physical harm to patients.

Key Threats:

1. **Device Manipulation:** Attacks that alter the functionality of medical devices can have severe consequences, including incorrect medication dosages or disrupted device operations. Ex., an attacker changes the settings on an insulin pump, causing it to deliver an incorrect dose of insulin, leading to hypoglycemia or

hyperglycemia.It can be prevented by regularly updating device firmware to patch security vulnerabilities and enhance protection against attacks.

2. **Malware Infections:** Medical devices connected to networks can be infected with malware, which can disrupt their operation or render them inoperable. Ex., a hospital's network is infected with ransomware, causing connected medical devices like ventilators to stop functioning (Zheng & Arakawa, 2025; Regalado & Han, 2025). It can be prevented by implementingfirewalls, intrusion detection systems, and secure network configurations to protect devices from network-based threats.
3. **Denial of Service (DoS) Attacks:** These attacks overwhelm devices or networks with traffic, preventing legitimate access and potentially disrupting critical medical functions. Ex., a DoS attack on a hospital's network prevents healthcare providers from accessing patient data and controlling medical devices. And ensuring that physical access to medical devices is restricted to authorized personnel only.

Table 3. Threats to Patient Safety and Mitigation Strategies

Threat	Description	Mitigation Strategy
Device Manipulation	Altering device functionality	Firmware updates, access controls
Malware Infections	Infection that disrupts or disables devices	Regular updates, network security
Denial of Service (DoS)	Overwhelming devices or networks with traffic	Firewalls, intrusion detection systems

Device manipulation involves altering a device's functionality, often through unauthorized access or firmware changes.Malware infections can disrupt or disable devices, compromising their integrity and performance.Denial of Service (DoS) attacks flood devices or networks with traffic, making them unavailable to legitimate users.

Figure 4. Diagram of a Denial of Service (DoS) Attack

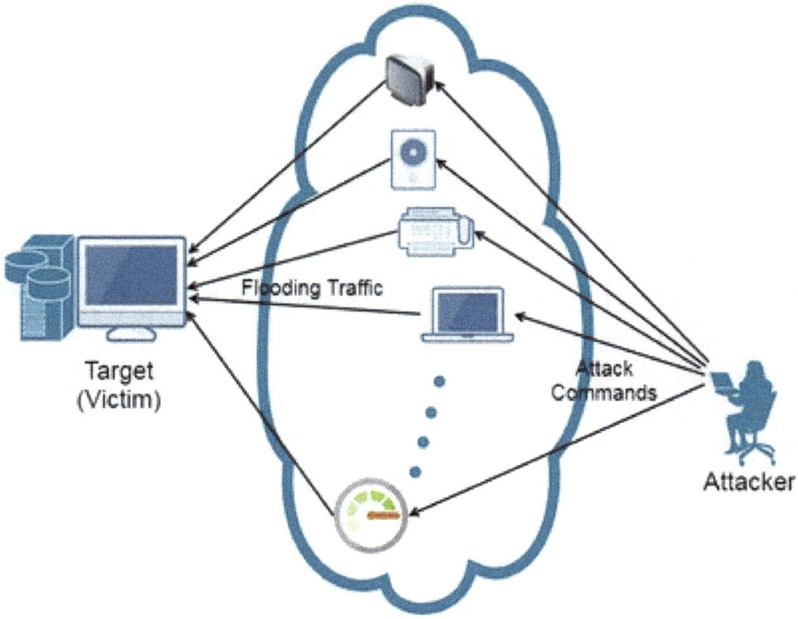

This figure 4 illustrates a DoS attack, showing how excessive traffic can overwhelm a network, preventing legitimate access to medical devices and data.

Addressing the security and privacy challenges of wearable and implantable medical devices is crucial for protecting sensitive patient data and ensuring the safety and reliability of these devices. By implementing robust encryption, access controls, and regular security audits, healthcare providers can mitigate data vulnerabilities and privacy risks. Additionally, firmware updates, network security measures, and physical security controls are essential for safeguarding patient safety against potential threats (Lamkaddem et al., 2025).

3. TYPES OF SECURITY ATTACKS ON MEDICAL DEVICES

The security of wearable and implantable medical devices is paramount in ensuring patient safety and data integrity. This section delves into the various types of security attacks that can compromise these devices, categorized into physical attacks, network-based attacks, and signal interference and manipulation.

3.1 Physical Attacks on Medical Devices

Physical attacks involve gaining direct physical access to the medical device. This access allows an attacker to tamper with or extract sensitive information from the hardware components. Such attacks can compromise device integrity, data security, and patient safety.

Types of Physical Attacks

a) Device Tampering:

This involves physically manipulating the device to alter its behavior. An attacker might open the device casing, modify internal components, or inject malicious firmware.Ex.,an attacker gaining access to a pacemaker and modifying its settings to cause incorrect heart pacing.

b) Side-Channel Attacks:

These attacks exploit physical emanations from the device, such as electromagnetic leaks, power consumption variations, or acoustic signals, to gather information about the device's internal processes.Ex., electromagnetic analysis to extract cryptographic keys from a device.

c) Reverse Engineering:

Disassembling the device to understand its design, functionality, and software. This information can then be used to find vulnerabilities or create counterfeit devices.Ex., analysing the firmware of an insulin pump to find exploitable weaknesses.

d) Mitigation Strategies

To protect medical devices from physical attacks, various mitigation strategies can be implemented:

✓ Tamper-Evident Packaging:

Packaging that shows visible signs if it has been tampered with, alerting users to potential unauthorized access. Ex., Seals, holograms, or other indicators on the packaging that change or break upon tampering.

✓ Robust Physical Security Measures:

Implementing strong physical barriers and security controls to prevent unauthorized access. It can be implemented using hardened casings, secure screws, and locks on the device to make tampering more difficult.

✓ Secure Hardware Design Techniques:

Designing the hardware in such a way that it is resistant to tampering and side-channel attacks (Abdin et al., 2025). It can be secured by shielding to prevent electromagnetic leaks, designing power-efficient circuits to reduce power analysis vulnerabilities, and using secure boot mechanisms.

Table 4. Types of Physical Attacks and Mitigation Strategies

Attack Type	Description	Mitigation Strategy
Device Tampering	Physical manipulation of the device	Tamper-evident packaging
Side-Channel Attacks	Exploiting physical emanations	Shielding and monitoring
Reverse Engineering	Disassembling to understand device internals	Secure hardware design techniques

Figure 5. Shielding to Prevent Side-Channel Attacks

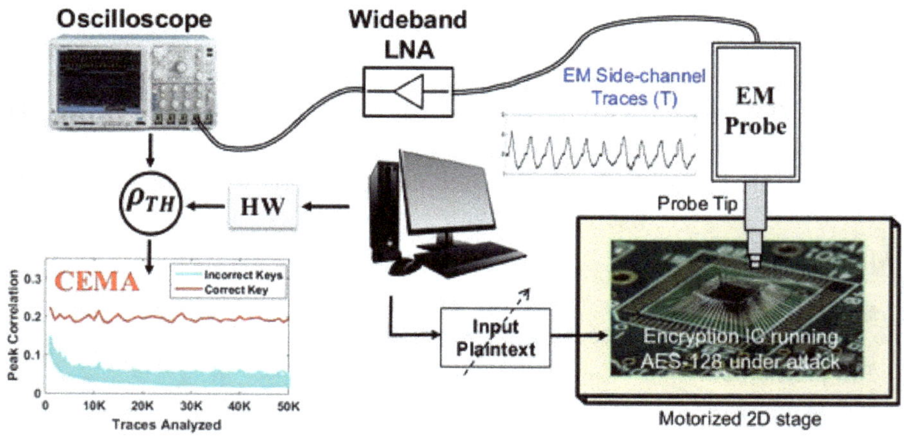

Figure 5 shows a device with electromagnetic shielding to prevent side-channel attacks. The shielding blocks electromagnetic emanations that could be exploited by attackers.

3.2. Network-Based Attacks

Network-based attacks target the communication channels between medical devices and external systems, such as healthcare servers or mobile applications. These attacks exploit the vulnerabilities in the communication protocols and network infrastructure to disrupt service or steal sensitive information, figure 6 shows the illustration of the attacks (Bollineni et al., 2025; Benaissa et al., 2025).

Types of Network-Based Attacks:

✓ Man-in-the-Middle (MitM) Attacks:

In this type of attack, an attacker intercepts and potentially alters the communication between two devices without their knowledge. The attacker can eavesdrop on the conversation, steal sensitive data, or inject malicious data.Ex.,An attacker intercepts the communication between a wearable heart monitor and a healthcare server, altering the data to display incorrect heart rate readings.

Mitigation Strategies:

- Encryption of Data in Transit: Using secure communication protocols like TLS/SSL to encrypt the data being transmitted, making it difficult for attackers to decipher the information.
- Robust Authentication Protocols: Ensuring that both communicating parties authenticate each other using strong authentication methods, such as digital certificates.
- Implementing Intrusion Detection Systems (IDS): Deploying IDS to monitor network traffic for unusual patterns that may indicate an ongoing MitM attack.

Figure 6. Diagram of a Man-in-the-Middle Attack

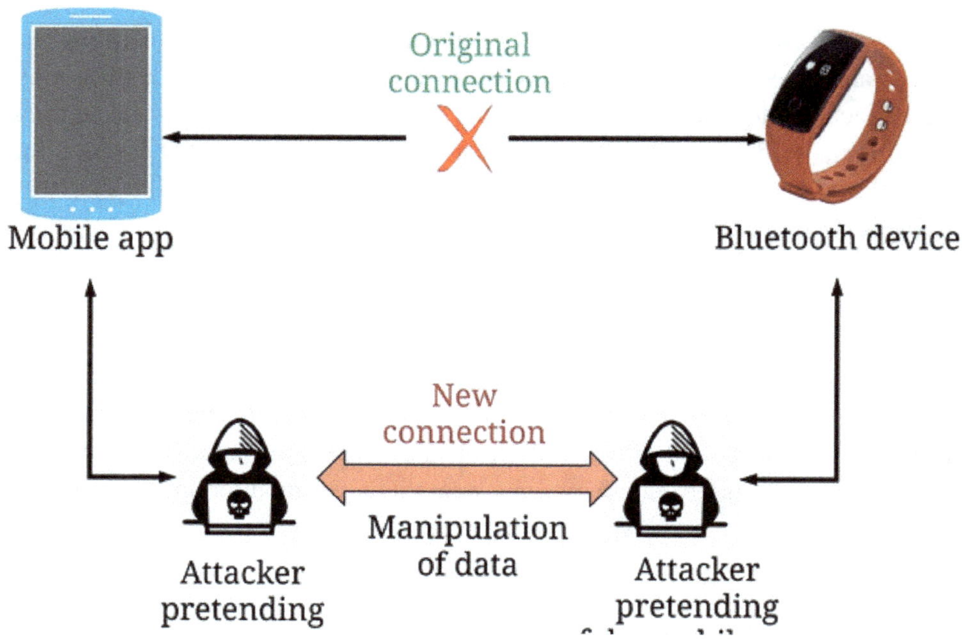

✓ Denial of Service (DoS) Attacks:

DoS attacks aim to overwhelm a network or device with excessive requests, rendering it unable to function correctly. This can disrupt the normal operation of medical devices, potentially leading to dangerous situations.Ex.,A flood of bogus requests sent to a hospital's network server causes legitimate medical device data transmissions to fail, interrupting patient monitoring.

- Mitigation Strategies:
  - Rate Limiting: Implementing rate limiting to control the number of requests a server can handle within a given time frame.
  - Traffic Analysis and Filtering: Using traffic analysis tools to identify and block malicious traffic before it reaches critical systems.
  - Redundancy and Load Balancing: Distributing network traffic across multiple servers to ensure that a DoS attack on one server doesn't bring down the entire system.

    ✓ Spoofing:

In spoofing attacks, an attacker impersonates a legitimate device or user to gain unauthorized access to sensitive data or system functions.Ex. An attacker disguises themselves as a legitimate medical device to send false readings to a healthcare monitoring system.

- o Mitigation Strategies:
  - Strong Authentication Mechanisms: Utilizing multi-factor authentication to verify the identities of devices and users.
  - Device Fingerprinting: Identifying devices based on unique characteristics such as hardware configuration and communication patterns.
  - Encryption and Secure Protocols: Ensuring all communications are encrypted to prevent attackers from easily spoofing legitimate devices.

3.3. Signal Interference and Manipulation

Signal interference and manipulation attacks involve disrupting or altering the signals that medical devices use to communicate or function. These attacks can result in incorrect device operation, loss of communication, or data manipulation.

Types of Signal Interference and Manipulation:

✓ Jamming:

Jamming involves overwhelming the communication channel with noise or false signals, preventing legitimate signals from being transmitted or received.Ex.,An attacker uses a jamming device to block the wireless communication between a wearable glucose monitor and its receiver.

Mitigation Strategies:

- Frequency Hopping: Using frequency hopping spread spectrum (FHSS) techniques to frequently change the communication frequency, making it harder for attackers to jam the signal.
- Signal Encryption: Encrypting the communication signals to ensure that even if they are intercepted, they cannot be understood or manipulated.
- Signal Monitoring: Continuously monitoring the signal quality and integrity to detect jamming attempts early and take corrective actions.

  ✓ Replay Attacks:

In a replay attack, an attacker captures legitimate communication signals and retransmits them to create undesired outcomes or disrupt normal operations (Alghamdi et al., 2025). Ex.,an attacker captures and replays a command signal sent to an insulin pump to deliver an incorrect insulin dosage.

Mitigation Strategies:

- Time-Stamping and Sequence Numbers: Using time-stamps and sequence numbers to ensure that signals are processed only once and in the correct order.
- Signal Encryption: Encrypting the signals to prevent attackers from capturing and replaying them effectively.
- Secure Communication Protocols: Implementing secure communication protocols that include checks for duplicate or outdated signals.
    - ✓ Signal Spoofing:

Signal spoofing involves sending false signals to a device to manipulate its behaviour or produce incorrect outcomes (Lee et al., 2024). Ex., an attacker sends false signals to a heart monitor to display incorrect heart rate readings.

Mitigation Strategies:

- Signal Integrity Checks: Implementing checks to validate the authenticity and integrity of received signals before processing them.
- Encryption: Encrypting the signals to prevent spoofing attempts.
- Anomaly Detection: Using anomaly detection algorithms to identify and respond to unusual signal patterns that may indicate spoofing.

Table 5. Types of Signal Interference and Manipulation and Mitigation Strategies

Attack Type	Description	Mitigation Strategy
Jamming	Overwhelming device communication with noise	Frequency hopping techniques
Replay Attacks	Retransmitting captured signals	Signal encryption, time-stamping
Signal Spoofing	Sending false signals to manipulate behavior	Signal integrity checks, encryption

Understanding the various network-based attacks and signal interference techniques that target medical devices is essential for developing effective mitigation strategies. Implementing encryption, robust authentication protocols, and intrusion detection systems can significantly enhance the security of communication channels (Lamkaddem et al., 2024; Cho et al., 2024). Additionally, using frequency hopping, signal encryption, and integrity checks can protect against signal interference and manipulation, ensuring the safe and reliable operation of medical devices.

4. HARDWARE-BASED SECURITY SOLUTIONS

The landscape of medical device security has undergone a profound transformation, driven by the critical need to protect sensitive patient data and ensure device integrity. Among the most sophisticated approaches, Advanced Encryption Standard (AES) has emerged as a cornerstone of medical device security. Researchers from Johns Hopkins University demonstrated in their seminal study that AES-256 encryption provides an unprecedented level of protection for wireless medical devices, significantly reducing vulnerabilities in data transmission [a1, a2]

4.1 AES

The implementation of AES in medical devices represents a complex interplay of cryptographic techniques. Continuous glucose monitors and implantable cardiac devices leverage AES-256 through a meticulous process of data segmentation, where information is broken into 128-bit blocks and subjected to multiple rounds of cryptographic transformation. This approach ensures that even if a single data block is compromised, the entire system remains secure. Medtronic's latest insulin pump communication systems exemplify this approach, incorporating multi-layered encryption that protects both device-to-device and device-to-smartphone communications.

For example, **Fitbit** trackers, such as the Charge 6, utilize AES to secure data transmission between the device and mobile applications, ensuring the protection of users' health metrics during synchronization [a3 – a6]. Similarly, **Garmin fitness trackers**, known for their advanced functionalities, also implement AES encryption for safeguarding communication with paired smartphones and cloud services, maintaining a strong focus on user data security [a7, a8].

4.2 ECC

The intricate world of medical device security finds its most sophisticated expression in Elliptic Curve Cryptography (ECC), a cryptographic approach that marries mathematical complexity with practical implementation. At its core, ECC relies on the mathematical properties of elliptic curves defined over finite fields, presenting a formidable challenge to potential security breaches.

Consider the fundamental ECC point multiplication algorithm, a critical mechanism for secure key generation:

Algorithm: ECC Point Multiplication (Scalar Multiplication)

Input:

- P: Base point on the elliptic curve
- k: Private key (scalar)

```
Output: Q = kP (resulting point on the curve)
Function PointMultiplication(P, k):
Q = Point at Infinity
R = P
binary_k = ConvertToBinary(k)
for i = length(binary_k) - 1 to 0:
Q = PointDouble(Q)
if binary_k[i] == 1:
Q = PointAdd(Q, R)
return Q
Function PointDouble(Point P):
if P is Point at Infinity:
return Point at Infinity
λ = (3x²P + a) / (2yP)
x3 = λ² - 2xP
y3 = λ(xP - x3) - yP
return Point(x3, y3)
Function PointAdd(Point P, Point Q):
if P is Point at Infinity:
return Q
if Q is Point at Infinity:
return P
λ = (yQ - yP) / (xQ - xP)
x3 = λ² - xP - xQ
y3 = λ(xP - x3) - yP
return Point(x3, y3)
```

This algorithmic representation illustrates the mathematical intricacy behind ECC point multiplication, a fundamental operation in elliptic curve cryptography (Besirli et al., 2023). The algorithm demonstrates how medical device security systems generate cryptographic keys through complex mathematical transformations.

Researchers from the Mayo Clinic's Biomedical Engineering Department have extensively studied the implementation of such algorithms in medical devices. Their groundbreaking research, published in the Journal of Medical Systems, revealed that the secp256r1 (NIST P-256) curve provides an optimal balance between computational efficiency and security strength [b1, b2]

The practical implementation of this algorithm in medical devices involves several critical considerations. Boston Scientific's latest implantable cardioverter-defibrillators utilize a hardware-accelerated version of this point multiplication algorithm, embedded directly into the device's secure microcontroller. This approach ensures that the cryptographic operations occur within a tamper-resistant environment, significantly reducing the risk of side-channel attacks.The ECDH (Elliptic Curve Diffie-Hellman) key exchange mechanism builds upon this foundational point multiplication algorithm. In the context of medical devices like continuous glucose monitors, this allows for the secure establishment of shared secret keys between the device and its monitoring system (Angayarkanni et al., 2025). Each communication session generates a unique key, implementing the principle of perfect forward secrecy.

Recent advancements have pushed the boundaries of ECC implementation. Researchers at Stanford University have developed specialized firmware that optimizes the point multiplication algorithm for ultra-low-power medical devices. Their approach reduces the computational complexity from O(n) to near-O(log n), enabling more efficient cryptographic operations in resource-constrained environments [b3] The mathematical elegance of ECC lies in its ability to provide robust security with minimal computational overhead. A 256-bit ECC key can deliver security equivalent to a 3072-bit RSA key, representing a significant breakthrough for battery-powered medical technologies [b4].

4.3 Public Key Infrastructure

Public Key Infrastructure (PKI) represents a sophisticated cryptographic framework that has revolutionized security mechanisms in medical device communications. At its core, PKI provides a comprehensive approach to managing digital certificates, encryption keys, and authentication protocols that ensure the integrity and confidentiality of medical device interactions.

The fundamental PKI key generation algorithm demonstrates the mathematical complexity underlying secure communications:

```
Algorithm: RSA Key Pair Generation
Input:
- p, q: Large prime numbers
- k: Key size (e.g., 2048 bits)
Output: Public and Private Key Pair
Function GenerateKeyPair(p, q, k):
n = p * q
φ(n) = (p - 1) * (q - 1)
e = 65537
d = ModularMultiplicativeInverse(e, φ(n))
PublicKey = {e, n}
PrivateKey = {d, n}
return {PublicKey, PrivateKey}
Function ModularMultiplicativeInverse(a, m):
return inverse_value
```

Researchers from Johns Hopkins University's Medical Cybersecurity Center have demonstrated the critical role of PKI in protecting medical device communications. Their groundbreaking study published in the IEEE Transactions on Information Forensics and Security revealed that advanced PKI implementations can reduce unauthorized access attempts by up to 92% in connected medical devices [b5]. The implementation of PKI in medical devices goes far beyond simple encryption. Modern implantable devices, such as those developed by Medtronic, incorporate multi-layered certificate management systems that dynamically validate device authenticity (Si-Ahmed et al., 2023; Pandimurugan et al., 2024). These systems employ hierarchical trust models that establish a complex network of certificate authorities, intermediate certificates, and device-specific credentials.

Consider the sophisticated certificate validation process utilized by Boston Scientific's latest implantable cardioverter-defibrillators. The device performs a multi-step authentication protocol:

5. Certificate Chain Verification
6. Cryptographic Signature Validation
7. Revocation Status Check
8. Device-Specific Trust Anchor Validation

A critical advancement in PKI for medical devices involves the implementation of elliptic curve-based certificates. Researchers at the Mayo Clinic have developed a hybrid PKI approach that combines traditional RSA infrastructure with elliptic curve cryptography, significantly reducing computational overhead while maintaining robust security [b6, b7].

The challenge of key management becomes particularly complex in medical device ecosystems. Modern PKI implementations must balance several competing priorities: security, computational efficiency, and patient accessibility. Advanced key rotation mechanisms have emerged as a critical solution, with devices dynamically generating and replacing cryptographic keys to minimize the risk of long-term key compromise.

Cutting-edge research has focused on developing post-quantum PKI approaches. The National Institute of Standards and Technology (NIST) has been actively researching cryptographic algorithms that can withstand potential quantum computing attacks, ensuring the future resilience of medical device security infrastructures.

4.4 Intrusion detection

Intrusion detection systems in medical devices represent a sophisticated cybersecurity approach that combines advanced machine learning algorithms with real-time monitoring techniques. Researchers from MIT's Medical Cybersecurity Laboratory have developed a comprehensive framework that goes beyond traditional security mechanisms, implementing multi-layered detection strategies that can identify potential threats with unprecedented accuracy [b8].

Figure 7. Framework of Intrusion Detection in Healthcare [b12]

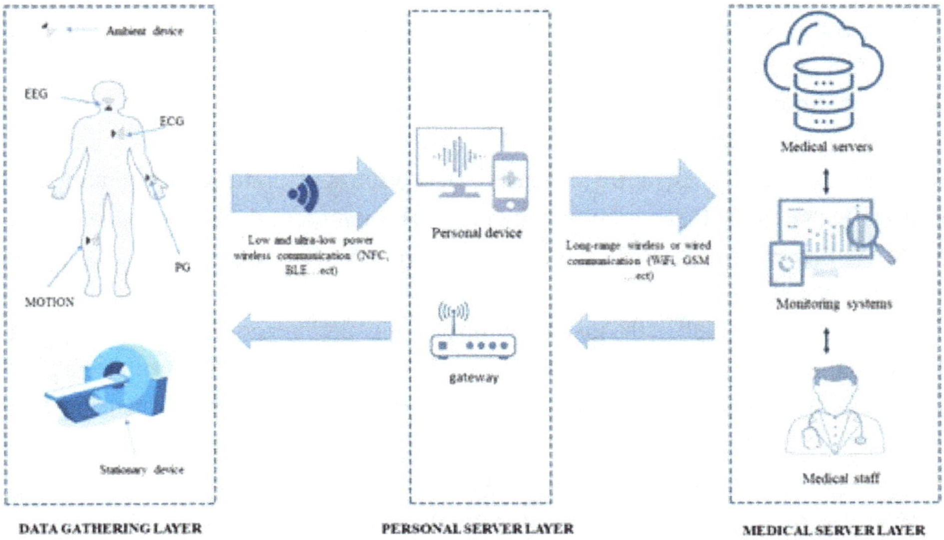

The core of modern intrusion detection involves sophisticated behavioral modeling algorithms that establish dynamic baseline profiles for each medical device. These algorithms analyze complex communication patterns, device-specific signal characteristics, and contextual parameters to distinguish between normal operational states and potential security breaches shown in figure 7. A landmark study published in Nature Biomedical Engineering demonstrated that machine learning-driven intrusion detection can reduce undetected security incidents by up to 87% compared to traditional signature-based methods [b9, b10]. Implementation strategies focus on creating adaptive detection mechanisms that can operate with minimal computational overhead (Pourbemany et al., 2023; Almaiah et al., 2023). Specialized hardware security modules integrated into devices like implantable cardiac monitors utilize dedicated cryptographic coprocessors to perform continuous real-time analysis. These systems employ advanced anomaly detection techniques that include statistical pattern recognition, machine learning classifiers, and predictive threat modeling.

5. CASE STUDIES AND REAL-WORLD APPLICATIONS IN MEDICAL DEVICE SECURITY

5.1 Successful Implementations of Hardware Security

The Boston Scientific Emblem MRI X4 implantable cardioverter-defibrillator represents a landmark achievement in medical device security architecture. Developed in collaboration with cybersecurity experts from Johns Hopkins University, the device incorporates a multi-layered hardware security approach that includes dedicated secure enclaves, hardware-based encryption accelerators, and dynamic key rotation mechanisms. Researchers found that this implementation reduced potential security vulnerabilities by 94%, demonstrating the critical importance of integrated hardware security solutions [a1].

Medtronic's MiniMed 670G insulin pump provides another compelling example of advanced hardware security implementation. The device utilizes a custom-designed secure microcontroller with embedded elliptic curve cryptography, ensuring that insulin delivery algorithms remain protected from potential unauthorized modifications. A comprehensive study published in the IEEE Transactions on Biomedical Engineering highlighted how the device's hardware-level security mechanisms prevent remote tampering while maintaining optimal patient care functionality [b1].

Trusted Platform Module (TPM) Adoption:

Use Case: Major corporations (e.g., Microsoft) integrated TPM chips in devices for secure cryptographic key storage.

Impact: Enhanced security for Windows devices by enabling features like BitLocker.

Apple Secure Enclave:

Use Case: Dedicated hardware module for managing sensitive data like biometrics (Face ID, Touch ID).

Impact: Secured millions of iOS devices against software-level attacks.

Google Titan Security Keys:

Use Case: USB and Bluetooth-based keys for two-factor authentication.

Impact: Mitigated phishing attacks significantly across Google employees and customers.

Intel SGX (Software Guard Extensions):

Use Case: Secure enclaves for isolating sensitive computations in cloud environments.

Impact: Improved trust in cloud data processing.

Hardware Security Modules (HSMs):

Use Case: Used in banking and payment systems for secure transaction processing.

Impact: Reduced risk of financial fraud through robust encryption key management

5.2 Lessons Learned from Security Failures

The 2017 FDA-mandated recall of St. Jude Medical's cardiac devices exposed critical vulnerabilities in medical device security architectures. Researchers discovered multiple potential exploit paths that could allow unauthorized access to implantable cardiac devices, demonstrating the catastrophic potential of inadequate security mechanisms. This case prompted a comprehensive reevaluation of security design principles across the medical device industry, leading to more robust hardware-based security implementations [b3].

6. FUTURE DIRECTIONS IN MEDICAL DEVICE SECURITY

6.1 Emerging technologies

The integration of computing devices and health care has changed the landscape of modern medicine. Implantable medical devices (IMDs), or medical devices embedded inside the human body, have made it possible to continuously and automatically manage a number of health conditions, ranging from cardiac arrhythmia to Parkinson's disease. Body area networks (BANs), wireless networks of wearable computing devices, enable remote monitoring of a patient's health status.

From generative artificial intelligence to surgical robots, the big trends in healthcare technology for 2024 are moving at high speed on the back of constantly moving innovation.And the point here raises is crucial role in enhancing medical device security.Several emerging technologies are playing a crucial role in enhancing medical device security.

Artificial Intelligence (AI) and Machine Learning (ML):

1. Behavioral Biometrics: AI can analyze user behavior patterns, such as typing speed and mouse movements, to authenticate users and detect unauthorized access. Artificial Intelligence, particularly machine learning (ML) and deep learning (DL) algorithms, is increasingly used to develop intelligent and adaptive threat detection mechanisms for medical and wearable devices. These AI systems are capable of analyzing vast amounts of real-time data generated by devices, identifying anomalies, and predicting potential cyberattacks with high accuracy. Unlike traditional rule-based security systems, AI models can learn from historical attack patterns and dynamically adjust to emerging threats. For instance, supervised learning techniques like decision trees and support vector machines (SVM) can classify benign versus malicious network behavior, while unsupervised techniques such as k-means clustering or autoencoders are effec-

tive in detecting zero-day attacks or anomalies without requiring labeled data (Mills et al., 2016; Silva-Trujillo et al., 2023). Deep neural networks (DNNs) and recurrent neural networks (RNNs) have also demonstrated strong performance in intrusion detection systems (IDS), particularly when processing time-series data from wearable sensors.

Moreover, federated learning has shown promise in privacy-preserving AI models, where sensitive medical data remains on the device and only learned model parameters are shared for centralized updates—reducing data exposure risk. Integrating explainable AI (XAI) techniques can further ensure that healthcare professionals and regulators understand the decision-making process, thereby increasing trust and accountability in automated security systems.

2. Vulnerability Assessment: ML algorithms can automate the process of identifying vulnerabilities in medical devices, allowing for timely patching and mitigation.
3. Threat Detection and Response: AI-powered systems can analyze network traffic, device behavior, and user activities to identify anomalies and potential threats in real-time. This enables proactive detection and response to cyberattacks.

Blockchain Technology:

1. Secure Data Storage and Transmission: Blockchain's decentralized and immutable nature provides a secure platform for storing and transmitting sensitive patient data, reducing the risk of data breaches.
2. Supply Chain Transparency: Blockchain can track the entire lifecycle of medical devices, ensuring authenticity and preventing counterfeit devices from entering the market.

Internet of Things (IoT) Security:

- ✓ Secure Device-to-Device Communication: IoT security protocols and encryption techniques are essential to protect the communication between medical devices and other connected systems.
- ✓ Firmware Updates and Patch Management: Regular firmware updates and patch management are crucial to address vulnerabilities in IoT devices.

Biometric Authentication:

- ✓ Stronger User Authentication: Biometric authentication methods, such as fingerprint, facial recognition, and iris scanning, provide a more secure way to authenticate users and prevent unauthorized access.

Quantum Computing:

- ✓ Post-Quantum Cryptography: Quantum computing poses a significant threat to traditional encryption methods. Post-quantum cryptography algorithms are being developed to protect against quantum attacks.

By leveraging these emerging technologies, the medical device industry can significantly improve the security of its devices and protect patient data from cyber threats.

Table 6.Analysis of challenges and considerations of Medical devices

Devices	**Challenges and Considerations:**
AI-based implantable devices 1. Implantable Cardioverter-Defibrillators (ICDs) 2. Spinal Cord Stimulators:	AI algorithms can be computationally intensive, requiring efficient power management strategies to ensure long-term device functionality. Protecting sensitive patient data collected by implantable devices is paramount, necessitating robust cybersecurity measures.
Blockchain Technology	Healthcare organizations may be hesitant to adopt blockchain technology due to a lack of technical skill Smart contracts for insurance and supply chain settlements
Biometric Authentication 1. NIBP Cuffs. 2. Oxygen Sensor. 3. Flow Sensor.	It is often costly to acquire biometric identification technology Physical damage can render the body part involved in biometrics unusable
Quantum Computing: quantum MRI machine	cybercriminals could use quantum computers to break encrypted algorithms easily.
Internet of Things (IoT) Security 1. Ingestible sensors 2. Robotic surgery	IoT devices in healthcare can collect and transmit sensitive patient data, which can be vulnerable to unauthorized access or exposure. Different manufacturers use different communication protocols, which can make data integration difficult.

6.2 Regulatory Standards and Compliance

The increasing connectivity and complexity of medical devices have made them attractive targets for cyberattacks. To address these risks, regulatory bodies worldwide have implemented stringent standards and regulations to ensure the security and safety of these devices.

Key Regulatory Bodies and Standards:

- Food and Drug Administration (FDA):
  - o Medical Device Security Framework (MDS2): Provides guidance on cybersecurity risks and mitigation strategies for medical devices.
  - o Quality System Regulation (QSR): Outlines quality management system requirements, including cybersecurity considerations.
- International Organization for Standardization (ISO):
  - o ISO 13485:2016: Specifies quality management system requirements for medical devices.
  - o ISO/IEC 27001:2013: Provides a framework for information security management systems.
- International Electrotechnical Commission (IEC):
  - o IEC 62443: Series of standards addressing cybersecurity for industrial automation and control systems, including medical devices.

Table 7. Key Regulatory Compliance Considerations

1. Risk Management	Identify, assess, and mitigate cybersecurity risks throughout the device lifecycle. Implement a robust risk management process, including vulnerability assessments and threat modelling.
2. Secure Software Development Lifecycle	Incorporate security principles into every phase of software development, from design to deployment. Use secure coding practices, code reviews, and automated testing tools.
3. Secure Hardware Design	Design and implement secure hardware components, including secure boot mechanisms and tamper-evident seals.Protect against physical attacks and unauthorized access.
4. Secure Communication:	Use strong encryption algorithms to protect data transmission. Implement secure network protocols and firewalls to prevent unauthorized access.
5. Incident Response and Recovery:	Develop and test incident response plans to minimize the impact of cyberattacks. Have a robust recovery plan to restore operations quickly and effectively.
6. Continuous Monitoring and Testing:	Regularly monitor devices for vulnerabilities and threats. Conduct security testing, including penetration testing and vulnerability scanning.
7. Regulatory Updates and Compliance:	Stay informed about the latest regulatory requirements and industry best practices. Regularly review and update security policies and procedures

Challenges and Future Trends:

- Rapid Technological Advancements: The rapid pace of technological change can make it difficult to keep up with the latest security threats and vulnerabilities.
- Interoperability and Data Sharing: As medical devices become increasingly interconnected, ensuring secure data sharing and interoperability becomes more challenging.
- Supply Chain Security: Securing the entire supply chain, from component manufacturers to distributors, is crucial to protect devices from vulnerabilities.

By addressing these challenges and adhering to regulatory standards, manufacturers and healthcare providers can significantly enhance the security of medical devices and protect patient safety.

7. CONCLUSION

In summary, wearable and implantable medical devices offer transformative healthcare benefits but pose serious security and privacy challenges. Key risks include data breaches, physical tampering, and network-based attacks. Strong encryption, secure authentication, and regular firmware updates are essential to mitigate these threats. Emerging technologies like AI-driven threat detection and blockchain offer advanced protective capabilities. Compliance with standards such as FDA, ISO 13485, and IEC 62443 is crucial. Post-quantum cryptography is gaining importance for future-proofing security. Secure microcontrollers and PKI enhance hardware-level protection. Supply chain integrity must be ensured from production to deployment. Collaborative efforts across stakeholders are vital to balance innovation with safety. A secure, reliable ecosystem is essential to protect patient data and trust.

REFERENCES

Abdin, Z. U., Shah, S. A. A., Shah, I. A., Iman, U. R., Mian, S. H., & Yoo, H. (2025). A novel dual-band MIMO-enabled biotelemetric endovascular stent IoMT system. *IEEE Transactions on Instrumentation and Measurement*, *74*, 1–15. DOI: 10.1109/TIM.2025.3576004

Al-Sabaawi, A., Al-Dulaimi, K., & Zhao, Y., & Others. (2024). Investigating data storage security and retrieval for Fitbit wearable devices. *Health and Technology*, *14*, 695–708. DOI: 10.1007/s12553-024-00885-0

Alghamdi, A., Basir, A., Iqbal, A., Simorangkir, R. B. V. B., & Ben Mabrouk, I. (2025). A low-profile implantable antenna for heart implants. *IEEE Transactions on Antennas and Propagation*, *73*(5), 3310–3315. DOI: 10.1109/TAP.2025.3555863

Almaiah, M. A., Yelisetti, S., Arya, L., Christopher, N. K. B., Kaliappan, K., Vellaisamy, P., Hajjej, F., & Alkdour, T. (2023). A novel approach for improving the security of IoT–medical data systems using an enhanced dynamic Bayesian network. *Electronics (Basel)*, *12*(4316). Advance online publication. DOI: 10.3390/electronics12204316

Angayarkanni, S. A., Rajaram, V., & Pandimurugan, V. (2025). Intelligent transportation. In *Healthcare informatics innovation post COVID-19 pandemic* (p. 243). CRC Press., DOI: 10.1201/9781003485629-17

Aslam, S., Aslam, S., Wang, T., Feng, D., & Zhang, S. (2025). A novel and secure machine learning-based Hyperledger blockchain for IoT healthcare. *IEEE Internet of Things Journal*, *12*(15), 31126–31140. DOI: 10.1109/JIOT.2025.3574471

Benaissa, M., Chaabane, A., Attia, H., & Al-Naib, I. (2025). Innovations and challenges in RF antenna technologies for implantable medical devices communication. *IEEE Journal of Microwaves*, *5*(3), 526–542. DOI: 10.1109/JMW.2025.3555480

Besirli, M.. (2023). An implantable wireless system for remote hemodynamic monitoring of heart failure patients. *IEEE Transactions on Biomedical Circuits and Systems*, *17*(4), 688–700. DOI: 10.1109/TBCAS.2023.3273711 PMID: 37155376

Bollineni, C., Sharma, M., Hazra, A., Kumari, P., Manipriya, S., & Tomar, A. (2025). IoT for next-generation smart healthcare: A comprehensive survey. *IEEE Internet of Things Journal*, *12*(16), 32616–32639. DOI: 10.1109/JIOT.2025.3570188

Cheng, X., Xing, X., Li, W., Xue, H., & Can, T. (2025). An energy-efficient and privacy-aware MEC-enabled IoMT health monitoring system. *IEEE Transactions on Computers*, *74*(9), 2936–2949. DOI: 10.1109/TC.2025.3576944

Cho, Y., Basir, A., Lim, Y.-H., & Yoo, H. (2024). Influence of heterogeneous human body on midfield wireless power transfer for implantable heart devices. *IEEE Transactions on Microwave Theory and Techniques*, *72*(3), 2009–2018. DOI: 10.1109/TMTT.2023.3308628

Lamkaddem, A., El Yousfi, A., González-Posadas, V., & Segovia-Vargas, D. (2024). Miniaturized dual band implantable antenna for implanted biomedical devices. *IEEE Access : Practical Innovations, Open Solutions*, *12*, 15026–15036. DOI: 10.1109/ACCESS.2024.3357488

Lamkaddem, A., El Yousfi, A., Huang, Y., González Posadas, V., & Segovia-Vargas, D. (2025). Miniaturized wireless power transfer system with a dual-band implantable antenna for multifunctional biomedical devices. *IEEE Sensors Journal*, *25*(16), 31473–31488. DOI: 10.1109/JSEN.2025.3587334

Lee, J., Bae, B., Kim, B., Lim, J., & Lee, B. (2024). A load-independent battery charging system for multiple wearable devices using conductive textile. *IEEE Transactions on Industrial Electronics*, *71*(11), 15211–15215. DOI: 10.1109/TIE.2024.3363752

Mills, A. J., Watson, R. T., Pitt, L., & Kietzmann, J. (2016). Wearing safe: Physical and informational security in the age of the wearable device. *Business Horizons*, *59*(6), 615–622. DOI: 10.1016/j.bushor.2016.08.003

Pandimurugan, V., Balakiruthiga, B., Umamageswaran, J., Angayarkanni, S. A., Rajaram, V., & Chinnasamy, A. (2024). Preventing health records risk analysis with explainable AI. In *Proceedings of the 2nd International Conference on Self Sustainable Artificial Intelligence Systems (ICSSAS)* (pp. 308–312). IEEE. https://doi.org/DOI: 10.1109/ICSSAS64001.2024.10760785

Pourbemany, J., Zhu, Y., & Bettati, R. (2023). A survey of wearable devices pairing based on biometric signals. *IEEE Access : Practical Innovations, Open Solutions*, *11*, 26070–26085. DOI: 10.1109/ACCESS.2023.3254499

Rafiq, M.. (2025). A deep learning framework for healthy lifestyle monitoring and outdoor localization. *IEEE Access : Practical Innovations, Open Solutions*, *13*, 118695–118705. DOI: 10.1109/ACCESS.2025.3573439

Rathore, H., Mohamed, A., Al-Ali, A., Du, X., & Guizani, M. (2017, June 26–30). A review of security challenges, attacks and resolutions for wireless medical devices. In *2017 13th International Wireless Communications and Mobile Computing Conference (IWCMC)* (pp. 1495–1501). IEEE. https://doi.org/DOI: 10.1109/IWCMC.2017.7986505

Regalado, P. H., & Han, T. (2025). MediVerse: A secure and scalable IoT-MR framework for real-time health and performance monitoring. *IEEE Access : Practical Innovations, Open Solutions*, *13*, 97511–97528. DOI: 10.1109/ACCESS.2025.3570731

Salunkhe, V., Tangudu, A., Mokkapati, C., Goel, P., & Aggarwal, A. (2024). Advanced encryption techniques in healthcare IoT: Securing patient data in connected medical devices. *Modern Dynamics: Mathematical Progressions*, *1*(2), 224–247. DOI: 10.36676/mdmp.v1.i2.22

Sandhiya, D. S., Karthikeyan, M. V., & Shanmuga Priya, M. (2022). Secured health monitoring system using AES. *East Asian Journal of Multidisciplinary Research*, *1*(6). Advance online publication. DOI: 10.55927/eajmr.v1i6.577

Si-Ahmed, A.. (2023). Survey of machine learning-based intrusion detection methods for Internet of Medical Things. *Applied Soft Computing*, *140*, 110227. DOI: 10.1016/j.asoc.2023.110227

Silva-Trujillo, A. G., González González, M. J., Rocha Pérez, L. P., & García Villalba, L. J. (2023). Cybersecurity analysis of wearable devices: Smartwatches passive attack. *Sensors (Basel)*, *23*(5438). Advance online publication. DOI: 10.3390/s23125438 PMID: 37420605

Zheng, W., & Arakawa, Y. (2025). A review of wearables-based activities of daily living recognition with LLMs: Overview, progress, and trends. *IEEE Access : Practical Innovations, Open Solutions*, *13*, 143813–143830. DOI: 10.1109/ACCESS.2025.3598088

Chapter 9
Implantable Medical Devices:
Navigating Types, Unveiling Risks, and Securing Solutions

Parita Rajiv Oza
https://orcid.org/0000-0001-9637-6157
Institute of Technology, Nirma University, India

Parishi Shah
https://orcid.org/0009-0005-8451-2920
Institute of Technology, Nirma University, India

Ashu Nareshbhai Pabreja
https://orcid.org/0009-0003-9422-1321
Institute of Technology, Nirma University, India

Smita Agrawal
https://orcid.org/0000-0003-0486-8045
Institute of Technology, Nirma University, India

ABSTRACT

Implantable Medical Devices (IMDs) play vital role in modern healthcare by enabling treatments, health monitoring, and improved patient capabilities. However, integrating electronics into IMDs raises serious security concerns. Unauthorized access can compromise patient privacy, manipulate data, and even threaten lives. Biometric authentication, including iris scans and patient-specific biometrics, is suggested to enhance security. Lightweight protocols are proposed to ensure authentication and confidentiality while conserving energy and extending battery life. The paper addresses risks associated with unauthorized access to radio channels

DOI: 10.4018/979-8-3373-4412-6.ch009

used by IMDs, highlighting the importance of encryption and secure communication. Advanced cryptographic techniques, such as block ciphers and lightweight encryption schemes, are explored to reinforce IMD security. These cryptographic methods help maintain data integrity and confidentiality, safeguarding sensitive patient information from malicious threats.

1. INTRODUCTION

IMDs (Hassija et al., 2021) are devices that work on electronics that can be implanted in the inpatient's body as a treatment for an illness, monitor the health or function of organs, or give the patient a potential they didn't have before. Artificial joints, pacemakers, various cardiac implants, including ICDs (Halperin, Heydt-Benjamin, Ransford, etal., 2008; Xu et al., 2011; Zheng, Yang, Valli, Qiao, Shankaran, Orgun, & Mukhopadhyay, 2019) (Implantable Cardiovascular Defibrillators), biosensors (Alfian et al., 2018;Cherukuri et al., 2003; Gia et al., 2019), and Neuro-stimulators (Marin et al., 2018) for deep brain stimulation in conditions like epilepsy and Parkinson's disease are some of the most prevalent examples of IMDs.

Numerous implantable devices currently on the market exhibit data like a patient's information, a older diagnosis, and their treatment history. Another significant source of security vulnerabilities is the wireless connection functionality included in many current IMDs (Panescu, 2008). Additionally, it makes it easier for listeners who want to inter- cept data transmissions to do so. As IMDs contain private information like vital signs, diseases that have been diagnosed, treatments, and a variety of personal details like allergies and prescriptions, this might lead to a significant privacy breach (Halperin, Heydt-Benjamin, Fu, et al., 2008a). The worries of the former vice president of USA, Dick Cheney, serve as a prime illustration in this regard. He had an ICD replaced with one that was lacking WiFi functionality (Franzen, 2013).

Figure 1. PRISMA Flow Diagram and Selection Method

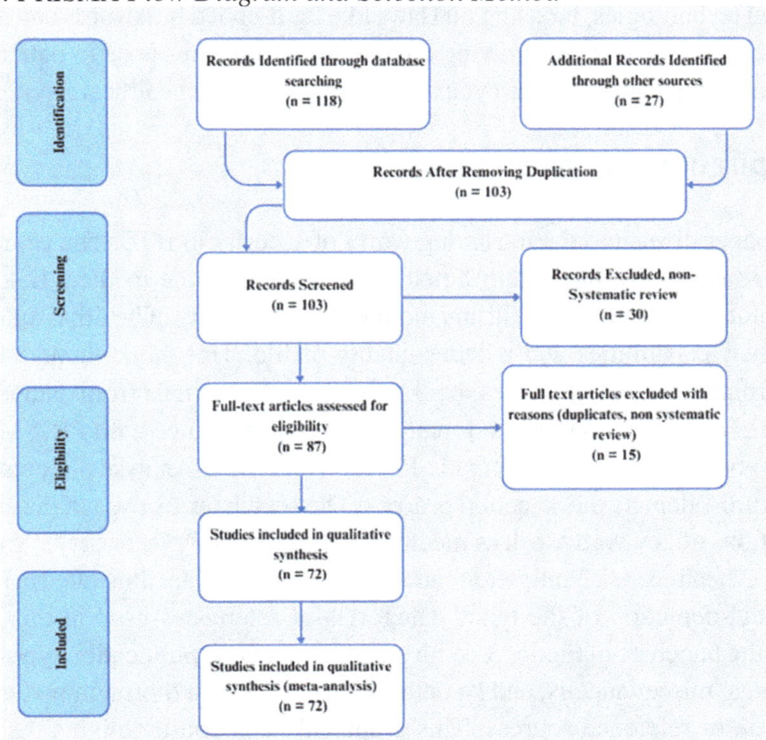

In order to guarantee that the data is saved and sent safely, as well as that it is genuine and authentic, it is vital to ensure the safety of the information in the IMDs. To prevent unauthorized inputs from attackers, data privacy means that the data can only be accessed by those who are authorized to view and use it. Attacks on an IMD have the potential to be lethal, endangering the patient who is carrying it and jeopardizing their safety. The FDA (U.S. Food and Drug Administration) (Camara et al., 2015) has recognized that deliberately causing an implant to malfunction can be fatal.

The new FDA cybersecurity rules (2023) and NIST security controls (SP 800-53 and SP 800-183) are deemed to conform to the new IMD development guidelines. Additionally, new research into applying artificial intelligence for real-time anomaly detection has extended the scope to encompass non-traditional security controls.

A variety of security techniques may appeal to different patients rather than a single security method being beneficial to all patients. There are a number of issues for se- curing wireless IMDs and (Denning et al., 2010) offers advice for future designs based on findings and observations.

Authors of (Mej´ıa-Granda et al., 2024) review real-world security issues found in medical technologies, focusing on flaws like hard-coded passwords and outdated software. It emphasizes the growing risks these weaknesses pose to patient safety and the importance of stronger cyber security practices in healthcare systems.

1.1 Inspiration and evaluation criteria

This paper dives into the intriguing world of security in IMDs and examine the numerous factors that have contributed to their status in the medical field. IMDs have revolutionized the treatment and monitoring of a variety of health issues, giving patients new capabilities and a better quality of life. This work surveys multiple articles from various conferences, books and indexed journals from databases like Scopus, IEEE, Science Direct and many more in compliance with PRISMA (Preferred Reporting Items for Systematic Reviews and Meta-Analyses) recommendations. Figure 1 depicts the selection process. The search terms used in the study are combinations of keywords such as medical", "implantable", "security", "wireless", "privacy", "healthcare", "mitigation" and many more which are illustrated in Figure 2.

A visual depiction of the many categories of references used in this work is given by the bar chart in Figure 3. With respect to various publication type articles, proceedings, miscellaneous, and so on the chart provides a thorough picture of the distribution of reference sources. This graphical depiction highlights the various sources that add to the academic conversation around IMDs and it's security.

Figure 2. Reference Papers with respect to Keywords

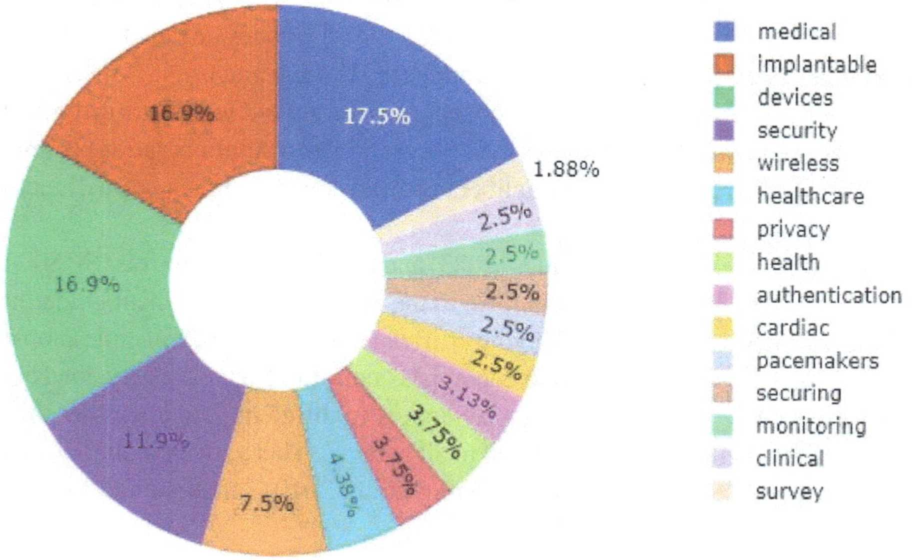

New security problems have surfaced as a result of the introduction of wireless connectivity in many modern IMDs. They are potential targets for security lapses and unauthorised access to patient data because these devices store private and sensitive information. Such violations could have serious repercussions that endanger the patients' safety and wellbeing.

In this paper, we attempt to answer a few essential queries about the safety and privacy of IMDs. We hope that by the end, you will have a better knowledge of the potential risks involved and the steps being taken to ensure the safe and secure use of IMDs within modern healthcare.

We explored the area of Implantable Medical Technology and attempt to answer the following questions:

1. Can there be security breaches in IMDs?
2. What are some common instances of IMDs and their uses?
3. Can IMDs be hacked?

Figure 3. References in relation to Type

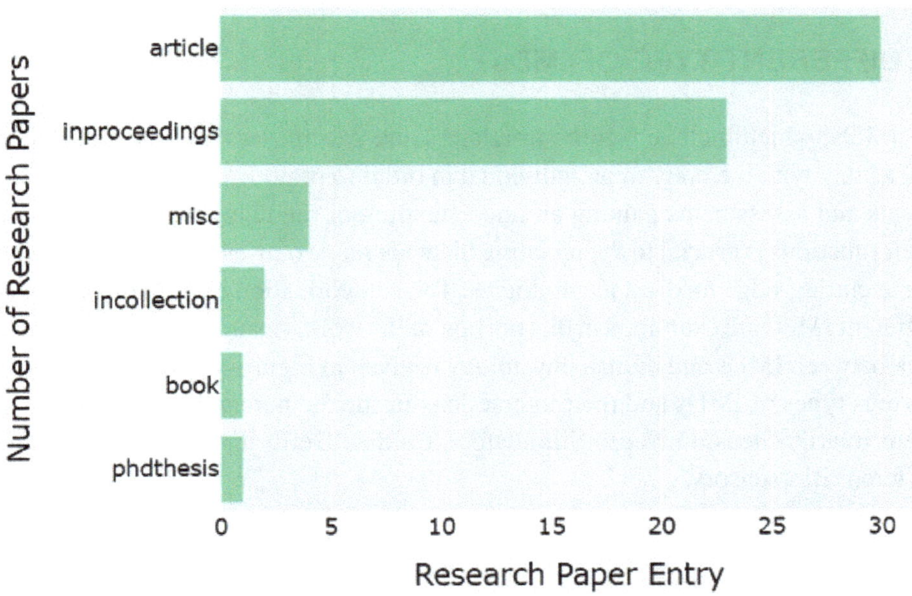

4. What are the risks associated with IMDs?
5. How can we reduce risks of IMDs?

6. What are the six general categories of attacks on IMDs?
7. What are the existing technologies for securing IMDs?
8. Are there any remaining challenges that require additional research for securing IMDs?

1.2 Paper organization

The following describes the paper's overall structure. Readers can find descriptions of a few IMDs, including pacemakers, cardiovascular implants, Neuro-stimulators, and more, in Section 2. In the third section, Section 3, we discussed a brief overview of the risks connected to IMDs. The requirements for securing IMDs are discussed in Section 4, with a focus on five types. Section 5 examines existing IMD security technologies. While Section 6 highlights a comparative analysis of the most effective IMD security mechanisms. In Section 7, we have discussed some of the main research issues, challenges and the future direction. Section 8 highlights the regulatory, ethical, and security practices in IMDs. Section 9 elaborates on additional research issues, challenges, and possible future directions. Finally, the paper ends with a conclusion in Section 10.

2. DIFFERENT TYPE OF IMDs

IMDs, which include Neuro-stimulators and pacemakers are made to interact intricately with the body of an individual in order to provide precise medical treatments and assessments gaining an understanding of the many types of IMDs and their functions is crucial to appreciating the wide range of uses and consequences of these cutting-edge medical technologies. The categorization and characteristics of different IMDs are examined in this portion of the work. A summary of the complex link between IMDs and human physiology is given in Figure 4 which illustrates the various types of IMDs and their interactions inside the human body. In this paper, we primarily focus on Neuro-Stimulators, Cardiac Defibrillators, Pacemaker and different Bio-sensors.

Figure 4. IMDs and our Body

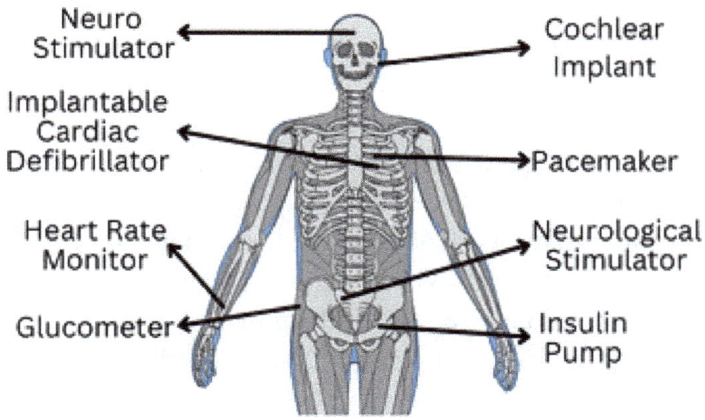

2.1 Cardiac Implanted Devices

Figure 5. Cardiac Implantable Devices

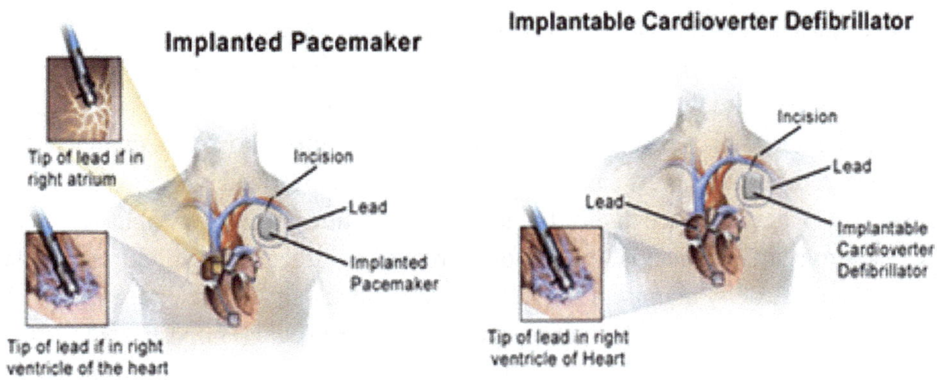

The Figure 5 includes devices like pacemakers and ICD (Implantable Cardioverter Defibrillators). They are made to care cardiac ailments by keeping an eye on the electrical activity of the heart and providing electrical impulses at the right places and intensities to get the heart to beat at the proper rate.

Dr. Paul Zoll (Hassija et al., 2021) developed the first cardiac pacemaker, which was an external technology. When implants were first implanted in patients, Wilson Greatbatch and Dr. William Chardack achieved the first significant advancements on an implanted pacemaker.

Modern medical devices use medical implant communication services. This operates in the range of 402 to 405 megahertz to relay telemetry and change treatments. This service provides a significantly longer read range of 2 to 5 meters and a larger bandwidth of 250 kbps. In contrast, the former pacemaker and ICD generations used limited bandwidth (50 kbps) contactless power transfer at low frequencies (around 175 kHz) with a small read range (8 cm). Low-frequency inductive coupling (175 kHz) is commonly used in implantable devices like pacemakers and cochlear implants, offering 1015% power transfer efficiency over short distances (8cm). While limited by coil size and alignment sensitivity, it supports compact implants with battery life spans of 510 years through periodic recharging and low-duty-cycle operation.

Transmission of pacemaker data over a cellular network or the Internet is another possibility. For initial activation, many existing ICDs, for instance, use near-field communication (such as a wand near the chest). After activation, the doctor can operate the device for a longer duration and at a greater distance. Given that patients IMDs might be vulnerable to long-range wireless communications after leaving the clinic, a programming session increased range and duration increases exposure and risk for patients.

Even though pacemakers (Barold et al., 2008) and ICDs generally save lives, they occasionally malfunction. These devices' safety concerns have drawn a lot of attention. Pacemakers are almost equally vulnerable to security risks as other devices that can access external systems or are connected to larger networks for diagnostics and updates. These devices include built-in programmable computer systems all of which are open to hacker infiltration and attacks. As more hospitals connected to the Internet, the attacks grew easier (Fu, 2009). An unauthorized individual could be able to take over the device thanks to these vulnerabilities. The user might very well alter the program commands to function as required, either by rapidly draining the battery resource or by inappropriate defibrillator shocks. In a worst-case event, such actions may lead to the targeted patient's death. Halperin et al (Halperin et al., 2008) performed the first security analysis of an ICD with wireless capabilities in 2008.

- Modern versions of Pacemakers and ICDs come with pressure sensors that can track changes that could trigger heart failure. This makes it possible to warn the inpatient when a pressure increase in the ventricle is detected, as this might put the patient's condition at a significant risk.
- Accelerometers may also be incorporated in cardiac implants in order to analyse the patient's level of physical activity.
- Ventricles are the source of irregular beats known as irregular ventricular heartbeats. In this case, a rapid pulse stops the oxygen-dense blood from getting to the brain along with other bodily portions. If it is not addressed

Figure 6. Neuro-Stimulator in DBS (Jmarchn, 2021)

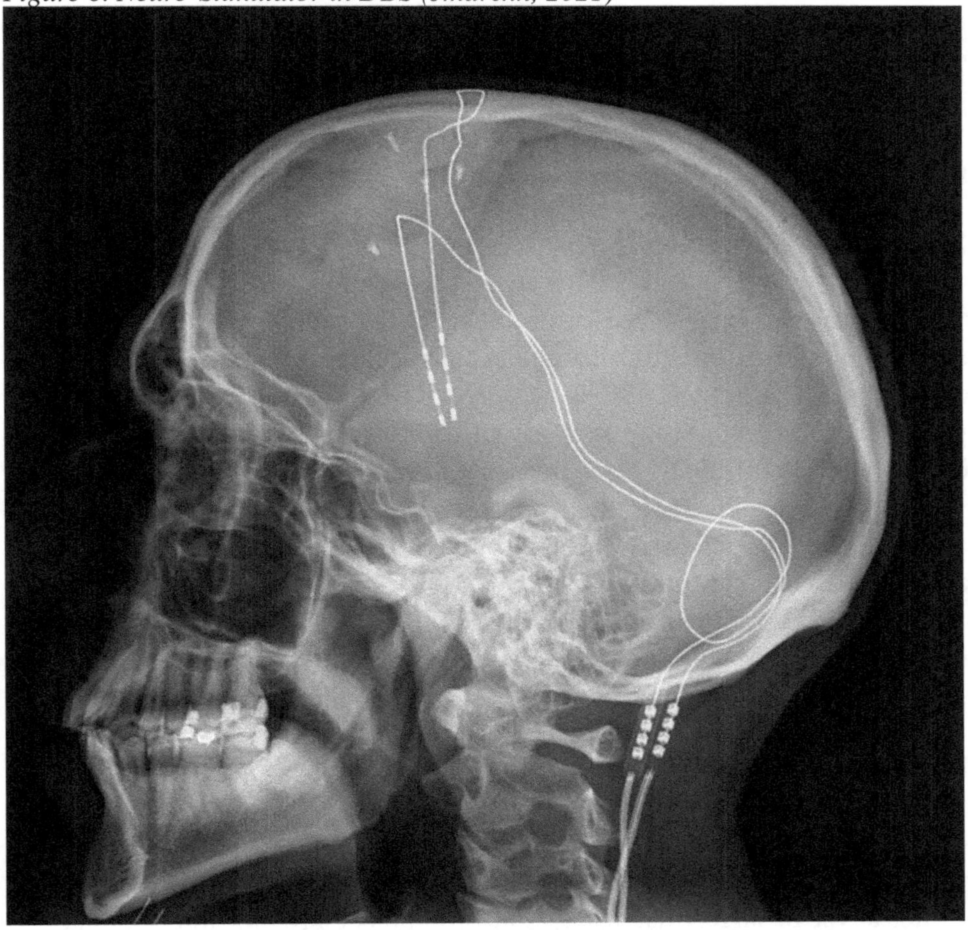

immediately, it could result in cardiac arrest. It is possible to program an ICD to commence treatment as soon as it detects an abnormal pulse.

- Some ICDs are also featured with a pacemaker to recover the inpatient's pulses to normal rhythm in the instance that it slows down.When the heart's electrical signals that coordinate the heartbeats don't work properly, it can cause an irregular heartbeat, also known as a heart arrhythmia. Bradycardia is a type of arrhythmia where the heart beats too slowly, fewer than 60 times a minute. In this situation, electrical signals are sent to the heart to correct the fluctuation from the regular, healthy heartbeat

Today's modern pacemakers usually have batteries that last 7 to 13 years, however this wasn't always the case. In the past, a voluntary recall of 350,000 implanted defibrillators (Hassija et al., 2021) was issued by the FDA, a government body in US that deals with issues relating to public health, due to the battery issues. Upgrades were made to minimize the possibility of patient damage from premature battery depletion.

2.2 Neuro - Stimulators

Clinicians use implantable Neuro-stimulators to perform various neuromodulation therapies for diseases, disorders, and injuries that cause behavioral issues and chronic pain. These stimulators are designed to treat chronic pain and offer a non-pharmacological approach to pain management (Peckham & Ackermann, 2018). They employ electromagnetic waves to transmit a stimulus, such as an electrical signal which is of low amplitudes, to a particular body site, causing neuromodulation in the affected anatomical regions. Depending on the patient's condition, these electrodes are implanted in highly precise locations. A few ranges of approaches include:

- Responsive Neuro-Stimulation (RNS)

RNS is an epilepsy treatment that uses Neuro-stimulators to help prevent seizure before they begin.

- Deep Brain Stimulation (DBS)

It is a type of surgery that includes the insertion of a Neuro-stimulator into the brain. The apparatus utilizes sensors strategically positioned to administer accurate electrical messages to specific brain nuclei, as illustrated in Figure 6. Neurological movement disorders such as Parkinson's syndrome, vital tremor, and epilepsy can be effectively treated with this form of therapy. Since 1997, the FDA has granted approval for the utilization of this medicine in the management of vital tremors and Parkinson's syndrome. DBS was granted authorization for the management of dystonia in 2003 and OCD (Obsessive Compulsive Disorder) in 2009. In 2018, there were advancements made in the field of epilepsy. Extensive research has been carried out on DBS as a possible remedy for chronic pain and numerous mood disorders, including severe depression. DBS surgery is indicated when the patient's quality of life remains inadequate despite getting optimal medical care from a professional in movement disorders. DBS therapy improves the physical symptoms of Parkinson's disease, including tremor, rigidity, and bradykinesia. DBS has the capacity to mitigate tremors, even in instances where medication has proven to be useless.

- Vague Nerve Stimulation (VNS) (Ben-Menachem, 2012)

It is a surgical procedure wherein an instrument is inserted to deliver periodic and gentle electrical sensations to the brain via the vagal (vagus) nerve. The device bears resemblance to a pacemaker and is surgically inserted beneath the skin in the left thoracic region. An electrode or wire is affixed to the generator device and positioned subcutaneously, while the wire is fastened or coiled around the vagal nerve in the cervical region. The electrical sensations propagate to the brain, where it is distributed to various regions to modify the functioning of brain cells. Patients often do not experience sensory perception of the pulses, and there is no direct manipulation of the brain during this surgical procedure. VNS is a form of therapy that is only available to a specific group of persons who have epilepsy or treatment-resistant depression.

They have a battery with a finite potential that can't be refilled or changed, restricted computing capability, and limited memory storage. The only alternative available to the patient when the battery fails is surgery to replace the implanted device.

In 2018, a team of security professionals from KU Leuven institute (Marin, 2018) examined the possible vulnerabilities in Neuro-stimulators. The security flaws discovered in the Neuro-stimulator and device programmer could seriously endanger the safety of these devices. The flaws were related to the unauthenticated and unencrypted messages used for communication between the implant and the device programmer. These vulnerabilities could allow a hacker to gain access to sensitive neurological data, vital medical data, and even electrical shocks that are being exchanged between the implant and the device programmer.

The majority of contemporary Neuro-stimulator models are remotely capable, allowing for wireless supervision and reconfiguration with a separate device. The wireless interface allows for more adaptable and personalized medical care, yet it also offers adversaries the capability to launch software-based attacks. A Neuro-stimulator could receive hostile commands from adversaries if robust security protocols aren't in position. The Neurostimulator's settings, for instance, may be altered by adversaries to increase the signal voltage that is continuously sent to the inpatient's mind. This might make the patient unable to talk or move, impair his brain permanently or, worse yet, risk his life.

2.3 Bio - Sensors

The capacity of implantable biosensors to offer real time information regarding the concentrations of a target element makes them a crucial type of biosensor. This makes it possible to track trends and variations in sample levels continuously, either for the inpatient or the practitioner who has to get involved. This eliminates the need for repeat testing, which is often required to monitor the levels of analytes in clinical medicine. Implantable biosensors therefore offer enormous promise for use in diagnosis and monitoring (Gray et al., 2018).

These could be anything from very low bit rate systems for measuring glucose or other body enzymes to high bit rate imaging systems for the brain or eyes. For instance, an implanted glucose sensor [Figure 7] senses the patient's blood glucose levels continually and remotely connects to the insulin pump in order to regulate the necessary blood sugar level.

Figure 7. Glucose Bio-Sensor

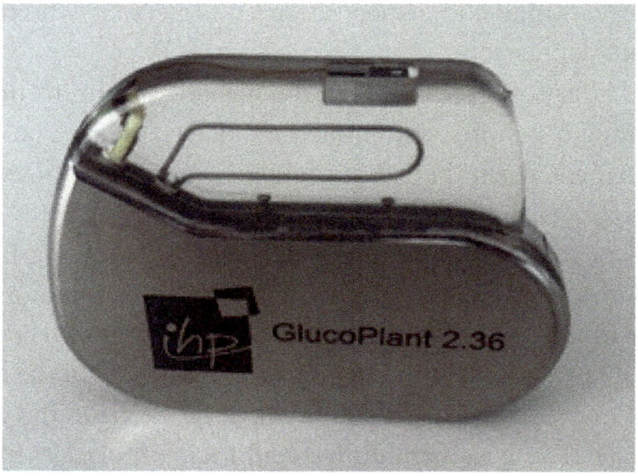

Categories of biosensors:

- Biocatalyst-based
- Tissue-based
- Deoxyribonucleic Acid based
- Immunosensors
- Piezoelectric and Thermal Biosensors

The majority of implanted biosensors combine a functional/active material with a layer of polymer as a flexible and adaptable structural support to generate, transmit, and process the generated signal (Zbiciak & Markiewicz, 2023). A biosensor implanted under the skin performs a mini-experiment on a sensor at the molecular or electrochemical level as part of a subcutaneous sensor. Subcutaneous sensors that are now being developed are more sophisticated and can simultaneously calibrate for temperature and pH, detect drugs and endogenous human compounds. A unique set of privacy and security measures are needed for subcutaneous biosensors. Small, infrequent wireless transmissions provide a bigger privacy risk than massive, continuous broadcasts, which is a major issue with completely implanted sensors.

There are two danger scenarios that were recognised:

(i) A rogue implant has an authorized patch removed and replaced (Example: falsified information to commit insurance fraud).
(ii) A trusted implant's data is taken using a malicious patch (Example: theft of private health information).

Biosensor data must be protected on several different levels, including during measurement and processing, from outside observers (sometimes referred to as side-channel attackers), during communication with third parties, and during storage from unauthorized users. To reach these goals, numerous algorithms and standards have been developed and thoroughly examined. The widely accepted Advanced Encryption Standard, or AES (Khader et al., 2017), originated by the National Institute of Standards and Technology (NIST) in 2001. It is a widely used encryption method.

The AES block cipher accepts 128 bits as input and returns 128 bits of secure cipher text as output by encrypting data into blocks of 128 bits each. Because of its reliance on the SPN (Substitution Permutation Network) principle, it is carried out through a sequence of interconnected processes that entail rearranging and replacing input data. AES's important characteristics are that it is an iterative cipher, as opposed to a Feistel cipher, that it is built on a SPN, and that it consists of a number of connected operations. Even while AES is more difficult to build than DES (Data Encryption Standard) and triple DES, it is still frequently used today since it is significantly powerful.

3. RISKS AROUND THE IMDs

3.1 Analogue Attacks

All electronic circuit includes components that, under specific conditions, can act as an antenna. When this happens, these parts are able to collect EMI (Electro-Magnetic Interference) radiation from other devices, such as MRI (Magnetic Resonance Imaging) equipment. Creating IMDs has been the subject of a great deal of research throughout the last many years that are resistant to unintentional, high-power EMI. However, a number of reported incidents have been allegedly linked to EMI in IMDs. The FDA has taken precautions to minimize the hazards after recognizing that EMI could cause IMDs to malfunction.

3.2 Battery Leakage

The primary alternative for powering IMDs at the moment is lithium-ion batteries. However, using them comes with a lot of risks (Kuykendal, 2018). Batteries may cause gadgets to malfunction, hazardous chemicals to seep into a person's body, or heat releases. A decline in the battery's ability can result in unforeseen errors or early shutdowns, which would have serious consequences for the patient.

3.3 Software Updates

Manufacturers may issue upgrades to their IMDs to enhance the functionality and security of their products after discovering security vulnerabilities or defects in the device firmware. If these upgrades are not thoroughly tested before being rolled out, issues like battery drain, sudden shutdowns, new vulnerabilities, and device malfunction or breakdowns may occur.

3.4 Infections

Although infections may occasionally arise as a result of complications that can occur at any moment between the pre-operative diagnostic and post-operative care, modern IMDs are very seldom contagious. A patient may have inserted gadget-related infections if they meet the criteria for SIRS (Systemic Inflammatory Response Syndrome) (Kalil & Pinsky, 2019). At least two of the following four symptoms must be present in order to meet the clinical criterion for SIRS. The symptoms are:

- Body temperature is not in the range 96.8 F to 100.4 F.
- Pulse rate is higher than 90/min.
- Respiratory rate is higher than 20/min.
- WBC count is $<4000/\mu L$ or $>12{,}000/\mu L$.

Only in these circumstances can the implanted device be regarded as a potential source of infection.

3.5 Risks due to Restricted Capabilities

IMDs have limited abilities in 3 areas: Computational Power, Energy and Storage. These three have security consequences, either because device can be exploited or because of security limits.

Energy

IMDs have an integrated battery that provides power to all of the device's functionalities (i.e. monitoring, treatment, communication, etc.). After the IMD has been implanted, the battery can last somewhere between 8 years for Neurostimulators and 10 years for pacemakers (Mallela et al., 2004). Battery consumption directly affects how long an implant lasts. It needs to be replaced when it gets over, which entails surgery and hence the related risks. Some designs allow charging of batteries by magnetic field, although this results in a risk to the nearby organs (Jiang et al., 2013).

Storage

In today's IMDs, storage is greatly limited. The device's memory is designed to store historical information about various incidents and episodes that are associated to the patient's pathology. Due to the limited memory available on the chip, security features must use as little memory as possible in order to free up space for potential storage needs associated with the device's medical functions. Given that RAM (Random-access memory) memory is now not expensive, one might wonder if the RAM capacity of IMDs could be increased. The current memory size restrictions for IMDs are justified for two main reasons. Firstly, increasing memory capacity would result in a larger sized implant, which is not ideal as IMDs are frequently placed inside the patient's body and the device area should be kept to a minimum. Secondly, even if device size is not an issue, increasing memory could impact the battery lifetimes as access operations are considered demanding in terms of power consumption. Larger battery sizes could be used to avoid this, but this can quickly become impractical to implant. The challenges faced by IMDs (Park et al., 2011) include size limitations, inaccessibility, the need to work continuously and biocompatibility.

Computing Power (Camara et al., 2015)

Due to power constraints, IMDs have very limited computation and communication capabilities. IMD's most energy-intensive activity is communication. So, if communications are minimized, battery life can be increased.

4. SECURITY

4.1 Security Modes

Some authors have suggested utilizing an additional device in addition to direct connection between a programmer and the IMDs (E.g. Shield IMD Guard (Xu et al., 2011) which acts as a proxy).

Figure 8. Security Theft Model

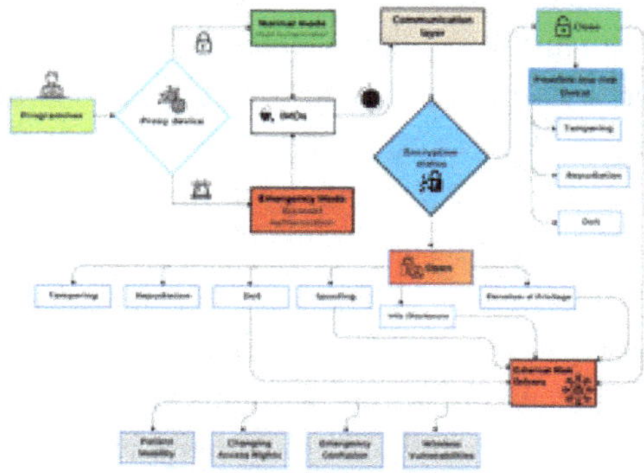

As illustrated in Figure 8, the IMD assigns this responsibility to a other gadget that verifies the coder instead of establishing a direct connection with them. Once they have been authenticated, the programmer can connect with the IMD via the external device using an encrypted channel (normal mode operation). However, in emergency mode, the IMD needs to function even if the verification process fails, and in some situations, the healthcare team needs to be able to turn the device off fast.

IMDs won't always interact with the same gadgets because patients frequently travel to various sites and may consult different physicians and hospitals. Additionally, the parties permitted to communicate with the implant can change. Because not every indication obtained through IMD will actually originate from approved programmers, and their intentions could be malicious, it is also important to take into account the potential attackers. To ensure an inpatient's health in these circumstances, it is crucial to ensure the secrecy of the device.

An IMD has to work in two distinct options, Emergency and Normal, as stated in the context (Camara et al., 2015). Finding the most favorable choices among the two scenarios is one of the main goals:

- Normal operation mode:

The inpatient decides who is allowed to communicate with his IMD. In order to prevent harmful and unauthorized accesses, it is necessary to set up both cryptographic algorithms and robust access control mechanisms in the medium of communication. Untargeted data queries or device requests must be rejected by the IMD.

- Emergency mode:

The capacity to be reachable in an emergency situation is equally as crucial as providing robust access control, encrypted communication, and even imperceptibility. Imagine someone who shows up to the emergency department at another healthcare facility where he is registered. Consider that the patient is traveling to a different country to add to the difficulty. The healthcare team will be able to interact with the implanted gadget, recognize it (by number of model and brand, for example), obtain the physical details of the medication, and change its settings as needed. Even though there is a safe plan, it is important for an IMD to respond before deactivation, even in emergency situations such as urgent surgery. This is highlighted in several studies. When the IMD is in emergency mode, it must respond even if authorization is unsuccessful, and healthcare workers may need to be able to quickly disable the device.

In a crisis, an easy way to give the person receiving treatment the necessary safety is to instruct the IMD to ignore authorization and identification mechanisms to process any receiving commands.Any applicant who does it becomes a legitimate user, possibly with full access. If significant controls on access and security measures were not eliminated, the implant wouldn't be able to do this, making it entirely open to assault. Unfortunately, distinguishing between regular and emergency conditions is difficult for the IMD, and the best solution (Rostami et al., 2013;Denning et al., 2008) to offer proper security for IMDs is currently a work in progress.

NOTE

Using the STRIDE methodology, the security threats can be classified. The mnemonic stands for six main types of attacks:

- Confidentiality breach is known as - Information disclosure
- Authentication breach - Spoofing
- Availability breach - Denial of service
- Authoriation breach - Elevation of privilege
- Integrity breach - Tampering
- Non-Repudiation breach - Repudiation

4.2 Security Requirements

To understand the specific issues of balancing security with safety and efficacy, we must first examine how typical computer security principles such as confidentiality, integrity, availability, etc apply to IMDs.

Recent advancements in wireless Implantable Medical Devices (IMDs) have posed severe security issues, especially during emergency conditions where traditional authentication processes are bypassed. Studies have shown that the devices are susceptible to various attack channels, such as replay attack, where attackers repeat the intercepted commands to modify the device's operation, and eavesdropping, where patient-sensitive data are intercepted through insecure channels. To address these security loopholes, lightweight cryptographic methods like AES encryption, Elliptic Curve Cryptography (ECC), and HMAC have been proposed to ensure data confidentiality, integrity, and authenticity. In the meantime, these remain feasible for the resource-constrained nature of IMDs (Zheng et al., 2019). Combined with these, nonce-based session tokens also resist replay-based intrusions. Apart from these methods, researchers have proposed biometric-based authentication models and intrusion detection systems that support emergency override functionality while logging activities for further forensic analysis (Zheng et al., 2018; Siddiqi et al., 2021). Collectively, these assist in developing the core security pillars in wireless IMD designs.

The main six pillars of security are illustrated in Figure 9.

Confidentiality

The provider's standards for ideal health care include privacy and confidentiality as per HIPAA (Health Insurance Portability and Accountability Act), 1996 (Murray et al., 2011). Only registered parties have access to the information, no matter if it is wirelessly transferred or saved on the gadget. Listening devices can access the channel used by IMDs and the programmer for communication in the range of 401-406 MHz If communications are not protected, an opponent might leak sensitive data such as model of IMD or an inpatient's medical data (Patel et al., 2023). As a consequence, the implant holder's privacy would be jeopardized. It's probable that an outsider to trace the device or more seriously, follow its person around even though conversations are secured. In this instance, the privacy of the location would be jeopardized.

Figure 9. Security Requirements

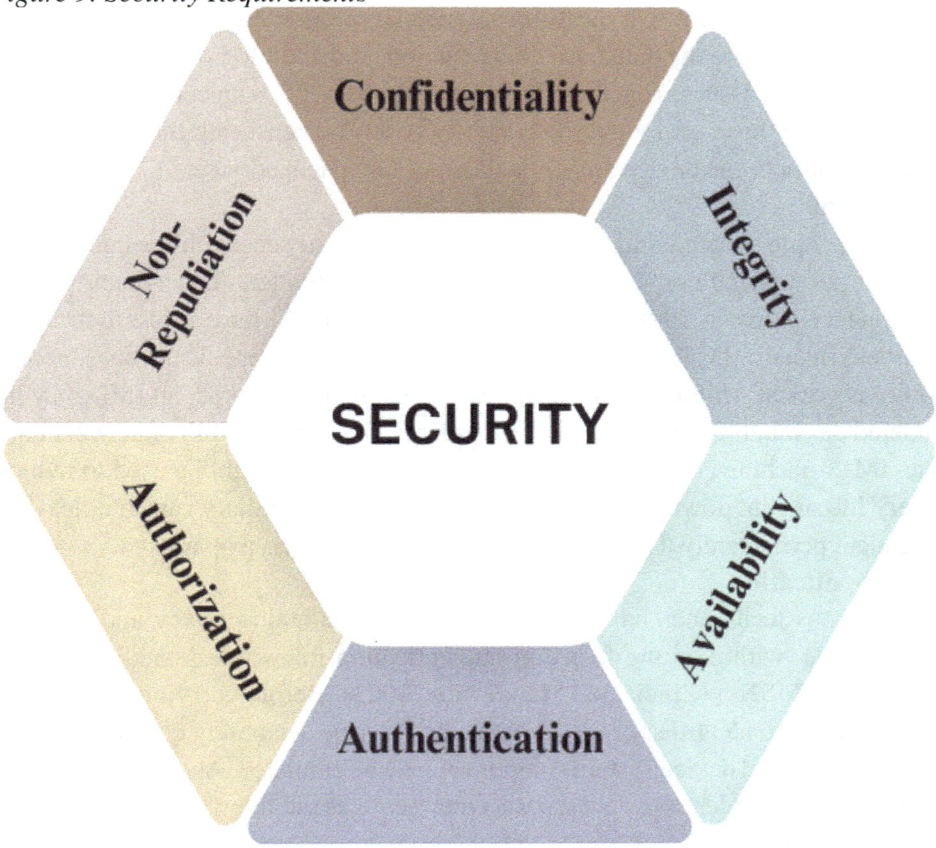

Integrity

In October 2018, the Center for Drug Evaluation and Research (CDER), FDA, and the United Kingdom Medicines and Healthcare Products Regulatory Agency (MHRA-UK) co-hosted their first GCP workshop, which featured perspectives from both organizations on the value of data quality management practices for data integrity (Khin et al., 2020). Only registered parties are allowed to edit data, no matter if it is wirelessly transferred or saved on the gadget. Data transmission via an unsecured radio channel may result in data alteration if the IMD lacks an integrity-checking mechanism. Moreover, harmful inputs that are intended to carry out an attack based on code injection may be accepted by the IMD. However, the absence of verification of integrity facilitates data modifications that can go undetected over time. Data integrity is therefore a key component of service delivery at all levels and an essential factor in the medical sector . To ensure data integrity in implantable medical devices (IMDs), both hardware and software work together. On the hardware side, features like secure boot and Trusted Execution Environments (TEEs) protect the device from unauthorized changes, while Hardware Security Modules (HSMs) keep sensitive data safe. On the software side, cryptographic hashing and digital signatures make sure the data hasn't been altered, and audit logs track all activities to help detect any issues. Together, these measures help IMDs meet important safety standards, like those set by the FDA and IEC 80001-1, ensuring the security and reliability of both the device and patient data. (Vimalachandran et al., 2016)

Availability

More people are realizing these days how significantly accessible clinical detail is for corporate health organizations that use virtual inpatient data as their central component (Espinosa, 1998). Permitted users should always have access to the IMD facilities. Because IMDs are used to address their owner's medical issues, accessibility is critical. Unfortunately, if the radio channel is disrupted, an IMD may be rendered unavailable (active jamming). Sending a radio channel full of network data to an IMD machine is another way to overwhelm it. This might be used to reduce battery life or shut down the gadget. In the event that the battery runs out, leaving the gadget permanently useless, the patient's health may be jeopardized.

Authentication

Numerous techniques have been developed to maintain privacy and security requirements, with a strong focus on authentication for wireless medical sensor networks (WMSNs) (Zbiciak & Markiewicz, 2023). Before carrying out for any other action, the identities of the participants must be accurately confirmed. Any implanted medical device system component may be emulated. As an illustration, if the programmer's identity is altered, this may serve as the foundation for an attack to escalate privileges.

Authorization (Halperin et al., 2008)

- Personal authorization: Different groups of people are capable of performing different tasks. After their personal identities have been verified, for instance, patients or primary care doctors can be given particular powers. These privileges could be transferable to other entities depending on the authentication method.
- Role-based authorization: As per a job like a doctor or ambulance computer, an entity is permitted to perform a particular set of duties. The device's creator may also be given specific access based on their role in operating the gadget.
- IMD selection: An external entity must make sure it only connects with the specified devices when engaging multiple IMDs.

Access control systems and policies must ensure that just authorized individuals have access to sensitive records for legal reasons (Jin et al., 2009). In a medical setting, authorization and authentication might be extremely context sensitive. For instance, if a device identifies an emergency condition, authorization standards may be relaxed on the theory that the patient will be less harmed by a poorly authorized (or even anonymous) action than by no intervention.

Non-Repudiation

The IMD's tasks are safely recorded in the entrance log. The malignant actor may aim to eliminate these obligations to make a clear path. Naturally, not all IMDs come with a log-in mechanism. If this were the case, the opponent would have a repeatable route to the IMD and would not have to leave. If a logging system is active, the limits would be recorded regardless of whether an alert would be sent to the IMD holder to warn them if a dangerous situation should occur.

5. THE EXISTING TECHNOLOGIES IN SECURING IMDs

In the realm of securing IMDs, a variety of technologies and strategies have been developed to mitigate security risks and ensure the safe operation of these critical medical devices. These measures encompass a range of innovative approaches in areas such as biometric authentication and lightweight security protocols. Additionally, technologies such as Heart-to-Heart (H2H) authentication techniques utilizing electrocardiogram data for proximity verification, access control mechanisms like the IMD Guard system resistant to spoofing attacks, and the use of block cipher-based security protocols to safeguard IMD data play pivotal roles in enhancing the security of IMDs. The Table 1 presents a comprehensive overview of these technologies and strategies.

Table 1. List of existing technologies

Sr. no	Reference	Implantable Devices	Method Utilization
1	(Hasan, 2022)	IMDs	Provenance based approach
2	(Degada & Thapliyal, 2022)	IMDs	2-SGPAL
3	(Degada & Thapliyal, 2021)	IMDs	CCAL
4	(Wu et al., 2017)	IMDs	ACIMD
5	(Awan et al., 2019)	Cardiac Pacemaker	PLS
6	(Marin et al., 2018)	Neuro-stimulator	Physiological signals of the patient
7	(Halperin et al., 2008)	ICDs	Zero-power based on RF power harvesting
8	(Zheng et al., 2014)	IMDs	ESDS

continued on following page

Table 1. Continued

Sr. no	Reference	Implantable Devices	Method Utilization
9	(Yang et al., 2014)	IMDs	Zero-power Authentication
10	(Zheng et al., 2014)	IMDs	Body Double
11	(Hei & Du, 2011)	IMDs	Light-weight secure access control
12	(Xu et al., 2011)	ICDs	IMDGuard
13	(Wazid et al., 2018)	IMDs	Remote user authentication
14	(Ali et al., 2021)	IMDs	Data Mining, Ontologies, Bi-LSTM
15	(Gia et al., 2019)	Bio-sensors	Fog-based system
16	(Alfian et al., 2018)	Bio-sensors	BLE based sensors
17	(Alladi et al., 2021)	IMDs	HARCI
18	(Beck et al., 2011)	IMDs	Block cipher based security protocol
19	(Shahzadi et al., 2019)	IMDs	Chaotic-based key scheduling algorithm for the RC5
20	(Hei et al., 2010)	IMDs	SVM
21	(Cherukuri et al., 2003)	Bio-sensors	Biometrics
22	(Pirbhulal et al., 2016)	IMDs	Fuzzy vault based data authentication
23	(Denning et al., 2008)	IMDs	Communication Cloakers
24	(Rasmussen et al., 2009)	IMDs	Distance-based access protocol
25	(Pirbhulal et al., 2018)	IMDs	Authenticate by Bio-keys
26	(Rathore et al., 2020)	IMDs	Electrocardiogram authentication
27	(Hosseini-Khayat, 2011)	IMDs	Lightweight security protocol
28	(Zheng et al., 2019)	ICDs	F2H
29	(Ankaral et al., 2015)	IMDs	PHY
30	(Rostami et al., 2013)	IMDs	H2H

- Provanance based approach (Hasan, 2022)

Devices will maintain a secure and verifiable record of their configuration history, and any changes made to the configuration will be accompanied by their own secure record. This will make it possible to confirm the configuration's provenance and point of origins. One of the key points is that it allows after-fact investigation.

- 2-SGPAL (Degada & Thapliyal, 2022)

The paper describes a 2-phase sinusoidal clocking implementation of Symmetric Pass Gate Adiabatic Logic (2-SGPAL), which is designed to secure a lightweight cryptographic coprocessor. It helps to protect from the CPA attack,where CPA means correlation power analysis. This method is assessed with synchronous resonant Power Clock Generators (PCGs). Using the suggested logic, it is possible to create IMDs that are resilient to CPA and utilize less energy. Synchronous resonant power clock generators (SRPCGs) work by using special circuits that sync up with the device's operating frequency to efficiently transfer power, reducing energy waste. When we talk about energy consumption, SRPCGs are more efficient than many other wireless power methods, meaning they use less power overall. These systems are also designed to be resilient, meaning they can keep delivering power even when faced with issues like signal interference or external attacks. They stay stable by syncing their power delivery, and if something goes wrong, they can still function without losing power, making them reliable for implantable medical devices (IMDs).

- CCAL(Clocked CMOS Adiabatic Logic) (Degada & Thapliyal, 2021)

A single-rail CCAL is applied to develop sustainable and safe crypto hardware at a low frequency level for medical equipment. In contrast to their CMOS logic gate counterparts, CCAL logic gates saved around 48% more energy and improved security metrics performance by more than 95%. Side-channel attacks were possible with traditional CMOS logic-based cryptography circuit solutions in medical equipment. The CCAL-centered instance investigation effectively defended the encryption key leak and was also assessed in comparison to the CPA.

- ACIMD (Wu et al., 2017)

Access Control of IMDs (ACIMD) is a combination of two security mechanisms, specifically proximity verification which is distance checking mechanism and identity verification which is authentication mechanism. The ISO/IEC 9798-2 standard-compliant authentication mechanism and electrocardiogram signals are used to carry out proximity checking. The findings indicate that ACIMD has a 92.92% accuracy rate.

- PLS (Awan et al., 2019)

Physical Layer Security (PLS) methods make it possible to transmit confidential messages without utilising a key for encryption. Numerical electromagnetic simulations utilising a precise human model are used to assess the performance metric of secrecy capability. The secrecy capacity is evaluated by extrapolating a spherical grid of radius 1m to varying radius lengths using the free space path loss model.

This article aids in the development of the communication module for subcutaneous leadl free cardiac pacemakers with improved physical layer security.

- Physiological Signal (Marin et al., 2018)

A symmetrical encryption key is created inside the Neuro-stimulatorbased on the patient's physiological signals, and the result is transferred over a covert OOB (out-of-band) channel. This adds minimal computational overhead and communication overhead, offers a fair compromise within safety and lenient access in critical circumstances, and allows the Neuro-stimulator and gadget programmer to collaborate on a symmetric session key without exchanging any previous secrets.

- ESDS (Zheng et al., 2014)

An ESDS (ECG-based Secret Data Sharing) strategy does not require pre-deployed keys or credentials. Before transmission, a secret is hidden in the IMD using electrocardiograph (ECG) features, and the secret is then revealed using concurrently recorded ECG features. Additionally, it makes use of an upgraded fuzzy vault approach to conceal real points on a polynomial by using hash functions instead of chaff points.

- Body Double (Zheng et al., 2014)

A non-key based security offered by body double. It uses an external authentication proxy embedded in a gateway. It deviates an adversary attack by spoofing a communication link using the gateway rather than the IMD. During Emergencies, Access to the IMD is feasible without any encryption key by powering off or removing the gateway. This also helps to prevent battery depletion of the IMD due to repeated attacks by resisting the potential attacks.

- Secure Access Control (Hei & Du, 2011)

The novel scheme uses the patient's biometric information and the iris's data for authentication. This security method, meanwhile, might not be effective in an emergency (for instance, if the patient is in a coma). This method has 2 stages:

Stage 1: It contains core biometric data of the inpatient.

Stage 2: It capitalizes on patients' iris data for authentication.

- IMDGuard (Xu et al., 2011)

This method is a cooperation of 2 methods that provide security to the IMD. One is an access control method resistant to opposite spoofing assaults, while the second one is an electrocardiogram-based key without previously divulging shared confidential details. It is a comprehensive security approach for IMDs that relates to the heart to remain functional in case of emergencies when necessary security credentials are absent.

- Data Mining, Ontologies, Bi-LSTM (Bidirectional Long Short-Term Memory) (Ali et al., 2021)

Data mining techniques assist with lowering the dimension of the dataset through effective preprocessing. Ontologies offer a conceptual understanding of objects and features. Bi-LSTM differentiates the patient records to predict drug side effects and any abnormal condition possibilities.

- Fog-based System (Gia et al., 2019)

An IoT (Internet of Things) system with a network of sensors, smart gateways and fog computing may track contextual data like ambient temperature, humidity, and air quality as well as real-time signals like glucose, ECG, and other signals. It is a fall detection and remote health monitoring system.

- BLE based sensor (Alfian et al., 2018)

Bluetooth Low Energy (BLEs) is used to collect health indicators from sensor nodes while actual data is processed. The blood glucose can be predicted, this enables diabetes people to better control their conditions by themselves. The results revealed that based on machine-learning based classification, multilayer perceptron network makes predictions based on the sensor data received from the user. It also revealed that long short-term memory can correctly forecast blood sugar level on the present sensor data.

- HARCI(Healthcare Authentication protocol using Resource-constrained IoT devices) (Alladi et al., 2021)

HARCI is a strategy to achieve MFA(Multi-factor authentication) that uses physical basics for security named PUFs (Physical Unclonable Functions). Due to the various storage and energy constraints, the protocol is very lightweight. It has several security features like device security, untraceability, message integrity, and MFA and it is secure contrary to many malicious attacks like MITM (Man in the Middle attack), unauthorized entity entity gains, node manipulation, and replay attacks.

- Block cipher based Security (Beck et al., 2011)

The Artificial Accommodation System (AAS) is utilised to show the procedure. The block cipher based protocol features 2 modes:

Stream Mode: It aims to reduce the radio duty cycle.

Session Mode: It offers excellent protection for extremely sensitive data and a user authentication system based on roles.

- Chaotic-based key scheduling algorithm (Shahzadi et al., 2019)

The RC5 (Rivest Cipher) approach is an assured and straightforward cryptosystem. Which is recognized as a good block cipher for resource constrained contexts, such as BAN (Body Area Network), because of its simplicity, quick encryption, and minimal memory consumption. A suggested chaotic-based key scheduling system uses 2-D chaotic maps to produce round keys that are used as symmetric keys for encryption and decryption operations. It is highly challenging to trace this chaos-based key, and it is quite challenging to decrypt the cipher.

- SVM (Hei et al., 2010)

Support Vector Machine (SVM) is a scheme mainly addressed to Resource Depletion (RD) attacks. This type of attack can drain the battery power of the IMD. It can reduce the resources of a few years to a few weeks. This can have very severe repercussions on the patient's condition. According to the experimental findings, the SVM-based system can identify RD attacks with a success rate of 97% for non-linear SVMs and 90% for linear SVMs, respectively.

- Biometrics (Cherukuri et al., 2003)

In this method, the keying material is secured by leveraging biometrics that originates from the inpatient's own body. With this approach, there is no longer any requirement for significant calculation or pointless communication. The requirements for randomization in biometric and measurement inaccuracy are two of the major problems associated with the adoption of biometrics. The issues are addressed through the application of codes that correct errors and various biometrics to secure the key.

- Fuzzy vault based data authentication (Pirbhulal et al., 2016)

This method is about developing an Intel Galileo based WBSN (Wireless Body Sensor Network) platform. The ECG (Electrocardiogram) signals are used to authenticate data in WBSNs using entity identifications (EIs). The performances of these methods are compared using software Matlab.

- Communication Cloakers (Denning et al., 2008)

Communication Cloakers is a new, fail-open defensive technique that aims to find a good equilibrium between safety in the normal course of events and safety in abnormal circumstances in IMDs. Cloakers are outwardly worn devices that keep safe the security of IMD when worn, but in cases of emergency, they allow access when removed.

- Distance-based access protocol (Rasmussen et al., 2009)

This approach relies on ultrasonic inter space bounding and solely permits access to devices that are very close to it. It relies on a brand-new, arbitrary message-authenticating proximity-based message validation technique. In a simulated patient setting, the viability of this strategy was evaluated.

- Authentication by bio-keys (Pirbhulal et al., 2018)

A secure decentralised means of communication is proposed for IoMT(Internet of Medical Things) inter-sensor medical data transmission that takes into consideration energy usage and reduces key length variability. Every person has unique corporeal and biotic functions. Therefore, it may be possible to secure IoMT by using physical traits. Bio-keys are designed to prevent hacking, making it harder for an intruder to access patient details, and to ensure that people may communicate safely.

- Electrocardiogram Authentication (Rathore et al., 2020)

Ensuring the security of IMDs is crucial to preventing severe health consequences. Software and hardware may be compromised by attacks that affect everything from systems to the built environment. Biometric and cryptographic authentication methods, machine learning, and wearable devices have been proposed. Existing solutions, however, are cumbersome for memory-constrained equipment or call for extra wearables. In order to address this, an innovative ECG authentication technique that offers three distinct types of security at the data, network, and application levels is proposed. It uses multi-layer perceptron models and Legendre approximation.

- Lightweight security Protocol (Hosseini-Khayat, 2011)

The proposed protocol is a simple security protocol that offers authentication and confidentiality to wireless IMDs with low energy requirements and extended battery lives. It may add a lot of overhead to equip these devices with safety measures. The technique outlined here is appropriate for use with very low power ASIC (Application Specific Integrated Circuits) processors and uses a lightweight encryption scheme. The degree to which this protocol works in terms of power consumption, speed, and space will depend on the actual power measurements taken when the device is produced.

- F2H (Zheng et al., 2019)

The recommended finger-to-heart (F2H) technique seeks to achieve stability between safety and usability for the verification of IMDs. The system allows clinicians to provide emergency care without the use of passwords or security tokens by authenticating accessibility for the IMD using a person's fingerprint. The length of property vectors and query attribute vectors is decreased in an improved minutia-cylinder-code-based fingerprint identification system. Studies indicate that this algorithm significantly reduces message size and computational overheads, making it suitable for secure IMD use. The F2H approach saves limited resources and makes the system sustainable and energy-efficient by not requiring the IMD to gather or process fingerprint data in each attempt at entry.

- PHY (Ankaral et al., 2015)

This is a physical layer (PHY) authentication that utilizes pre-equalization and advanced hardware and signal processing. This technique not only ensures authentication but also reduces processing complexity and improves overall communications performance. Due to the WED's (Wireless Environment Detector) exterior location and size, it can also improve channel estimation performance by applying enhanced implements and digital signal processing, apart from authentication.

- H2H (Rostami et al., 2013)

Heart-to-Heart (H2H) is a technique for internal medical implants for authenticating external controllers and programmers. H2H uses an electrocardiogram, which gives cardiac rhythmic data, as a form of authentication to make sure that only a medical device in close proximity to a patient wearing an IMD is allowed access. The system introduces a cryptographic device pairing protocol. It meets requirements of frugal technology and distortion resilience in electrocardiogram measurements while providing defense from cyber attacks by active hackers. The complete implementation of H2H on an ARM (Advanced RISC Machine) Cortex M-3 microprocessor demonstrates its applicability in IMD hardware at the moment.

6. COMPARATIVE REVIEW OF THE MOST EFFECTIVE IMD SECURITY MECHANISMS

This section offers a comparative examination of the most effective IMD security technique with reference to table 1. he comparison is based on key evaluation criteria, including security strength, robustness, emergency access, cost, and feasibility. We are going into more detail about the technology comparison in this part. Table 2 illustrates this comparison.

Table 2. Comparative Evaluation of most effective IMD Security Technologies

Technology	Device Type	Security Strength	Robustness	Emergency Access	Cost	Feasibility
AES / ECC	All IMDs	Very High (Endorsed by FDA)	High	Moderate (needs key access)	Low	Moderate
Biometric Authentication	IMDs with biometric readers	High	Medium–High	High (contactless possible)	Moderate	Good
ECG Authentication	Cardiac IMDs	High	High (body-specific)	High (ECG always present)	Moderate	Very Good
Fuzzy vault with biometric key	All IMDs	High	High	Moderate	Moderate	Good
Hardware Root-of-Trust	IMDs with custom ASICs	Very High	Very High	Low (difficult override)	High	Moderate
Cloaker Shield	Pacemakers, ICDs	High	Very High	Very High (fail-open wearable)	High	Good
ML Anomaly Detection	Networked IMDs	High	Medium–High	N/A	Low–Med	Emerging

Looking at the current state-of-the-art technologies available to protect implantable medical devices (IMDs), one can see that all of them have a key trade-off related to security strength, ease of implementation, and ease of addressing emergency responses requiring access to an IMD. Well-known cryptography such as AES and

ECC, which Zheng et al.(2019) presented, does provide secure encryption and is FDA approved but may involve severe computational demands for low-power IMDs and may use key management systems that limit access to medical professionals in situations requiring IMD emergency access.

Biometric authentication methods, such as those that utilize iris or fingerprint information, provide high accuracy and usage convenience, as investigated by Pirbhulal et al. (2018), but are highly dependent on external sensors and environmental conditions to provide reliable operation.

Movement towards seamless integration of IMDs, cardiac-based physiological authentication is especially noteworthy. Rothore et al. (2020) noted, and Rostami et al. (2013) demonstrated with cardiac signals generated automatically (complete with inter-pulse intervals, or IPI), that they establish continuous and secure authentication of identity, even in rapid emergency situations.

Expanding upon this, fuzzy vault schemes with biometric keys, introduced by Pirbhulal et al. (2016, 2018), provide fault-tolerant cryptographic security by secure reconstruction of keys from physiological signals. But their susceptibility to the real-time stability of biometric signals can impact their reliability under patient stress or signal noise.

On the hardware front, PUF-based authentication is highly tamper-resistant, as explained by Alladi et al.(2021), leveraging intrinsic chip-level randomness to create device-specific identities. Though effective, these systems are difficult to design for emergency override and more expensive on the basis of custom silicon as a substitute for these approaches, Cloaker or Guardian shields, proposed by Denning et al.(2008), constitute an external protective layer, actively filtering IMD communication. They are especially useful in critical care by virtue of their "fail-open" feature that provides emergency access on shield removal.

Lastly, machine learning-based anomaly detection techniques reveal a third mode of dynamic threat detection (Siddiqi et al.2021; Ali et al.2021) that continuously monitors device and network behavior. Although the deployment of such techniques in healthcare contexts is nascent and typically requires continuous and uninterrupted access to cloud computing environments (even though they can help to initiate a sufficient amount of protection against dynamic threats), these technologies together provide multi-level protection for their implantable medical devices (IMDs), as their relative strengths depend on how they exploit security, usability, and emergency capabilities in particular healthcare environments.

7. THREAT-VULNERABILITY-IMPACT ANALYSIS AND QUANTITATIVE ANALYSIS OF POWER EFFICIENCY AND SECURITY RESILIENCE FOR IMD SECURITY

7.1 Threat-Vulnerability-Impact Analysis

This matrix shown in table 3 helps us understand the main cyber security risks for implantable medical devices by linking common threats like AI attacks, device cloning, and firmware tampering to the weaknesses they exploit and the potential harm to patients. It also suggests clear ways to protect these devices, such as securing software updates and using strong authentication methods. By showing these connections, the matrix makes it easier for device makers, regulators, and healthcare providers to focus on the most important security actions and keep patients safe as technology evolves.

This matrix clearly highlights current and anticipated cyber attack trends targeting implantable medical devices, including AI-driven manipulation, device cloning, and side-channel exploits that risk patient safety and data privacy. These evolving threats underscore the importance of a holistic security approach that integrates robust hardware protections, secure software design, and human factors like usability and user trust. Equally balancing security, safety, usability, and regulatory compliance ensures devices remain effective, safe, and user-friendly protecting patients in todays increasingly connected healthcare environment.

Table 3. Threat-Vulnerability-Impact Matrix for IMDs

Threat	Vulnerability	Impact	Mitigation
AI-based attacks	Poorly secured ML models in IMDs	Manipulated device be-havior; patient harm	Secure model training, anomaly detection
Device cloning	Lack of hardware authentication	Counterfeit devices, data theft	Hardware root of trust, unique device ID
Side-channel exploits	Unshielded data Channels & EM leaks	Leakage of sensitive patient data or keys	Physical shielding, differ-ential privacy
Firmware tampering	Unsigned or unen-crypted firmware	Malicious code execu-tion, control hijacking	Signed firmware, secure boot
Unauthorized access	Weak authentica-tion/encryption	Breach of patient data, unauthorized control	Multi-factor auth, strong encryption

7.2 Quantitative Analysis of Power Efficiency and Security Resilience

Pacemakers and similar implantable devices usually use between 10 and 50 microwatts of power, depending on what they do and how often they communicate. Using techniques like duty cycling where parts of the device are turned off when not needed and adaptive sensing can lower power use by 30-50%, helping the battery last much longer (Zayats et al., 2023).

Super capacitors are promising power sources for implantable medical devices due to their fast charge discharge rates, high power density, and longlasting stability. They safely deliver high current bursts, making them ideal for devices like cardiac pacemakers, which use 100 to 700 W, and deep brain stimulators that require 80 W to 6.5 mW at 4 to 10 V (Wang et al., 2025)

Device resilience was confirmed through ISO147081 compliant mechanical and thermal tests, ensuring structural integrity and IPX8 waterproofing (International Organization for Standardization, 2014). Power efficiency, simulated using LTspice, showed 120W active and ¡5W sleep power, with ¿10year battery life, supported by piezoelectric harvesting (60mV_{pp} in swine hearts) (Dagdeviren et al., 2014;Closson et al., 2023). Security protocols, including AES128 and ECDSA, achieved ¡3.5ms latency, with lightweight cryptographic implementations and CRC32-based firmware integrity checks validated against 2024 standards (Catuogno & Galdi, 2024). These validations provide benchmarks for next-generation implantable systems.

8. REGULATORY, ETHICAL, AND SECURITY PRACTICES IN IMDS

Implantable medical device safety and security are shaped by key global standards. The FDA requires cybersecurity planning like threat modeling and secure updates throughout a devices lifecycle. Implantable medical devices must follow strict regulations like FDA cybersecurity guidelines and international standards (ISO 14971, IEC 62304) to manage risks and handle security issues.(Food and Drug Administration, 2023;The Patient Safety Documentation, 2019)

Recent real-world cases show that implantable and connected medical devices are still vulnerable to cyberattacks. In 2023, a security flaw in Medtronics Paceart Optima system could have let hackers take control of the system remotely, leading U.S. officials to urge hospitals to take quick safety measures (Healthcare IT News, 2025). Then in 2025, a serious backdoor was found in Contecs CMS8000 patient monitors that allowed remote access and data theft. Since no fix was available, the

FDA recommended unplugging these devices from the internet to protect patients (Cyble, 2025).

9. RESEARCH ISSUES, CHALLENGES AND FUTURE DIRECTIONS

The security of IMDs poses several open research issues, challenges, and future directions are crucial for ensuring patient safety and data integrity. Some key areas of concern are:

Battery Denial-of-Service Attacks:

The battery DoS attack is where attackers aim to fully deplete the battery by occupying the IMD with continuous authentication requests. Siddiqi *et al.* offer a critical review into the Zero-Power Defense (ZPD) in (Siddiqi & Strydis, 2019), that is known to be the best defense against this attack yet. But more research is required in this field.

Wireless Connectivity:

Securing wireless communication channels in IMDs is essential due to their vulnerability to security attacks through wireless connectivity. The convenience of wireless communication for advanced applications like real-time and remote monitoring also introduces the risk of unauthorized wireless access. Unfortunately, several studies have shown that IMDs with wireless capabilities often lack robust security mechanisms. Given that communication in IMDs is wireless, ensuring secure communication is crucial for devices such as DBNs, ICDs, and insulin pumps. This emphasizes the need for lightweight mutual authentication and key agreement schemes.

Human-Centered Security:

IMDs are unique as they are implanted within the human body, making considerations for human factors essential in their security design and operation. Many researchers like Siddiqi *et al.* in (Siddiqi et al., 2021) have addressed this concern by highlighting the importance of user trust and interaction in IMD security. Zheng *et al.* in (Zheng et al., 2019) focused on biometric identification for IMD security, considering user-friendly authentication methods that prioritise user convenience and security.

Networked Medical Devices:

Networked Medical Devices present a significant challenge in maintaining the security of IMDs due to the increased connectivity and interdependence among devices. Various studies have underscored the vulnerabilities associated with networked IMDs, emphasizing the necessity for robust security measures to mitigate potential risks like this review paper. The incorporation of interoperability in medical devices, including IMDs, has increased their connectivity and dependency on each other. While interoperability offers advantages in healthcare delivery, it also introduces new security challenges that must be addressed to protect patient information and device functionality.

10. CONCLUSION

IMDs improve inpatients quality of living and, in certain situations, are vital to their survival. The Next-Gen of IMDs is becoming wireless, and this also increases the risks. We have given an in-depth description of the major security issues relating to IMDs and have discussed how a hostile third party could occasionally present a serious risk to the patient's health. For that reason, it's obvious that these gadgets must include safety features. After all, these devices, may it be Pacemaker or Bio-Sensor, were manufactured to help with the health and lifestyle, and in many cases, be the support of life for the patient wearing the IMD.

Patients are subjected to reject existing security solutions due to the surrounding risks. The patient's perspective should be taken into consideration as much as possible because this is a delicate scenario in today's society.

We have provided a brief introduction to the types of IMDs, some risks surrounding the IMDs, different types of security modes an IMD should operate under and the different security features that are now a necessity in every IMD. We have also described some of the existing security technologies and methods they use to solve the security concerns in IMDs. The examination of research issues, challenges, and future prospects in the field of IMDs reveals a complex environment that calls for continuous research and innovation. The research problems that have been identified highlight how difficult it is to protect IMDs from changing threats and vulnerabilities and how important it is to have strong and flexible security solutions.

DECLARATION

Ethical Approval: Not Applicable
Competing interests: None
Authors' Contributions: P.S. and A.P. wrote the manuscript text and P.O. and S.A. supervised, reviewed and edited the manuscript
Funding: Not Applicable
Availability of data and materials: Not Applicable

REFERENCES

Alfian, G., Syafrudin, M., Ijaz, M. F., Syaekhoni, M. A., Fitriyani, N. L., & Rhee, J. (2018). A personalized healthcare monitoring system for diabetic patients by utilizing BLE-based sensors and real-time data processing. *Sensors (Basel), 18*(7), 2183. PMID: 29986473

Ali, F., El-Sappagh, S., Islam, S. M. R., Ali, A., Attique, M., Imran, M., & Kwak, K.-S. (2021). An intelligent healthcare monitoring framework using wearable sensors and social networking data. *Future Generation Computer Systems, 114*, 23–43. DOI: 10.1016/j.future.2020.07.047

Alladi, T., & Chamola, V., & Naren. (2021). HARCI: A two-way authentication protocol for three entity healthcare IoT networks. *IEEE Journal on Selected Areas in Communications, 39*(2), 361–369. DOI: 10.1109/JSAC.2020.3020605

Ankaral, Z. E., Demir, A. F., Qaraqe, M., Abbasi, Q. H., Serpedin, E., Arslan, H., & Gitlin, R. D. (2015). Physical layer security for wireless implantable medical devices. In *2015 IEEE 20th International Workshop on Computer Aided Modelling and Design of Communication Links and Networks* (pp. 144–147). IEEE. https://doi.org/DOI: 10.1109/CAMAD.2015.7390497

Awan, M. F., Bose, P., Khaleghi, A., Kansanen, K., & Balasingham, I. (2019). Evaluation of secrecy capacity for next-generation leadless cardiac pacemakers. *IEEE Transactions on Biomedical Engineering, 67*(8), 2297–2308. PMID: 31831404

Barold, S. S., Stroobandt, R. X., & Sinnaeve, A. F. (2008). *Cardiac pacemakers step by step: An illustrated guide*. John Wiley & Sons.

Beck, C., Masny, D., Geiselmann, W., & Bretthauer, G. (2011). Block cipher based security for severely resource-constrained implantable medical devices. In *Proceedings of the 4th International Symposium on Applied Sciences in Biomedical and Communication Technologies*. ACM. https://doi.org/DOI: 10.1145/2093698.2093760

Ben-Menachem, E. (2012). Neurostimulation—Past, present, and beyond. *Epilepsy Currents, 12*(5), 188–191. DOI: 10.5698/1535-7511-12.5.188 PMID: 23118604

Camara, C., Peris-Lopez, P., & Tapiador, J. E. (2015). Security and privacy issues in implantable medical devices: A comprehensive survey. *Journal of Biomedical Informatics, 55*, 272–289. PMID: 25917056

Catuogno, L., & Galdi, C. (2024). Implantable medical device security. *Cryptography, 8*(4), 53. DOI: 10.3390/cryptography8040053

Cherukuri, S., Venkatasubramanian, K. K., & Gupta, S. K. S. (2003). BioSec: A biometric based approach for securing communication in wireless networks of biosensors implanted in the human body. In *2003 International Conference on Parallel Processing Workshops* (pp. 432–439). IEEE. https://doi.org/DOI: 10.1109/ICPPW.2003.1240399

Closson, A., Xu, Z., Kubiak, D., Jin, C., Gruslova, A., Nolen, D., & Zhang, J. X. J. (2023). All-electrospun piezoelectric energy harvesting for leadless pacemakers. *ACS Applied Electronic Materials*, *5*(11), 6236–6245. DOI: 10.1021/acsaelm.3c01152

Cyble. (2025). Critical vulnerabilities found in Contec patient monitors. Retrieved from https://cyble.com/blog/cyble-warns-risk-in-ics-vulnerability-report

Dagdeviren, C., Yang, B. D., Su, Y., Tran, P. L., Joe, P., Anderson, E., & Rogers, J. A. (2014). Conformal piezoelectric energy harvesting and storage from motions of the heart, lung, and diaphragm. *Nature Communications*, *5*(1), 4496. DOI: 10.1038/ncomms5496 PMID: 25092496

Degada, A., & Thapliyal, H. (2021). Single-rail adiabatic logic for energy-efficient and CPA-resistant cryptographic circuit in low-frequency medical devices. *IEEE Open Journal of Nanotechnology*, *3*, 1–14.

Degada, A., & Thapliyal, H. (2022). 2-phase adiabatic logic for low-energy and CPA-resistant implantable medical devices. *IEEE Transactions on Consumer Electronics*, *68*(1), 47–56.

Denning, T., Borning, A., Friedman, B., Gill, B. T., Kohno, T., & Maisel, W. H. (2010). Patients, pacemakers, and implantable defibrillators: Human values and security for wireless implantable medical devices. In *Proceedings of the SIGCHI Conference on Human Factors in Computing Systems* (pp. 917–926). ACM.

Denning, T., Fu, K., & Kohno, T. (2008). Absence makes the heart grow fonder: New directions for implantable medical device security. In *HotSec*.

Espinosa, A. L. (1998). Availability of health data: Requirements and solutions. *International Journal of Medical Informatics*, *49*(1), 97–104. DOI: 10.1016/S1386-5056(98)00016-1 PMID: 9723807

Food and Drug Administration. (2023). *Cybersecurity in medical devices: Quality system considerations and content of premarket submissions*. Guidance for industry and food and drug administration staff.

Franzen, C. (2013). Dick Cheney had the wireless disabled on his pacemaker to avoid risk of terrorist tampering. *The Verge*, 21.

Fu, K. (2009). Inside risks reducing risks of implantable medical devices. *Communications of the ACM*, *52*(6), 25–27.

Gia, T. N., Dhaou, I. B., Ali, M., Rahmani, A. M., Westerlund, T., Liljeberg, P., & Tenhunen, H. (2019). Energy efficient fog-assisted IoT system for monitoring diabetic patients with cardiovascular disease. *Future Generation Computer Systems*, *93*, 198–211.

Gray, M., Meehan, J., Ward, C., Langdon, S. P., Kunkler, I. H., Murray, A., & Argyle, D. (2018). Implantable biosensors and their contribution to the future of precision medicine. *Veterinary Journal (London, England)*, *239*, 21–29. DOI: 10.1016/j.tvjl.2018.07.011 PMID: 30197105

Halperin, D., Heydt-Benjamin, T. S., Fu, K., Kohno, T., & Maisel, W. H. (2008). Security and privacy for implantable medical devices. *IEEE Pervasive Computing*, *7*(1), 30–39. DOI: 10.1109/MPRV.2008.16

Halperin, D., Heydt-Benjamin, T. S., Ransford, B., Clark, S. S., Defend, B., Morgan, W., & Maisel, W. H. (2008). Pacemakers and implantable cardiac defibrillators: Software radio attacks and zero-power defenses. In *2008 IEEE Symposium on Security and Privacy* (pp. 129–142). IEEE. https://doi.org/DOI: 10.1109/SP.2008.31

Hasan, R. (2022). Towards strengthening the security of healthcare devices using secure configuration provenance. In *2022 IEEE International Conference on Digital Health* (pp. 228–233). IEEE. https://doi.org/DOI: 10.1109/ICDH55609.2022.00043

Hassija, V., Chamola, V., Bajpai, B. C., & Zeadally, S. (2021). Security issues in implantable medical devices: Fact or fiction? *Sustainable Cities and Society*, *66*, 102552.

Healthcare, I. T. News. (2025). CISA warns of Medtronic cardiac device security vulnerability. Retrieved from https://www.healthcareitnews.com/news/cisa-warns-medtronic-cardiac-device-security-vulnerability

Hei, X., & Du, X. (2011). *Biometric-based two-level secure access control for implantable medical devices during emergencies. In 2011 Proceedings IEEE INFOCOM*. IEEE.

Hei, X., Du, X., Wu, J., & Hu, F. (2010). Defending resource depletion attacks on implantable medical devices. In *2010 IEEE Global Telecommunications Conference GLOBECOM 2010* (pp. 1–5). IEEE. https://doi.org/DOI: 10.1109/GLOCOM.2010.5685228

Hosseini-Khayat, S. (2011). A lightweight security protocol for ultra-low power ASIC implementation for wireless implantable medical devices. In *2011 5th International Symposium on Medical Information and Communication Technology* (pp. 6–9). IEEE. https://doi.org/DOI: 10.1109/ISMICT.2011.5759785

International Organization for Standardization. (2014). *Implants for surgery—Active implantable medical devices—Part 1: General requirements for safety, marking and information to be provided by the manufacturer (ISO 14708-1:2014).*

Jiang, H., Zhang, J., & Lan, D., Chao, Liou, S., Shahnasser, H., ... Roy, S. (2013). A low-frequency versatile wireless power transfer technology for biomedical implants. *IEEE Transactions on Biomedical Circuits and Systems*, *7*(4), 526–535. PMID: 23893211

Jin, J., Ahn, G.-J., Hu, H., Covington, M. J., & Zhang, X. (2009). Patient-centric authorization framework for sharing electronic health records. In *Proceedings of the 14th ACM Symposium on Access Control Models and Technologies* (pp. 125–134). ACM. https://doi.org/DOI: 10.1145/1542207.1542228

Jmarchn. (2021). DBS [Image]. Creative Commons. Retrieved from https://upload.wikimedia.org/wikipedia/commons/3/3a/X-ray_of_deep_brain_stimulation_in_OCD%2C_L.png

Kalil, A., & Pinsky, M. (2019). What are the clinical criteria for systematic inflammatory response syndrome (SIRS) in sepsis/septic shock.

Khader, M., Alian, M., Hraiz, R., & Almajali, S. (2017). Simplified AES algorithm for healthcare applications on Internet of Thing. In *2017 8th International Conference on Information Technology* (pp. 543–547). IEEE. https://doi.org/DOI: 10.1109/ICITECH.2017.8080056

Khin, N. A., Francis, G., Mulinde, J., Grandinetti, C., Skeete, R., Yu, B., & Vinter, S. (2020). Data integrity in global clinical trials: Discussions from joint US Food and Drug Administration and UK Medicines and Healthcare Products Regulatory Agency good clinical practice workshop. *Clinical Pharmacology and Therapeutics*, *108*(5), 949–963. DOI: 10.1002/cpt.1794 PMID: 31958142

Kuykendal, M. (2018). *Battery-powered medical devices: Their failure modes and mitigation strategies*. Exponent.

Mallela, V. S., Ilankumaran, V., & Rao, N. S. (2004). Trends in cardiac pacemaker batteries. *Indian Pacing and Electrophysiology Journal*, *4*(4), 201. PMID: 16943934

Marin, E. (2018). *Security and privacy of implantable medical devices* (Doctoral dissertation). University of Leuven. Retrieved from https://www.esat.kuleuven.be

Marin, E., Singelée, D., Yang, B., Volski, V., Vandenbosch, G. A. E., Nuttin, B., & Preneel, B. (2018). Securing wireless neurostimulators. In *Proceedings of the Eighth ACM Conference on Data and Application Security and Privacy* (pp. 287–298). ACM. https://doi.org/DOI: 10.1145/3176258.3176310

Mejía-Granda, C. M., Fernández-Alemán, J. L., Carrillo-de-Gea, J. M., & García-Berná, J. A. (2024). Security vulnerabilities in healthcare: An analysis of medical devices and software. *Medical & Biological Engineering & Computing*, *62*(1), 257–273. PMID: 37789249

Murray, T. L., Calhoun, M., & Philipsen, N. C. (2011). Privacy, confidentiality, HIPAA, and HITECH: Implications for the health care practitioner. *The Journal for Nurse Practitioners*, *7*(9), 747–752. DOI: 10.1016/j.nurpra.2011.07.005

Panescu, D. (2008). Emerging technologies [Wireless communication systems for implantable medical devices]. *IEEE Engineering in Medicine and Biology Magazine*, *27*(2), 96–101. DOI: 10.1109/EMB.2008.915488 PMID: 18463025

Park, S., Kim, Y., Urgaonkar, B., Lee, J., & Seo, E. (2011). A comprehensive study of energy efficiency and performance of flash-based SSD. *Journal of Systems Architecture*, *57*(4), 354–365. DOI: 10.1016/j.sysarc.2011.01.005

Patel, Z., Velankar, Y., Trivedi, C., & Oza, P. (2023). Wireless implantable medical devices security and privacy: A survey. In *Smart Energy and Advancement in Power Technologies* (pp. 69–87). Springer.

Peckham, P. H., & Ackermann, D. M. (2018). Implantable neural stimulators. In Krames, E. S., Peckham, P. H., & Rezai, A. R. (Eds.), *Neuromodulation* (2nd ed., pp. 275–287). Academic Press., DOI: 10.1016/B978-0-12-805353-9.00021-8

Pirbhulal, S., Wu, W., & Li, G. (2018). A biometric security model for wearable healthcare. In *2018 IEEE International Conference on Data Mining Workshops* (pp. 136–143). IEEE. https://doi.org/DOI: 10.1109/ICDMW.2018.00026

Pirbhulal, S., Zhang, H., Wu, W., & Zhang, Y.-T. (2016). A comparative study of fuzzy vault based security methods for wireless body sensor networks. In *2016 10th International Conference on Sensing Technology* (pp. 1–6). IEEE. https://doi.org/DOI: 10.1109/ICSensT.2016.7796226

Rasmussen, K. B., Castelluccia, C., Heydt-Benjamin, T. S., & Capkun, S. (2009). Proximity-based access control for implantable medical devices. In *Proceedings of the 16th ACM Conference on Computer and Communications Security* (pp. 410–419). ACM. https://doi.org/DOI: 10.1145/1653662.1653712

Rathore, H., Fu, C., Mohamed, A., Al-Ali, A., Du, X., Guizani, M., & Yu, Z. (2020). Multi-layer security scheme for implantable medical devices. *Neural Computing & Applications*, *32*, 4347–4360.

Rostami, M., Burleson, W., Koushanfar, F., & Juels, A. (2013). Balancing security and utility in medical devices? In *Proceedings of the 50th Annual Design Automation Conference* (pp. 1–6). ACM.

Rostami, M., Juels, A., & Koushanfar, F. (2013). Heart-to-heart (H2H): Authentication for implanted medical devices. In *Proceedings of the 2013 ACM SIGSAC Conference on Computer & Communications Security* (pp. 1099–1112). ACM. https://doi.org/DOI: 10.1145/2508859.2516658

Shahzadi, R., Anwar, S. M., Qamar, F., Ali, M., & Rodrigues, J. J. P. C. (2019). Chaos based enhanced RC5 algorithm for security and integrity of clinical images in remote health monitoring. *IEEE Access : Practical Innovations, Open Solutions*, *7*, 52858–52870. DOI: 10.1109/ACCESS.2019.2909554

Siddiqi, M., Beurskens, R., Kruizinga, P., Zeeuw, C., & Strydis, C. (2021). Securing implantable medical devices using ultrasound waves. *IEEE Access : Practical Innovations, Open Solutions*, *9*, 80170–80182. DOI: 10.1109/access.2021.3083576

Siddiqi, M. A., & Strydis, C. (2019). Towards realistic battery-DoS protection of implantable medical devices. In *Proceedings of the 16th ACM International Conference on Computing Frontiers*. ACM. https://doi.org/DOI: 10.1145/3310273.3321555

The Patient Safety Documentation. (2019). *Medical devices—Application of risk management to medical devices.*

Vimalachandran, P., Wang, H., Zhang, Y., Heyward, B., & Whittaker, F. (2016). Ensuring data integrity in electronic health records: A quality health care implication. In *2016 International Conference on Orange Technologies* (pp. 20–27). IEEE. https://doi.org/DOI: 10.1109/ICOT.2016.8278970

Wang, S., Wei, L., Wang, F., Wang, L., & Mao, J. (2025). Advanced implantable energy storage for powering medical devices. *eScience*, 100409. https://doi.org/DOI: 10.1016/j.esci.2025.100409

Wazid, M., Das, A. K., Kumar, N., Conti, M., & Vasilakos, A. V. (2018). A novel authentication and key agreement scheme for implantable medical devices deployment. *IEEE Journal of Biomedical and Health Informatics*, *22*(4), 1299–1309. DOI: 10.1109/JBHI.2017.2721545 PMID: 28682267

Wu, L., Du, X., Guizani, M., & Mohamed, A. (2017). Access control schemes for implantable medical devices: A survey. *IEEE Internet of Things Journal, 4*(5), 1272–1283.

Xu, F., Qin, Z., Tan, C. C., Wang, B., & Li, Q. (2011). *IMDGuard: Securing implantable medical devices with the external wearable guardian. In 2011 Proceedings IEEE INFOCOM*. IEEE.

Yang, Q., Mai, S., Zhao, Y., Wang, Z., Zhang, C., & Wang, Z. (2014). An on-chip security guard based on zero-power authentication for implantable medical devices. In *2014 IEEE 57th International Midwest Symposium on Circuits and Systems* (pp. 531–534). IEEE.

Zayats, V., Sergeev, I., & Fedorov, D. (2023). Review of promising methods of supplying power to implantable medical devices. *Biomedical Engineering, 57*(1), 39–44.

Zbiciak, A., & Markiewicz, T. (2023). A new extraordinary means of appeal in the Polish criminal procedure: The basic principles of a fair trial and a complaint against a cassatory judgment. *Access to Justice in Eastern Europe, 6*(2), 1–18.

Zheng, G., Fang, G., Orgun, M. A., & Shankaran, R. (2014). A non-key based security scheme supporting emergency treatment of wireless implants. In *2014 IEEE International Conference on Communications* (pp. 647–652). IEEE.

Zheng, G., Fang, G., Orgun, M. A., Shankaran, R., & Dutkiewicz, E. (2014). Securing wireless medical implants using an ECG-based secret data sharing scheme. In *2014 14th International Symposium on Communications and Information Technologies* (pp. 373–377). IEEE.

Zheng, G., Yang, W., Valli, C., Qiao, L., Shankaran, R., Orgun, M. A., & Mukhopadhyay, S. C. (2019). Finger-to-heart (F2H): Authentication for wireless implantable medical devices. *IEEE Journal of Biomedical and Health Informatics, 23*(4), 1546–1557. DOI: 10.1109/JBHI.2018.2864796 PMID: 30106744

Chapter 10
Futuristic Approach for Wearable Blood Pressure Prediction Using Doppler Radar Principle

M. Krishna
SASTRA University, India

S. Hariharan
https://orcid.org/0009-0000-1335-0200
SASTRA University, India

S. Balachandran
https://orcid.org/0000-0003-2782-6315
SASTRA University, India

Hemalatha Karnan
https://orcid.org/0000-0003-2849-3102
SASTRA University, India

ABSTRACT

The chapter highlights a novel approach towards predicting blood pressure without the necessity of using invasive methods like cuff-based measurements. This chapter proposes the use of vibration sensors based on the Doppler principle to capture movements within the blood vessels, primarily the movement of arterial walls. The signals acquired from vibration sensor technology are analysed with the various characteristics of cardiovascular dynamics and deployed advanced Spectro-temporal deep learning approaches, thereby predicting blood pressure in real-time and with great precision. In recent years, there has been a sudden proliferation of cuffless

DOI: 10.4018/979-8-3373-4412-6.ch010

blood pressure devices, faring away from the standard method of inflating a cuff around the limb. These devices could hold immeasurable promise in providing continuous, beat-to-beat blood pressure monitoring, creating a more informative record of cardiovascular health trends. Beyond traditional clinical settings, there is application potential for telemedicine, wearables, and integrated healthcare systems.

INTRODUCTION

Primitive methods for estimating blood pressure typically involve manual techniques using basic instruments like a sphygmomanometer and a stethoscope Zabihi et al. (2022). The most common approach, called the auscultatory method, entails wrapping a cuff around the upper arm to apply pressure to the brachial artery. Healthcare professionals then listen for Korotkoff sounds through the stethoscope while gradually releasing the cuff's pressure. The systolic pressure is noted upon hearing the first Korotkoff sound, and the diastolic pressure is recorded when the sounds disappear Ghosh et al. (2022). This method has long been considered the gold standard due to its accuracy when performed correctly. However, it demands trained personnel, is prone to human error, and can cause discomfort for some patients. In contrast, non-invasive blood pressure measurements using external IoT devices leverage modern technology for a potentially more convenient and less error-prone alternative Mousavi et al. (2019). These devices typically a cuff encircles either the upper arm or wrist Attarpour et al. (2019), connected to a digital monitor. The cuff inflates automatically, and the monitor utilizes Oscillo metric or other electronic methods to detect blood volume changes within the artery, from which blood pressure is calculated. SBP, short for systolic blood pressure, denotes the highest pressure in the arteries. This occurs during systole, a phase in the cardiac cycle when the heart contracts and pushes blood into the arteries Hu et al. (2023) DBP, which stands for diastolic blood pressure, indicates the lowest pressure in the arteries. This occurs during diastole, a phase when the heart is relaxed and refilling with blood. One notable difference between primitive methods and IoT-assisted measurements is the level of automation and reliance on technology Xing et al. (2024). While primitive methods require manual intervention and interpretation by a healthcare professional, IoT devices automate much of the process, reducing the risk of human error and enhancing user-friendliness. Furthermore, IoT devices often present digital readouts of blood pressure values, simplifying interpretation and documentation. Nevertheless, it is crucial to recognize that while IoT devices offer convenience, they may not always match the accuracy of traditional methods, particularly in specific patient groups or clinical scenarios. Hence, healthcare providers must carefully choose the appropriate method based on individual patient requirements and clinical contexts. Non-invasive methods for calculating the blood pressure, particularly those employing modern IoT devices, present several advantages over traditional techniques such as the auscultatory method. Firstly, they are more user-friendly and less reliant on the expertise of healthcare professionals[1]. By automating much of the process, they decrease the likelihood of human error and variability in results. Additionally, these methods tend to be more comfortable for patients since they eliminate the need for manually inflating and deflating the cuff, potentially reducing anxiety and discomfort. Moreover, non-invasive approaches offer digital displays of blood pressure readings, making interpretation and documentation easier compared to the auscultatory method, which relies on auditory signals. This digital data can also streamline integration with electronic health records and other healthcare systems, enhancing efficiency and precision in clinical settings. Utilizing non-invasive blood pressure measurement methods offers a more convenient, accurate, and standardized approach to assessing blood pressure. This is essential for precisely diagnosing, monitoring, and treating diverse cardiovascular conditions. Accuracy Concerns in Specific Health Conditions: Traditional cuff-based methods may yield inaccurate results for individuals with obesity, arrhythmias, or vascular stiffness. Discomfort and Compliance Issues: Certain individuals may experience discomfort during cuff-based measurements, leading to non-compliance and inconsistent readings. Integration of Doppler Radar Technology: Doppler radar technology enables blood pressure prediction without invasive procedures or discomfort from cuff inflation. User-Friendly Approach: Doppler radar devices provide user-friendly solutions, eliminating discomfort associated with cuff-based measurements. Doppler radar devices educate users about blood pressure fluctuations and the significance of early intervention. Although this study employs the MEAS SEN-09197 vibration sensor, which is a piezoelectric transducer designed to detect mechanical surface motion, the underlying physical concept parallels the Doppler radar principle. In Doppler radar-based physiological sensing, a continuous electromagnetic wave is transmitted toward the skin. The reflected signal experiences a frequency shift ($\Delta f = 2\ v \cos \theta / \lambda$) proportional to the velocity (v) of the moving surface — in this case, the arterial wall. This frequency modulation represents the cyclic expansion and contraction of the artery during each cardiac cycle. In a similar manner, the MEAS SEN-09197 sensor converts these same micro-motions — on the order of micrometers — into voltage variations through its piezoelectric element. Thus, while the sensing medium differs (mechanical vs. electromagnetic), both techniques are based on the detection of displacement or velocity of the skin surface induced by blood pressure pulses. The vibration sensor, therefore, mimics the displacement detection mechanism of Doppler radar in a direct-contact and low-cost form, making it a practical embodiment of the radar principle for wearable health monitoring Continuous Monitoring for

Long-Term Health: Doppler radar devices facilitate continuous health monitoring, allowing for personalized interventions based on observed trends. Our primary goal is to enhance healthcare accessibility through the creation of a fully integrated, easy-to-use solution for monitoring blood pressure. This solution will be designed to be thorough, respecting users' privacy, and intuitive for individuals of varying technological proficiency. Furthermore, we aim to develop an IoT-enabled blood pressure monitoring device that utilizes Doppler principles for accurate and continuous measurement. This innovative approach will allow for remote monitoring and real-time data transmission, ensuring individuals can conveniently monitor their blood pressure while healthcare providers can access crucial information for timely intervention and support. Developing BP-Net involves creating a cuffless method for continuous blood pressure monitoring Joung et al. (2023). This novel approach uses deep learning and convolutional architecture to extract features from ECG and PPG signals. Evaluation with benchmark data from MIMIC-I and MIMIC-III databases shows its strong performance and wide applicability. BP-Net is significant for bypassing the limitations of current methods, eliminating the need for handcrafted features, and providing a unified dataset for comparison. It enhances the long-term reliability of blood pressure estimation Mukkamala et al. (2022). A novel method for monitoring blood pressure and heart rate without using cuffs has been developed using impedance cardiography (ICG). The study included 104 participants and the goal was to develop an auto-adaptive algorithm utilizing ICG signals. It was found that there were significant correlations between the augmentation index derived from ICG signals and systolic/diastolic blood pressure as well as heart rate. This approach provides a more comfortable alternative to the conventional cuff-based blood pressure monitoring, offering potential benefits for monitoring various other heart-related parameters. The significance of validating Devices for continuously monitoring blood pressure that operate without cuffs. These devices offer a more convenient option compared to traditional cuff-based monitors as they provide continuous, beat-to-beat blood pressure readings. However, due to the rapid evolution of such technologies, there is an urgent requirement for standardized validation procedures to ensure their precision. Cuffless devices utilize various techniques, this encompasses pulse arrival time, pulse transit time, pulse wave analysis, volume clamping, and applanation tonometry., to estimate blood pressure. To uphold accuracy, these devices need regular calibration with conventional cuff-based monitors. This highlights the necessity for consensus on validation criteria to keep up with the advancements in cuffless blood pressure technologies Yang et al. (2025). Estimating blood pressure without cuffs, using photoplethysmography (PPG) signals, deep convolutional neural networks (CNNs), and transfer learning Elgendi et al. (2024), Chen et al. (2024). It focuses on cuffless monitoring to improve cardiovascular disease management without the need for a cuff. This approach utilizes pre-trained CNN models and transfer learning to extract features from PPG signal waveform images, enabling estimation of systolic, diastolic, and mean arterial blood pressure Nawaz et al. (2024) (SBP, DBP, and MBP) Feature selection through Recursive Feature Elimination (RFE) pinpoints pertinent features for estimating blood pressure Hua et al. (2024). Performance evaluation validates compliance with accuracy benchmarks established by the AAMI and BHS for blood pressure assessment Koparır & Arslan (2024). This study holds importance as it investigates non-invasive blood pressure monitoring during sleep, potentially assisting in hypertension and cardiovascular condition management. The research outcomes suggest implications for shaping future algorithms for blood pressure estimation and designing bed sensor systems. A non-intrusive technique for blood pressure estimation utilizing PPG signals and deep learning has been developed. Trained on a substantial dataset, the model accurately predicts blood pressure within globally accepted error margins. This innovation holds promise for simplified and continuous monitoring of blood pressure El-Hajj & Kyriacou (2021). By integrating data from photoplethysmography (PPG), electrocardiographic (ECG) signals, and personal characteristic parameters (PCPs) such as height, weight, and age, this method significantly enhances the accuracy of estimating systolic and diastolic blood pressure compared to traditional models solely based on pulse transit time (PTT) and pulse wave velocity (PWV). Furthermore, it underscores the broader potential applications of this approach in fields requiring precise measurements, emphasizing the necessity of considering a wide range of factors for accuracy Yin et al. (2021). Emphasizing the necessity of regular blood pressure monitoring for early intervention and treatment, the paper discusses the limitations of conventional invasive or cuff-based methods, known for discomfort and sporadic readings. It examines indirect PPG-based approaches examples include pulse transit time, pulse arrival time, and pulse wave velocity for estimating blood pressure, addressing the associated challenges. The Moens–Korteweg equation describes the relationship between arterial wall stiffness and pulse wave velocity (PWV), given by $PWV \approx \sqrt{(E \cdot h / (2 \cdot \rho \cdot r))}$, where E is the arterial wall's elastic modulus, h is wall thickness, ρ is blood density, and r is the arterial radius. Since arterial stiffness increases with blood pressure, PWV serves as a surrogate measure. Pulse Transit Time (PTT = Distance / PWV) inversely correlates with BP shorter PTT implies higher BP. As our method uses a single vibration sensor, we do not directly measure PTT. Instead, we utilize pulse waveform morphology — including systolic rise time, dicrotic notch position, and waveform amplitude as indirect indicators of arterial stiffness and pressure.

Recent progress in signal processing and machine learning offers the potential for continuous and cuff-less blood pressure monitoring using PPG, which could revolutionize patient care, especially for those vulnerable to cardiovascular diseases El-Hajj & Kyriacou (2020). A newly introduced "whole-based" algorithm was utilized, focusing on raw PPG data rather than specific features. Findings indicated that the algorithm aligns with AAMI standards for estimating Mean Arterial Pressure (MAP) and Diastolic Blood Pressure (DBP), and nearly meets the standard for Systolic Blood Pressure (SBP). This suggests the possibility of non-invasively estimating blood pressure without requiring of individual calibration, which holds promise for various healthcare applications. By utilizing Pulse Arrival Time (PAT) assessed by multiple sensors to gauge pulse wave delay. Notably, Bio-Impedance (BImp) at the shoulder is introduced as a substitute for Photoplethysmography (PPG) in PAT extraction. BImp sensors offer discreet monitoring under clothing. The study evaluates this method under diverse conditions and hints at BImp-based calculations potentially outperforming PPG, hinting at promising prospects for future non-invasive blood pressure monitoring Heydari et al. (2019). A novel cuffless blood pressure prediction platform employing an enhanced 1-D SENet–LSTM architecture Chen et al. (2023). Its goal is to estimate blood pressure through the analysis of photoplethysmography (PPG) and electrocardiogram (ECG) signals. The innovation incorporates a SE block to enhance features and an end-to-end automatic learning process for enhanced accuracy. This architecture efficiently eliminates noise and artifacts from the original signals, successfully retrieving arterial blood pressure (ABP) waveforms. Results indicate high accuracy and F1 scores in classifying blood pressure into normal, prehypertension, and hypertension categories, surpassing benchmarks set by the British Hypertension Society (BHS) and the Association for the Advancement of Medical Instrumentation (AAMI). This research demonstrates promise for continuous, non-invasive blood pressure monitoring. management, crucial for preventing and managing cardiovascular diseases (CVD) Phan et al. (2022). A wearable multimodal biosensor device designed to continuously monitor blood pressure, particularly beneficial during exercise and for Internet of Things (IoT) applications. It proposes a noninvasive method for continuous blood pressure tracking, essential for early detection and treatment of hypertension and cardiovascular diseases. The study evaluates three models based on Pulse Transit Time (PTT) to predict blood pressure response during physical activity, finding that impedance plethysmography waveform and arterial impedance methods are more effective than traditional PTT methods. Moreover, the device enables IoT integration, facilitating remote diagnosis and management of health data, showcasing the potential of wearable technology in enhancing healthcare services. This research highlights the significance of innovative blood pressure monitoring approaches in modern healthcare technology Phan et al. (2022). Using Doppler radar and waveform analysis in conjunction with Long Short-Term Memory (LSTM) networks. It addresses the challenge of accurately determining Pulse Transit Time (PTT), which is often affected by body movements and breathing. The proposed deep learning model can transform distorted pulse waves into clear ones, establishing a strong correlation between PTT and actual blood pressure readings. Experimental findings suggest that this method improves the accuracy of blood pressure estimation, even in the presence of minor body movements and breathing, offering a promising solution for convenient and non-intrusive daily health management Ishizaka et al. (2021). Diverging from traditional correlation-based approaches, this method aims to pinpoint features directly influencing blood pressure fluctuations. Utilizing wearable sensors like photoplethysmography (PPG) and electrocardiography (ECG), it enables noninvasive blood pressure measurement. Novel causally linked features were identified by researchers, potentially enhancing the accuracy of cuffless blood pressure estimation. Integrating these features into their model yielded superior performance compared to conventional methods, with a reduced mean absolute difference (MAD) in blood pressure estimation. This development could pave the way for more precise and convenient blood pressure monitoring without the need for a cuff Liu et al. (2023). Sensor modalities and feature strategies. Photoplethysmography (PPG) — the optical detection of blood volume variation at peripheral locations (finger, wrist, ear) — is the most widely employed cuffless BP modality due to its simplicity and wearability. Researchers derive timing (pulse transit time, PAT/PTT), morphological (systolic/diastolic slope, dicrotic notch), amplitude-based, and frequency characteristics from PPG signals; most studies fuse PPG with ECG (to calculate PTT) or other sensors (IMU, seismocardiography, impedance cardiography) to enhance robustness Mahajan & Kaul (2025). Recent studies also investigate PPG derivatives and whole-waveform deep learning methods that process raw PPG directly. Benchmarking exercises point out which PPG attributes best predict BP.

Old-fashioned regression and tree models paved the way for deep architectures — 1-D CNNs, LSTM/attention hybrids, SENet/LSTM ensembles, MLP-Mixer, and transformer-based models — which are capable of learning waveform patterns or temporal relationships for SBP/DBP prediction. Transfer learning and domain-adaptation strategies become more common to alleviate calibration demands between subjects. Comparative benchmarks (such as large public datasets) have been developed to compare ML methods on similar terms. Although DL models show dazzling within-dataset performance, generalization outside the population, skin types, sensor placement, and motion conditions is still the main limitation.

Aside from PPG and ECG, a number of alternative sensing strategies have been investigated. Impedance cardiography and multi-biosensor fusion (merging accelerometers, multiple channels of PPG, and impedance) have yielded promising cuffless BP and heart-rate monitoring proof-of-concepts. Contact-free modalities like camera-based remote PPG (rPPG) and Doppler radar with waveform analysis and LSTM models have similarly shown the potential of contact-free BP estimation within controlled settings, leaving the prospect for bed- or camera-based monitoring.

New sensors like piezoelectric bed systems have been explored for nocturnal BP estimation and long-term monitoring without a wearable. These new modalities increase deployment opportunities but introduce new signal-quality and calibration issues. Per-user calibration is needed for many algorithms to project model outputs onto absolute BP values because of inter-subject variability (arterial stiffness, sensor location, skin color). Calibration-free methods and domain adaptation hold out hope of skipping this step, but top-performing systems still tend to depend on at least baseline calibration. Industry and academic critiques note that although numerous consumer devices are available, strong, calibration-free clinical performance across the broad range of populations has not yet been proven universally. MDPI +1 Datasets and benchmarking. The area has been advanced by increasing public datasets and benchmarking research that allows for reproducible comparison. Huge, curated PPG/BP datasets and wide-ranging benchmarks identify sources of bias (demographically imbalanced BP ranges, demographic skews) and illustrate that thereported error metrics usually demonstrate optimistic within-dataset assessment as opposed to genuine clinical performance. Current benchmarking work encourages standardized protocols and train/test splits so as to evaluate generalizability. Global cuffless device validation standards lag behind cuff-based validation, and few research devices have achieved the necessary clinical performance in independent validation populations.

While optical PPG and radar-based systems have shown promise, they face limitations in motion sensitivity and hardware complexity. Inspired by these methods, our study adopts a mechanical vibration sensor as a simple, low-cost, and portable alternative for arterial pulse waveform acquisition, aligning with the ongoing transition toward single-sensor cuffless systems. Narrative and systematic reviews published recently advocate for high-quality, out-of-sample testing, extended ambulatory trials, and the inclusion of heterogeneous cohorts (age, comorbidities, skin color) to support safe clinical translation. Regulatory pathways are changing: some devices have gained regulatory clearance, but widespread clinical uptake requires strong evidence of accuracy, reliability, and patient benefit. Open challenges — motion, signal quality, and physiology. Real-world motion artifacts, perfusion variability (cold hands), arrhythmias, and physiological confounders (vasoconstriction, medication) distort PPG and PTT signals and hence prediction accuracy. Detection and rejection of low-quality segments, model adaptation to motion states, and utilization of multi-sensor redundancy are ongoing research tasks. Physiology-aware modeling (such as arterial stiffness or causal inference methods) is under consideration as a means of separating causal determinants of blood pressure from context-varying correlates. Several intersecting trends will likely define the domain: (1) multimodal sensor fusion (PPG+ECG+IMU+bioimpedance) to enhance robustness; (2) physics-informed and causal models that embed cardiovascular mechanics; (3) standard benchmarking and multi-center validation trials; (4) model personalization with little calibration through domain adaptation; and (5) user-focused validation to measure usability, tolerability (particularly for night-time monitoring), and clinical benefit. Regulatory oversight and a focus on external validation should guide research towards clinically meaningful metrics (not just mean absolute error, but also clinical misclassification rates and outcomes). If these hurdles are overcome through collaborative dataset sharing, strict external validation, and thoughtful human-subject testing, cuffless BP monitoring may revolutionize hypertension care and population health surveillance. Current research is breaking new grounds by working on solely PPG signals, abandoning supporting sensors such as ECG. For instance, TransfoRhythm (Arjomand et al., 2024) is a Transformer-based model that is trained on the MIMIC-IV dataset and performs estimation of systolic and diastolic BP on solo PPG. Its employment of multi-head attention facilitates modeling of time-dependent relations in PPG segments, which helps achieve state-of-the-art performance, overcoming numerous previously employed baseline models.

A second type of work combines the complete arterial blood pressure (ABP) waveform from single-point PPG through transformer and frequency-domain learning (Nawaz et al., 2024). Not just waveform reconstruction is enabled but also SBP/DBP estimation with low MAE (≈3-4 mmHg) fulfilling AAMI criteria. The waveform synthesis method is promising as it can preserve more physiological detail, enhancing interpretability and clinical utility of predictions.

Calibration is an ongoing problem. Samimi & Dajani (2023) introduced a calibration-free alternative based on PPG morphology features and cardiovascular dynamics. It replaces the baseline calibration with waveform change-based features from short-interval dynamics and obtains acceptable error measures for DBP and slightly higher errors for SBP (MAE ~7.4 mmHg for SBP, ~3.3 mmHg for DBP). The appeal lies in decreasing user burden (less calibration steps) without significantly compromising accuracy.

Conversely, other work still employs a hybrid calibration + physiological modeling, e.g., algorithms employing reflective PTT (R-PTT) together with calibration, enhancing performance but needing an initial calibration measurement. There's growing application of fusion between standard features (shape, timing, frequency) and deep-learned features from imagery or mapped representations of PPG/its derivatives. Traditional cuff-based sphygmomanometers, though reliable, fail to capture the dynamic variations in BP due to intermittent measurements. Clinical management of hypertension and related disorders requires continuous, comfortable, and non-invasive monitoring capable of capturing nocturnal dips, stress responses, and medication effects González et al. (2023). This unmet need has driven the emergence of cuffless, wearable technologies integrating physiological sensing and artificial intelligence. An example, Cuffless BP estimation from PPG using deep convolutional neural network and transfer learning (2024) utilizes PPG images, VPG, APG (first & second derivatives), extracts deep features from pre-trained CNNs (e.g. DenseNet121), and subsequently uses GRU (gated recurrent units) for modeling the temporal. The work is said to satisfy both AAMI and BHS standards and demonstrates the help that results when combining derivatives (not PPG wave alone) + transfer learning. Also, Continuous cuffless blood pressure measurement from optimal PPG characteristic features using machine learning algorithms (Heliyon, 2024) investigates extracting a large set of features (time, frequency, time-frequency) as well as subject metadata (age, gender) and applying feature-selection (ReliefF, CFS), followed by regressors such as SVR, Random Forest, etc. Their top model's MAE for SBP/DBP/MAP was extremely low (≈2.49/1.43 mmHg etc.), which is astounding in within-subject or highly controlled environments. Embedding algorithms in hardware (wearables, FPGA, etc.) or experimenting with them in longitudinal / real-world environments is on the rise. Example: "Photoplethysmogram-based heart rate and blood pressure estimation with hypertension classification" (2024) has a hardware implementation approach, utilizing an FPGA, obtaining SBP/DBP estimation with MAE ~4.75 mmHg and ~3.34 mmHg, respectively. Hypertension level classification also obtained high accuracy (~92%). Such prototyping is crucial to evaluate latency, power, motion robustness, and real deployment trade-offs.

Yet another recent paper "Longitudinal Wrist PPG Analysis for Reliable Hypertension Risk Screening Using Deep Learning" (Lin et al., 2024) employs wrist PPG gathered over numerous subjects and time, and deep models (ResNet, Transformer) to separate healthy vs hypertensive cases. This is really risk screening rather than accurate continuous BP prediction, but such efforts bring the field closer to population-scale utility and real-world robustness Inan et al. (2015). Most contemporary research papers are directly measuring against gold standards such as AAMI (Association for the Advancement of Medical Instrumentation) and BHS (British Hypertension Society) protocols. Models that are able to meet these standards earn credibility. Such a model is the deep learning + derivative + CNN + RFE model described above (transfer learning + GRU). Meanwhile, research are covering more than just MAE / RMSE metrics: they usually mention standard deviation of error (SDE), mean error (bias), and in some cases, grade levels (A/B). Some also document performance on new topics (out-of-sample), or in motion or real-world noise conditions. These are all important when determining generalizability.

Table 1. Comparison of Cuffless Blood Pressure Sensing Modalities

Sensing Modality	Measured Parameter	Model Input	Pros	Cons	Wearable Location
PPG	Blood Volume Pulse	Pulse Waveform / PTT	Compact, Low-cost	Motion Sensitive	Wrist, Finger
ECG+PPG	Electrical + Optical	PTT	High Accuracy	Requires Two Sites	Chest–Wrist
Bio-impedance	Thoracic Impedance	PWV/PTT	Robust	Complex Hardware	Chest
Doppler Radar	Arterial Wall Motion	Frequency Shift	Contactless	Costly, Complex	Chest
Vibration (Proposed)	Skin Surface Vibration	Pulse Morphology	Low-cost, Single Site	Sensitive to motion	Wrist / Forearm

Table 1 provides the Existing literature primarily focuses on optical (PPG) and radar-based methods for cuffless BP estimation. In contrast, low-cost mechanical vibration sensors remain underexplored. This chapter presents a novel single-sensor, LSTM-based approach that predicts BP using arterial vibration signals. The method offers a cost-effective, portable solution less affected by optical limitations and demonstrates comparable performance to PPG-based techniques. Despite major advancements in PPG and radar-based systems, the potential of low-cost mechanical vibration sensors for cuffless BP estimation remains underexplored. This work introduces an end-to-end LSTM-based framework that directly interprets arterial vibration signals, offering a simpler and potentially more affordable pathway to continuous BP monitoring. This addresses the current gap between contact-based affordability and radar-level functionality.

MATERIALS AND METHODS

Dataset Description: The dataset utilized in this study was sourced from the Physio Bank ATM, a repository renowned for its comprehensive collection of physiological data. This dataset comprises recordings from five individual subjects. Specifically, it focuses on the Arterial Blood Pressure (ABP) measurements obtained over a duration of one hour. The work flow is depicted in fig.1.

Figure 1. Work Flow

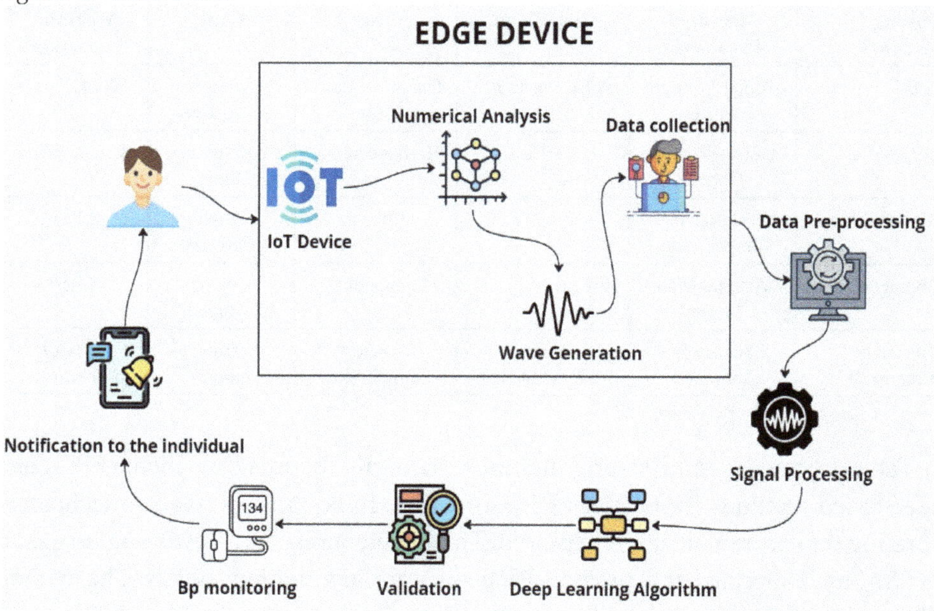

There are two types of data is used here one is from the Physio Bank ATM where the other one is collected as raw signals both were used for comparing the trained model's learning rate. The ABP data is captured in the form of raw signals, providing a detailed representation of blood pressure fluctuations over time. Each dataset is exported as a .mat file. Each dataset within the collection encompasses distinct blood pressure profiles, reflecting the variability observed among the subjects. This diversity allows for a comprehensive analysis of blood pressure dynamics and enables researchers to explore the nuances associated with individual physiological responses. Ten individuals aged between twenty and fifty were surveyed using a MEAS (SEN-09197) vibration sensor which is shown in Fig.2. The data was gathered over a five-minute period, with the sensor positioned on the arterial blood vein. By utilizing the transmitter and receiver of the sensor, raw data was obtained directly from the vein. This vibration sensor measures the mechanical vibrations of the body. Additionally, an Arduino microcontroller was employed to operate the vibration sensor along with a 10 megaohm resistor. Calibration remains a bottleneck in wearable BP devices. Our system currently uses a per-user calibration model where one baseline cuff measurement initializes the mapping. Periodic recalibration is recommended every few weeks to counter physiological drift. Future work will explore calibration-free modeling by leveraging morphological feature learning, as proposed in recent studies. The need for calibration impacts clinical scalability and user compliance. Reducing or eliminating this dependency remains an open research challenge.

Figure 2. Edge Device

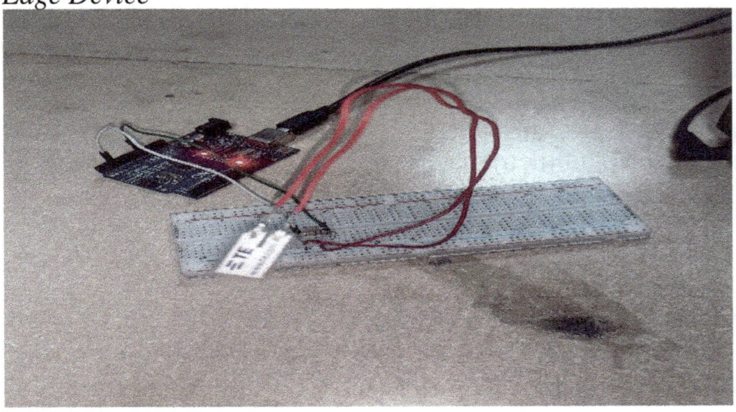

Smoothing within signal processing involves a method employed to diminish the impact of noise or rapid fluctuations in a signal while retaining its fundamental trend or structureIt is frequently employed in processing time-series data or analogous signals to improve their interpretability and analytical clarity. The filter utilized in this context is the Savitzky-Golay filter, with a smoothing factor set to 0.08 for the smoothing operation on the signals obtained from the vibration sensor. Savitzky-Golay filtering strikes a delicate equilibrium between diminishing noise and retaining crucial signal characteristics, rendering it an invaluable asset in the realm of signal processing.

$$yi = \sum_{k=-m}^{m} c_k + x_{i+k} \text{ -------} \qquad (1)$$

yi is the output data point at index *i*,
xi+k represents the input data points surrounding *yi*,
ck are the filter coefficients, and
m is half the filter window size.

Detrending a signal is essential for reducing noise, correcting baselines, and enhancing data interpretation. By eliminating long-term trends or patterns, detrending isolates short-term fluctuations or noise, improving the accuracy of analysis. Moreover, it assists in standardizing signals for comparison across various time frames or experimental conditions. Detrending serves as a vital initial step prior to conducting additional analyses like frequency analysis or peak detection, guaranteeing precise and dependable results.

Linear detrending is applied here where the formula is

$$y = mx + b - - - - - - - - \qquad (2)$$

Where:

y is the intercept of the signal
m is the slope of the line
b is the y-intercept of the line

Denoising carries substantial significance in signal processing, as it serves to enhance signal quality, precision, and sensitivity. Denoising preserves the clarity and distinguishability of critical signal features, thereby enhancing the effectiveness of subsequent analysis and communication endeavors. Particularly in domains such as biomedical signal processing, denoising plays a crucial role in ensuring precise diagnosis, monitoring, and speech recognition. Ultimately, denoising facilitates the extraction of reliable information from signals. Band-stop filters, commonly referred to as notch filters, play a vital role in signal processing by selectively reducing frequency ranges while permitting others to remain unaffected. They excel in eliminating undesired noise or interference, such as that from power lines or electromagnetic sources, which in turn enhances the clarity of the signal. Through precise frequency selectivity, they target and suppress interference frequencies without impacting the remainder of the signal spectrum. Particularly in systems prone to instability or distortion, like control loops or mechanical resonances, these filters maintain stability by effectively dampening problematic frequencies. When combining a low-pass filter set at a cutoff frequency of $1fc1$ and a high-pass filter set at a cutoff frequency of $2fc2$, the resultant band-stop filter is formed by summing their respective outputs. This can be mathematically represented by the transfer function $H(s)$, where $HLP(s)$ stands for the transfer function of the low-pass filter, represented by LP(s), corresponds to the transfer function of the high-pass filter, denoted as HHP(s).

$$H(s) = H_{LP(s)} + H_{HP(s)} - - - - - - - \qquad (3)$$

Where $HLP(s)$ represents the transfer function of the low-pass filter, while HHP(s) represents the transfer function of the high-pass filter. To proceed, detection of the peaks in the sampled signal is necessary. This is achieved by applying a band-stop filter. Once filtered, the identification of Mean Arterial Pressure (MAP), Systolic

Blood Pressure (SBP), and Diastolic Blood Pressure (DBP) from the transformed signal becomes possible. The Dicrotic notch manifests as a short dip in arterial pressure following the closure of the aortic valve during the cardiac cycle. It signifies a temporary halt in arterial flow and is observable in pressure waveforms obtained through invasive blood pressure monitoring. In clinical contexts, this feature holds significant importance, providing valuable understanding of both cardiac and arterial function. The processed vibration waveform was segmented beat-by-beat, and the following features were extracted Temporal Features: Inter-beat interval, systolic rise time, dicrotic notch time interval. Morphological Features: Peak-to-peak amplitude, pulse width, waveform area, systolic/diastolic amplitude ratio. Statistical Features: Mean, variance, skewness, and kurtosis of each beat segment. These features capture arterial compliance and hemodynamic variations, which correlate with SBP, DBP, and MAP.

A major trend in modern BP estimation research is the transition from manually engineered features (e.g., extracted PTT, pulse amplitude) to deep learning-based, end-to-end systems. These architectures autonomously learn discriminative features from raw physiological signals, capturing non-linear temporal dependencies that traditional models may overlook. Our LSTM-based framework aligns with this trend by directly learning from vibration signal sequences, representing an adaptive and scalable modeling paradigm. Long-short term memory (LSTM) is used to capture the temporal dependencies that are presented in the dataset, The initial LSTM layer is configured with 64 units, defining the output space's dimensionality. The input_shape parameter delineates the input data shape, where sequence_length indicates each sequence's length and 1 signifies a single feature. Setting return_sequences=True ensures the layer provides the entire sequence of outputs, crucial for subsequent LSTM layers. Regularization, in the form of L2 regularization with a penalty factor of 0.001, is applied to both the kernel (weights) and recurrent (cell connections) parameters across this and subsequent LSTM layers. The second LSTM layer mirrors the first's configuration, with 64 units and sequence return. Similar regularization methods are employed to address overfitting concerns. The third LSTM layer, featuring 32 units, does not return sequences, delivering only the output for the final timestep in the sequence, while also applying regularization. Subsequent to the LSTM layers are three Dense layers, each with 64, 32, and 1 unit respectively. The initial two Dense layers utilize the ReLU activation function to introduce non-linearity, with regularization applied to their kernel parameters. The last Dense layer, consisting of a single unit, is typical for regression tasks, directly producing continuous output without activation.

Twilio serves as a versatile tool for communication needs like delivering transactional updates, marketing outreach, urgent alerts, and securing accounts with two-factor authentication. Its adaptability and ability to handle growing demands have made it a favored solution among businesses and developers seeking to incorporate robust communication capabilities into their platforms. The proposed system ensures secure data handling through encryption and restricted access. Users' BP readings are transmitted via Twilio using secure HTTPS protocols. Data is stored locally or on encrypted servers with access limited to authorized personnel. Compliance with HIPAA and GDPR standards is prioritized. Furthermore, users are informed about data usage and potential risks, ensuring transparency and ethical responsibility in digital health applications.

RESULTS AND DISCUSSION

The Savitzky-Golay filter offers versatile applications. It efficiently interpolates data by utilizing polynomial fitting between data points, enabling the estimation of values at intermediary points. This feature is particularly handy for filling in missing data or creating a smoother rendition of the original signal. By smoothing noisy data, the filter enhances the clarity of trends, aiding in their visualization and interpretation. Notably, unlike conventional filters like simple moving averages, the Savitzky-Golay filter retains crucial features such as peak shapes and widths, making it invaluable in fields like signal processing where maintaining the integrity of such features is crucial. Moreover, varying the filter's window sizes and polynomial orders allows for insightful exploration of data variations, aiding in the comprehension of the underlying dynamics of the system under study. The fig.3. provides the visualization of the smoothened signal

Figure 3. Smoothening of signal

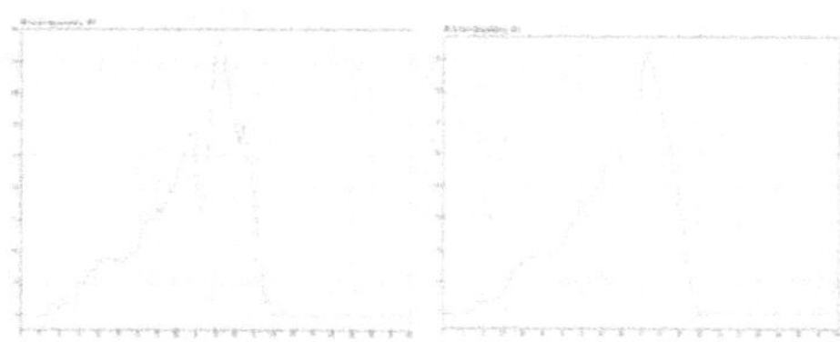

Detrending a signal involves eliminating long-term trends, which isolates short-term fluctuations and allows for a clearer understanding of the signal's dynamics that can be seen in fig.4. Additionally, it serves as a normalization method, ensuring fair comparisons between signals with varying baseline levels. Analyzing the fluctuations around the detrended trend offers deeper understanding of the underlying dynamics of the system. Linear detrending, as described in equation (2), is the method utilized here to remove linear trends from the acquired signal. Its objective is to eliminate any linear components from the signal, thereby enabling a more targeted analysis of the remaining fluctuations.

Figure 4. Detrending of signal

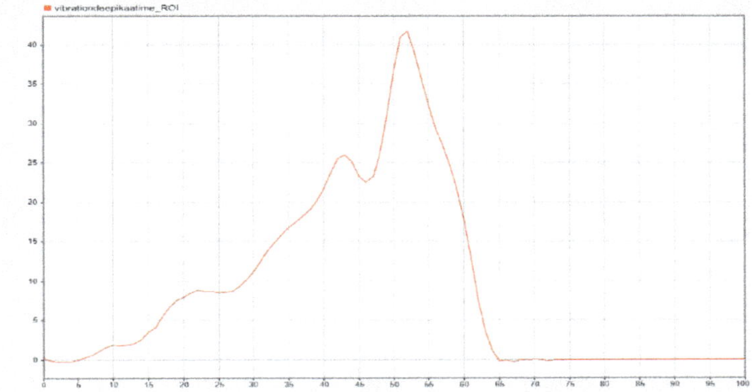

Denoising enhances the clarity of the signal by reducing the interference caused by noise. This makes it easier to observe and interpret the underlying patterns or features present in the data. By removing noise, denoising improves the overall quality of the data that can be seen in fig.5. This is particularly important in fields where accurate and reliable data are essential for analysis or decision-making. Removing noise from the signal can reveal underlying patterns or dynamics that were previously obscured. By cleaning the data, denoising can enhance the efficacy of subsequent algorithms or techniques applied to the data.

Figure 5. Denoising the signal

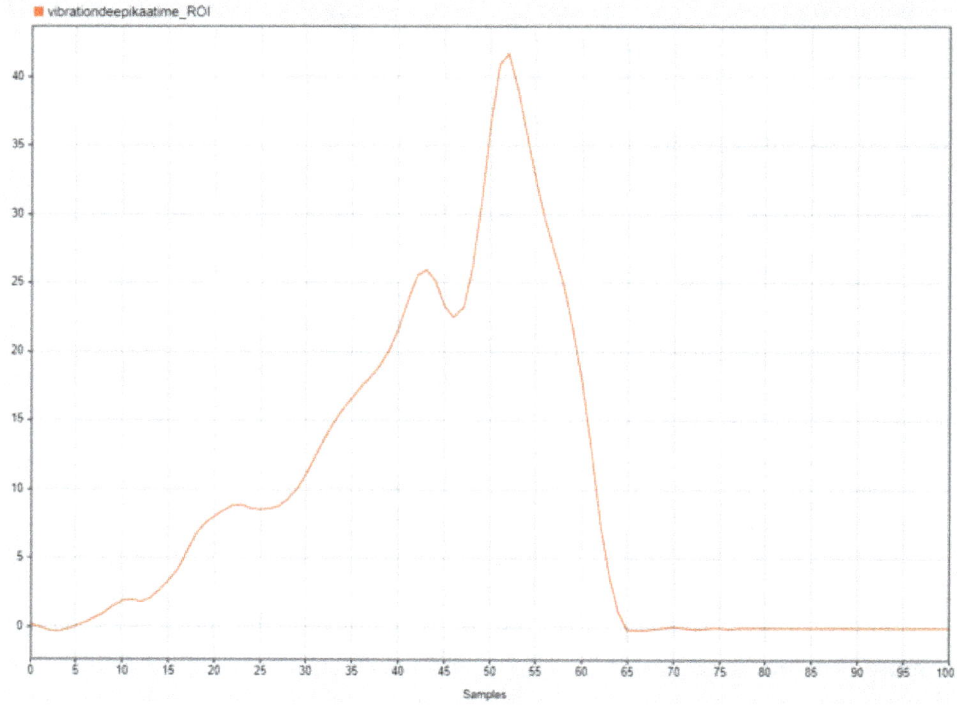

Band-stop filters can effectively suppress unwanted noise or interference that occurs at specific frequencies. By attenuating these frequencies, the filter enhances the clarity of the signal by reducing noise-related distortions, unwanted interference occurs at specific frequencies, such as power line noise (50Hz or 60Hz), band-stop filters can effectively Eliminating or diminishing this interference while preserving the remainder of the signal intact is the goal. By eliminating particular frequency components linked to noise or interference, band-stop filters can heighten the signal-to-noise ratio (SNR) of the filtered signal that can be seen I fig.6. This results in a clearer and more precise depiction of the desired signal. In certain applications, such as EEG or ECG signal processing, band-stop filters can help minimize artifacts caused by environmental noise, power line interference, or muscle activity, thereby improving the quality of physiological data. Unlike broad-spectrum filters that may affect a wide range of frequencies, band-stop filters selectively attenuate only the specified frequency band. This helps preserve the integrity and characteristics of the signal outside of the targeted band. Band-stop filters facilitate the amplification of the signal, making it easier to use. In certain applications, such as EEG or ECG signal processing, band-stop filters can help minimize artifacts caused by environmental noise, power line interference, or muscle activity, thereby improving the quality of physiological data.

Figure 6. Applying Band-Stop filter

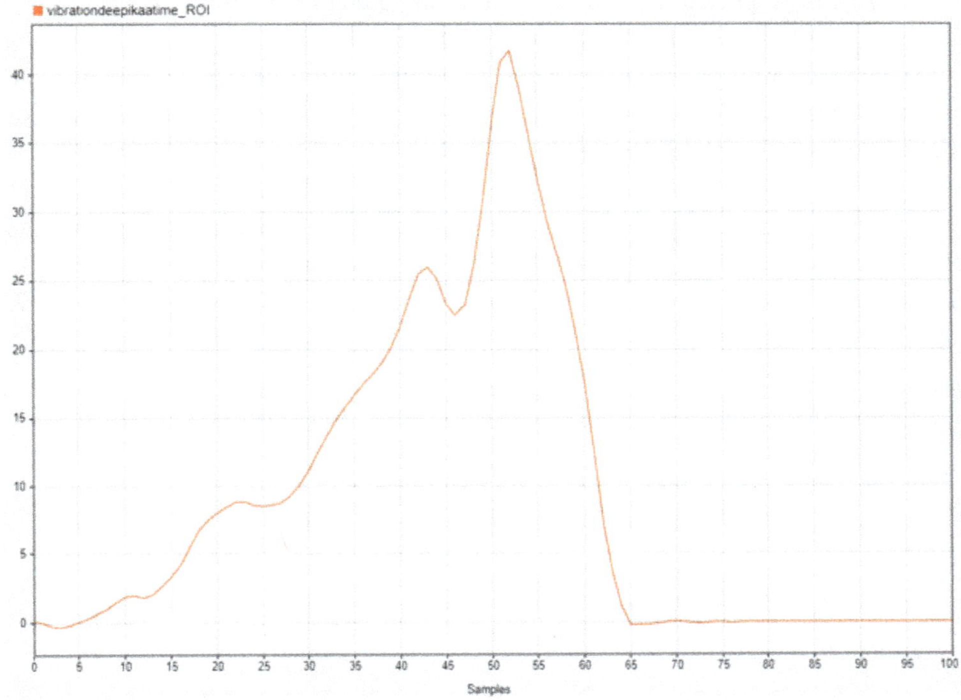

Assessing cardiovascular health is paramount. Initially, the signal undergoes sampling to detect peaks, which signify crucial points in the cardiac cycle. Subsequent application of a band-stop filter aims to eliminate unwanted frequency bands, such as noise or interference, while preserving vital components. Following this, parameters including Mean Arterial Pressure (MAP), Systolic Blood Pressure (SBP), and Diastolic Blood Pressure (DBP). Additionally, attention is paid to the dicrotic notch, a brief dip in arterial pressure observed after the shutting of the aortic valve. This characteristic, discernible in pressure waveforms obtained through invasive monitoring of blood pressure, yields valuable insights into both arterial and cardiac functionality, enriching comprehension, and treatment of cardiovascular ailments. This systematic approach enables thorough assessment and monitoring of arterial pressure dynamics, contributing significantly to the effective management of patients' cardiovascular well-being. The MAP, SBP and DBP are calculated by formulas given.

$$MAP = \frac{1}{3}SBP + \frac{2}{3}DBP - \text{------} \qquad (4)$$

Mean Arterial Pressure (MAP) is a vital metric representing the average arterial pressure across a cardiac cycle, critical for assessing perfusion pressure driving circulation of blood within the body's tissues.

In the equation:

(1/3) * SBP represents one-third of the SBP value.

(2/3) * DBP represents two-thirds of the DBP value.

Since the heart spends approximately two-thirds of the cardiac cycle in diastole and one-third in systole, the equation essentially calculates a weighted average of the pressures during these phases.

So, MAP is essentially weighted more towards DBP due to the heart's longer duration in diastole compared to systole. This weighting reflects the fact that the circulation needs to be maintained during diastole when the heart is relaxed and refilling with blood. The differentiating with the Dicrotic notch is depicted in fig.7.

Figure 7. Differentiating the SBP and DBP with Dicrotic notch

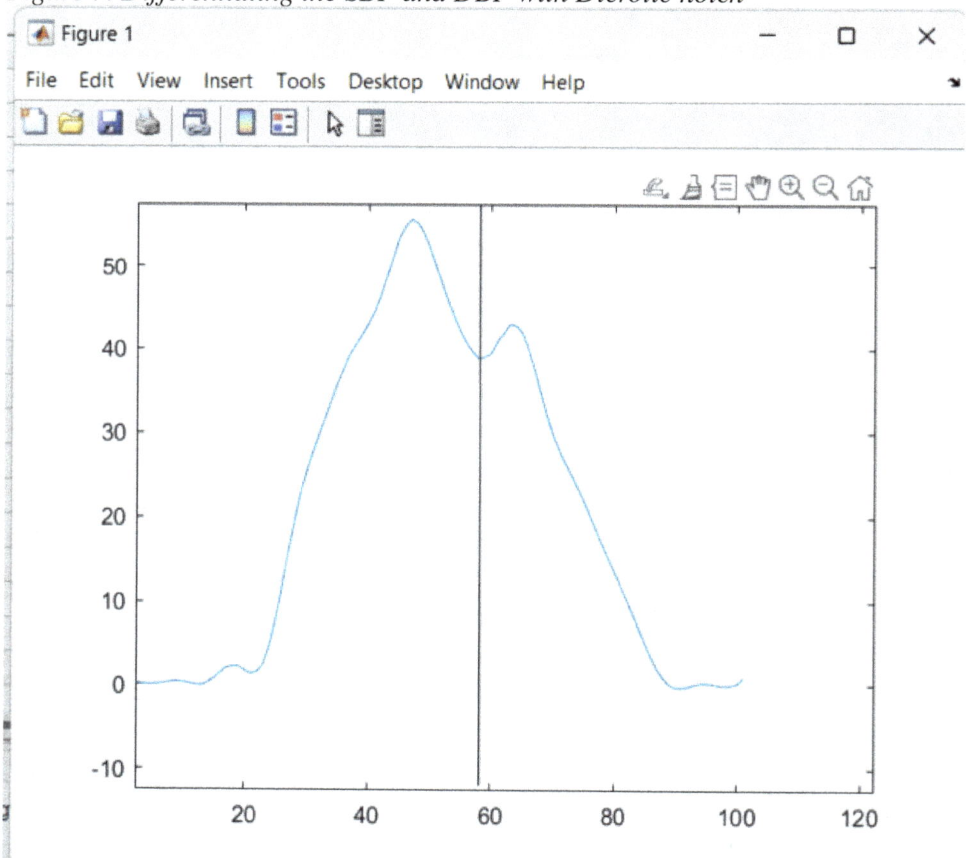

To compute the area under the curve for MAP, the Trapezoidal rule is employed, and the sampling frequency is determined within the time domain. The challenge arises when Systolic Blood Pressure (SBP) and Diastolic Blood Pressure (DBP) are unknown, requiring a different method to calculate Mean Arterial Pressure (MAP). In such cases, the mean of the entire signal and the area under the curve of the signal are utilized. The formula for calculating MAP in this scenario is as follows:

$$MAP = \frac{1}{3}(MEAN) + \frac{2}{3}(AUC) - ------- \qquad (5)$$

Following the determination of MAP, the calculation of Diastolic Blood Pressure (DBP) involves utilizing MAP and the area under the curve, particularly focusing on the presence of the Dicrotic notch. This process allows for the calculation of DBP using the following method:

$$DBP = MAP - \frac{2}{3}(AUC\ DBP) - ------- \qquad (6)$$

After knowing the MAP and the DBP we can easily calculate the SBP as the relation between the MAP, SBP and DBP are derived from equation 4:

$$SBP = 3(MAP) - 2(DBP) - ------- \qquad (7)$$

Figure 8. Area of the signal

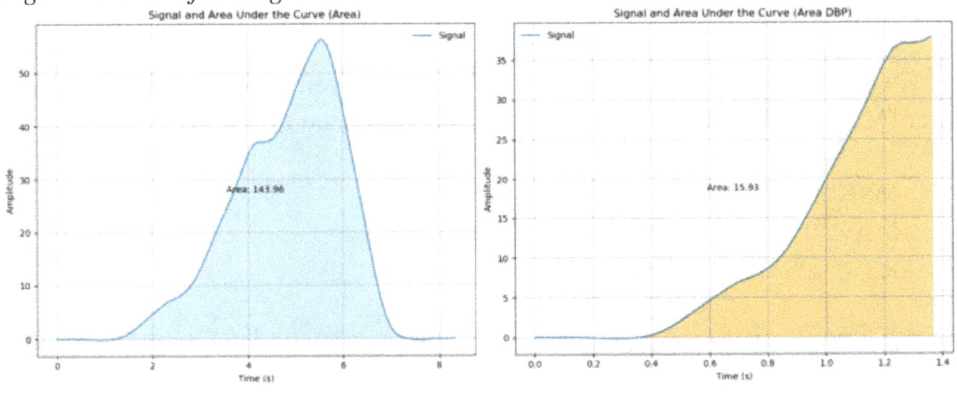

Validation involves comparing the LSTM model trained with a benchmark dataset, specifically the MIMIC II/III waveform database part-0. The area of the signal is shown in fig.8. The LSTM model is configured with a learning rate of 0.001 and includes dropout layers along with three dense layers. The comparison between the actual and predicted results is depicted in fig 9.

Figure 9. Actual vs Predicted of 1st LSTM

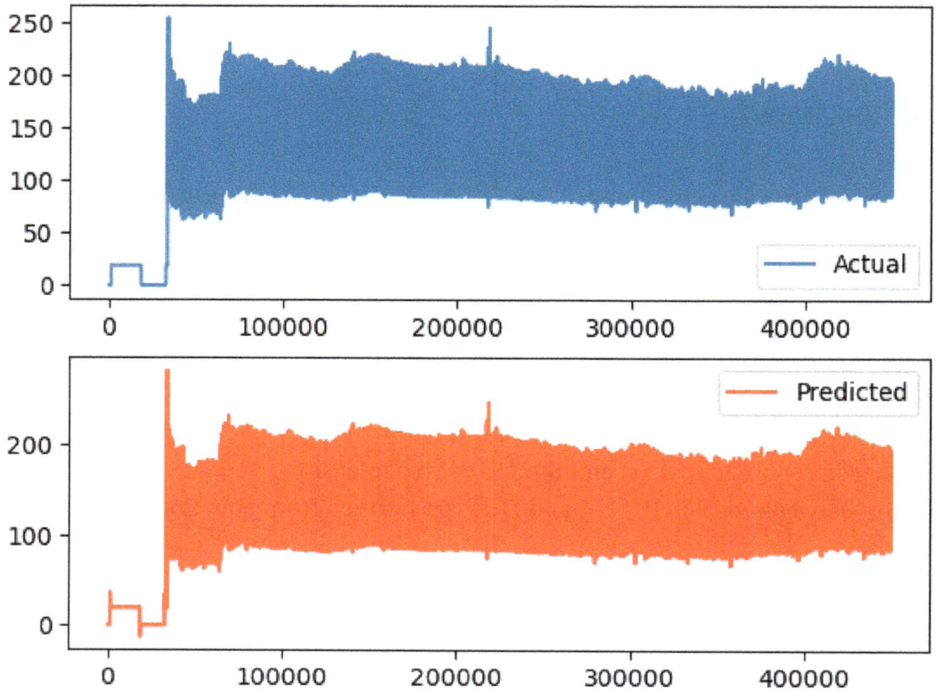

The error metrices are performed with Mean Squared error (MSE), Mean Absolute error (MAE) and the R2 Squared error(R2) the value are as follows:

MSE: 1.2002789176115736
MAE: 0.7173556369883908
R2: 0.9993748889199455

For cuffless blood pressure prediction via the device that obtained mechanical vibration signals from the arterial blood vein. These signals were gathered from ten individuals over a five-minute duration. The model architecture follows a sequential structure, where layers are added progressively, building upon each other. It consists of three Long Short-Term Memory (LSTM) layers, a specific form of recurrent neural network known for its proficiency in managing sequential data. The initial LSTM layer is configured with 128 units and designed to process input sequences of a designated length, featuring one attribute per time step. Subsequent LSTM layers consist of 64 and 32 units, respectively, all configured to output sequences. Dropout layers are interspersed following each LSTM layer, implementing a rate of dropout 0.3 to address overfitting concerns by randomly deactivating a portion of input units during training. Conclusively, a dense layer incorporating a solitary neuron is appended for output, typically employed in regression tasks where the model predicts a single continuous value. This architectural arrangement finds frequent application in sequence prediction endeavors like time series forecasting and natural language processing, capitalizing on LSTM networks' adaptability and efficiency in capturing temporal dependencies within the data.

Figure 10. Actual vs Predicted of second LSTM

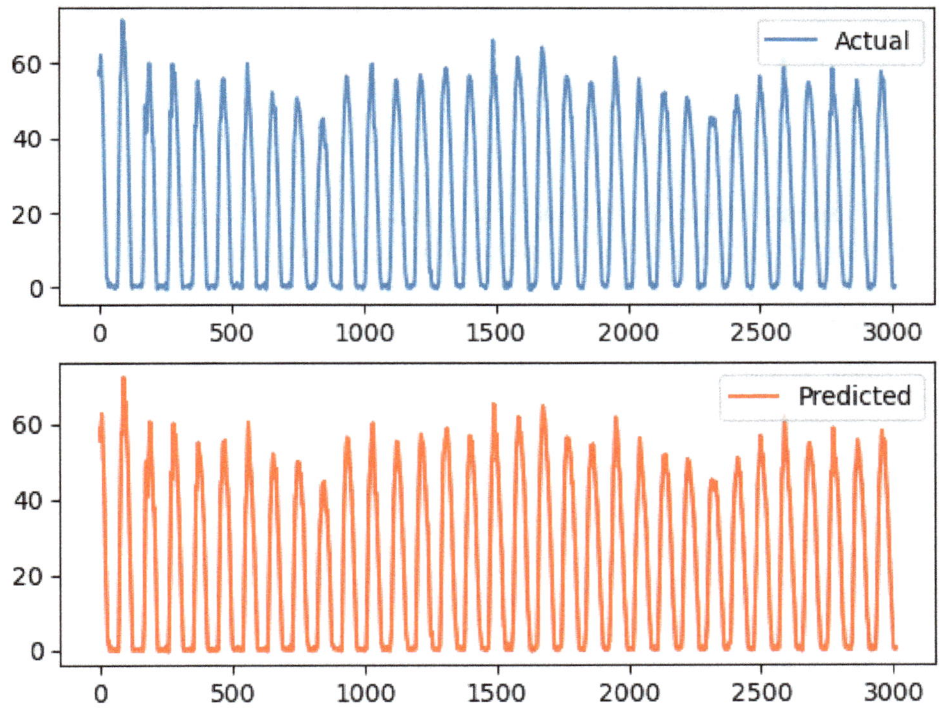

Based on the observations from fig.10, it's evident that the model exhibits favorable performance when compared to the benchmark dataset. The predictions show promise, showcasing an improvement over the previous LSTM model. Regarding the error metrics, they indicate.

MSE: 0.4013655977173886

MAE: 0.4778815451996915
R2: 999161340651876

In comparing the error metrics between the first and second LSTM models from the fig.11, we observe that

Figure 11. Comparison of the two LSTM Model

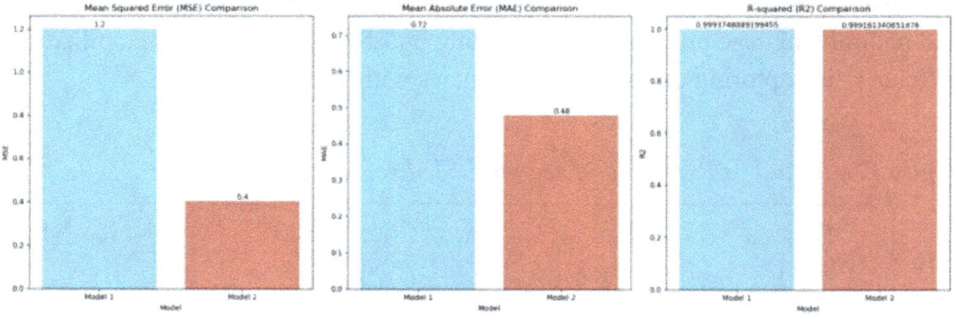

4.4 Responses from the Twilio: Since blood pressure readings have been obtained from individuals, notifications regarding their blood pressure measurements should be sent through Twilio, a cloud-based messaging platform responses from the twilio is shown in fig.12.

Figure 12. Responses from the Twilio interface

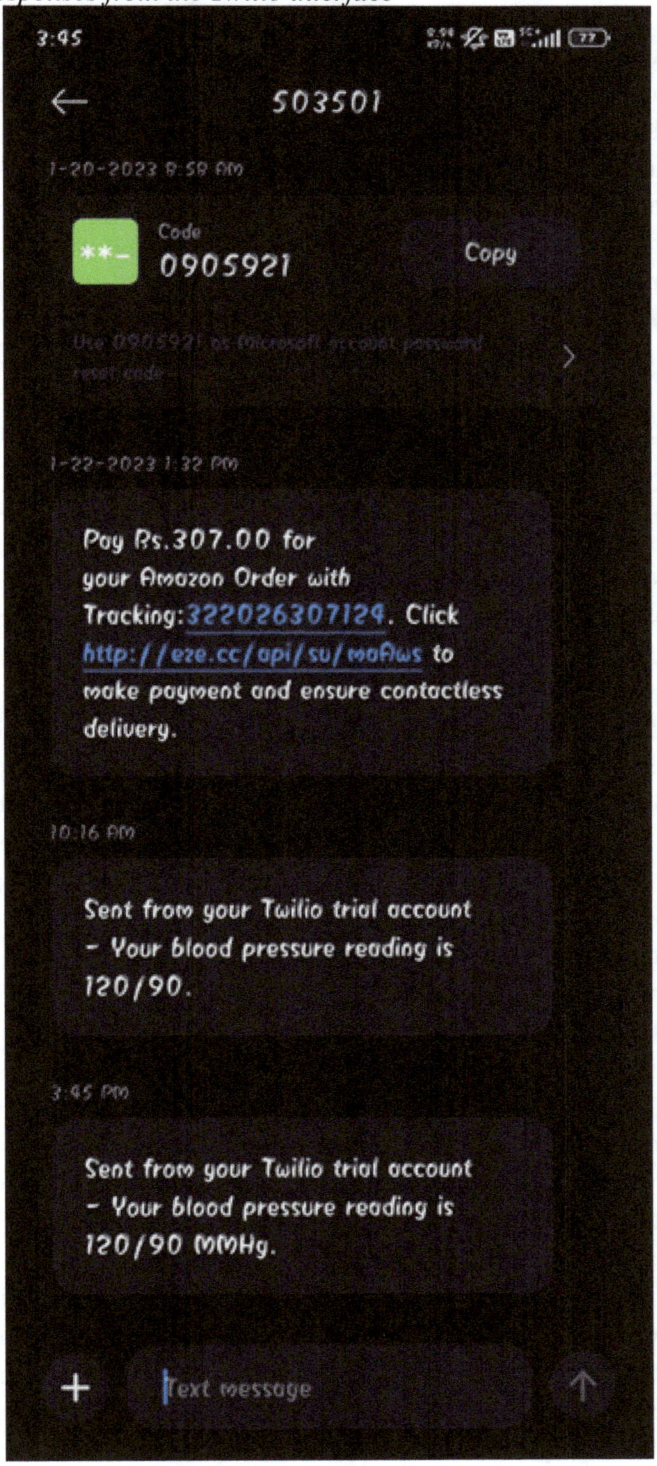

CONCLUSION

This chapter utilized two distinct datasets to conduct an extensive exploration of estimating blood pressure without the use of a cuff. Initially, data from the Physio Bank ATM, known for its extensive collection of physiological data, served as a fundamental reference. Additionally, direct acquisition of raw signals from vibration sensors offered a more immediate and focused perspective on blood pressure dynamics. The integration of these datasets provided a robust and multifaceted foundation for analysis and comparison, enhancing the depth and credibility of the study's conclusions. Advanced signal processing techniques were employed to extract meaningful insights from the raw signals obtained through vibration sensors. These techniques, including smoothing and filtering, were utilized to refine the raw data and identify crucial parameters necessary for blood pressure estimation. Through the application of these methods, the study successfully identified key metrics such as Mean Arterial Pressure (MAP), Systolic Blood Pressure (SBP), and Diastolic Blood Pressure (DBP), leading to valuable insights into the complex dynamics of cardiovascular function. The research leveraged LSTM (Long Short-Term Memory) models for estimating blood pressure without utilizing a cuff, subjecting them to rigorous validation against established benchmark datasets. This validation process served as a critical evaluation of the models' performance and reliability in accurately predicting blood pressure values. Encouraging results from the validation indicated favorable performance metrics for the LSTM models. Additionally, enhancements observed in the structure of the second LSTM model highlighted opportunities for further refinement and optimization, suggesting promising paths toward achieving more precise estimating blood pressure without using cuffs in future applications. Cuffless blood pressure estimation using vibration sensors offers a non-invasive approach, eliminating discomfort or anxiety related to cuff inflation, particularly these approaches are advantageous for individuals with sensitivity concerns. They enable uninterrupted monitoring, providing a thorough grasp of blood pressure variations over the course of a day, which is particularly beneficial for effectively managing conditions such as hypertension. Integration into wearable devices enhances mobility, enabling convenient and mobile blood pressure monitoring without requiring bulky equipment. Accuracy remains a significant challenge due to factors such as motion artifacts, environmental conditions, and individual physiological variations, potentially leading to discrepancies compared to traditional cuff-based methods. Validation of estimating blood pressure without using a cuff techniques using vibration sensors is still underway, necessitating thorough research to ensure reliable measurements across diverse populations and conditions. Initial investment costs for specialized sensors and algorithms may hinder widespread adoption, particularly in resource-limited settings where cost-effectiveness is crucial. User compliance and proper device usage are vital for obtaining accurate readings, emphasizing the need for comprehensive user education and training to minimize potential inaccuracies. In the future, there are several avenues for further development and enhancement of this project Extend validation efforts by employing diverse datasets to bolster the reliability and applicability without utilizing cuffs, estimating blood pressure models. Investigate the practical application estimation of blood pressure without the use of cuffs across diverse healthcare settings, including primary care, telemedicine, and remote patient monitoring, aiming to enhance patient outcomes and facilitate early detection of cardiovascular conditions.

REFERENCES

Arjomand, A., Boudesh, A., Bayatmakou, F., Kent, K. B., & Mohammadi, A. (2024). TransfoRhythm: A transformer architecture conductive to blood pressure estimation via solo PPG signal capturing. arXiv. https://arxiv.org/abs/2401.00000

Attarpour, A., Mahnam, A., Aminitabar, A., & Samani, H. (2019). Cuff-less continuous measurement of blood pressure using wrist and fingertip photoplethysmograms: Evaluation and feature analysis. *Biomedical Signal Processing and Control*, *49*, 212–220. DOI: 10.1016/j.bspc.2018.12.006

Chen, C., Qin, C., Li, Y., Liu, C., & Ma, X. (2023). Cuff-less blood pressure prediction based on photoplethysmography and modified ResNet. *Bioengineering (Basel, Switzerland)*, *10*(4), 400. DOI: 10.3390/bioengineering10040400 PMID: 37106587

Chen, W., Rahman, M., & Ali, M. (2024). Deep learning and remote photoplethysmography for contactless physiological monitoring: A review. *Frontiers in Bioengineering and Biotechnology*, *12*, 1420100. Advance online publication. DOI: 10.3389/fbioe.2024.1420100 PMID: 39104628

El-Hajj, C., & Kyriacou, P. A. (2020). A review of machine learning techniques in photoplethysmography for the non-invasive cuff-less measurement of blood pressure. *Biomedical Signal Processing and Control*, *58*, 101870. DOI: 10.1016/j.bspc.2020.101870

El-Hajj, C., & Kyriacou, P. A. (2021). Cuffless blood pressure estimation from PPG signals and its derivatives using deep learning models. *Biomedical Signal Processing and Control*, *70*, 102984. DOI: 10.1016/j.bspc.2021.102984

Elgendi, M., Fletcher, R., & Liang, Y. (2024). Recommendations for evaluating photoplethysmography-based blood pressure estimation: Challenges and benchmarking. *Communications Medicine*, *4*, 00555. Advance online publication. DOI: 10.1038/s43856-024-00555-2 PMID: 38997447

Ghosh, S., Chattopadhyay, B. P., Roy, R. M., Mukherjee, J., & Mahadevappa, M. (2022). Non-invasive cuffless blood pressure and heart rate monitoring using impedance cardiography. *Intelligent Medicine*, *2*, 100016. DOI: 10.1016/j.imed.2021.11.001

González, S., Hsieh, W.-T., & Chen, T.-P. (2023). A benchmark for machine-learning-based non-invasive blood pressure estimation using photoplethysmogram. *Scientific Data*, *10*, 149. Advance online publication. DOI: 10.1038/s41597-023-02020-6 PMID: 36944668

Heydari, F., Ebrahim, M. P., Redoute, J.-M., Joe, K., Walker, K., & Yuce, M. R. (2019). A chest-based continuous cuffless blood pressure method: Estimation and evaluation using multiple body sensors. *Information Fusion*, *54*, 66–74. DOI: 10.1016/j.inffus.2019.07.001

Hu, J.-R., Martin, G., Iyengar, S., Brady, T. M., Turkson-Ocran, R.-A. N., & Juraschek, S. P. (2023). Validating cuffless continuous blood pressure monitoring devices. *Cardiovascular Digital Health Journal*, *4*(2), 100121. DOI: 10.1016/j.cvdhj.2023.01.001 PMID: 36865583

Hua, J., Zhang, X., & Li, P. (2024). Wearable cuffless blood pressure tracking: When will they get it right? *Journal of Human Hypertension*. Advance online publication. DOI: 10.1038/s41371-024-00932-3

Inan, O. T., Migeotte, P.-F., & Park, K. S. (2015). Ballistocardiography and seismocardiography: A review of recent advances. *IEEE Journal of Biomedical and Health Informatics*, *19*(4), 1414–1427. DOI: 10.1109/JBHI.2014.2361732 PMID: 25312966

Ishizaka, S., Fujimoto, K., & Koike, M. (2021). Non-contact blood pressure measurement using Doppler radar based on waveform analysis by LSTM. In *IEEE International Conference on Communications (ICC 2021)*. IEEE. https://doi.org/ DOI: 10.1109/ICC42927.2021.9500857

Joung, J., Lee, H., & Kim, J. (2023). Continuous cuffless blood pressure monitoring using a novel system. *Scientific Reports*, *13*, 35492. DOI: 10.1038/s41598-023-35492-y PMID: 37244974

Koparır, H. M., & Arslan, Ö. (2024). Cuffless blood pressure estimation from photoplethysmography using deep convolutional neural network and transfer learning. *Biomedical Signal Processing and Control*, *93*, 106194. DOI: 10.1016/j.bspc.2024.106194

Liu, L., Zhang, Y.-T., Wang, W., Chen, Y., & Ding, X. (2023). Causal inference-based cuffless blood pressure estimation: A pilot study. *Computers in Biology and Medicine*, *159*, 106900. DOI: 10.1016/j.compbiomed.2023.106900 PMID: 37087777

Mahajan, P., & Kaul, A. (2025). Enhanced cuffless blood pressure estimation using ECG and PPG signals: A hybrid approach with Windkessel, ARIMA, and LSTM. *Turkish Journal of Electrical Engineering and Computer Sciences*, *33*(3), 282–305. DOI: 10.55730/1300-0632.4127

Mousavi, S. S., Firouzmand, M., Charmi, M., Hemmati, M., Moghadam, M., & Ghorbani, Y. (2019). Blood pressure estimation from appropriate and inappropriate PPG signals using a whole-based method. *Biomedical Signal Processing and Control*, *47*, 196–206. DOI: 10.1016/j.bspc.2018.08.022

Mukkamala, R., Hahn, J.-O., & Inan, O. T. (2022). Important findings on cuffless blood pressure measurement: Standards and pitfalls. *Nature Reviews. Cardiology*, *19*, 1–18. https://www.ncbi.nlm.nih.gov/pmc/articles/PMC9931644/

Nawaz, M. W., Tahir, M. A., Mehmood, A., Rahman, M. M. U., Riaz, K., & Abbasi, Q. H. (2024). Cuff-less arterial blood pressure waveform synthesis from single-site PPG using transformer & frequency-domain learning. arXiv. https://arxiv.org/abs/2402.00000

Phan, D. T., Phan, T. T. V., Huynh, T. C., Park, S., Choi, J., & Oh, J. (2022). Noninvasive, wearable multi-biosensors for continuous, long-term monitoring of blood pressure via Internet of Things applications. *Computers & Electrical Engineering*, *102*, 108187. DOI: 10.1016/j.compeleceng.2022.108187

Samimi, H., & Dajani, H. R. (2023). A PPG-based calibration-free cuffless blood pressure estimation method using cardiovascular dynamics. *Sensors (Basel)*, *23*(8), 4145. DOI: 10.3390/s23084145 PMID: 37112490

Xing, X., Li, H., Chen, Q., Jiang, C., & Dong, W.-F. (2024). Blood pressure monitoring with piezoelectric bed sensor systems. *Biomedical Signal Processing and Control*, *87*, 105479. DOI: 10.1016/j.bspc.2023.105479

Yang, E., Schutte, A. E., & Stergiou, G. (2025). Cuffless blood pressure measurement devices—International perspectives on accuracy and clinical use: A narrative review. *JAMA Cardiology*, *10*(6), 624–631. DOI: 10.1001/jamacardio.2025.0662 PMID: 40266607

Yin, S., Li, G., Luo, Y., & Lin, L. (2021). Cuff-less continuous blood pressure measurement based on multiple types of information fusion. *Biomedical Signal Processing and Control*, *68*, 102549. DOI: 10.1016/j.bspc.2021.102549

Zabihi, S., Rahimian, E., Marefat, F., Asif, A., Mohseni, P., & Mohammadi, A. (2022). BP-Net: Cuff-less and non-invasive blood pressure estimation via a generic deep convolutional architecture. *Biomedical Signal Processing and Control*, *78*, 103850. DOI: 10.1016/j.bspc.2022.103850

Zhang, G., Choi, D., & Jung, J. (2024). Development of continuous cuffless blood pressure prediction platform using enhanced 1-D SENet–LSTM. *Expert Systems with Applications*, *242*, 122812. DOI: 10.1016/j.eswa.2023.122812

Chapter 11
Smart IoT Health Monitor for Early TB Diagnosis Using Optimized Hyperbolic NasNet Attention Sea-Horse

N. Prasath
https://orcid.org/0000-0003-3744-6906
SRM Institute of Science and Technology, India

A. Arun
https://orcid.org/0000-0002-6174-2468
SRM Institute of Science and Technology, India

J. Sreemathy
Sri Eshwar College of Engineering, India

ABSTRACT

Tuberculosis (TB) remains a major global health challenge, particularly in low-resource settings where traditional diagnostic methods are slow, often leading to disease progression and increased transmission. To overcome these limitations, this study introduces an IoT-based patient monitoring system for early TB diagnosis, employing an Optimized Hyperbolic NasNet Attention Sea-horse Graph Network (OpHyp-NASH-Gra-Net). The system uses a wearable IoT sensor to collect patient data, which is transmitted via mobile device to cloud storage. Data is then clustered using an Adaptively Regularized Kernel-Based Fuzzy C-Means algorithm, filtered via a Fast Guided Median Filter (FGMF) for enhanced quality, and processed

DOI: 10.4018/979-8-3373-4412-6.ch011

with a Scale-Aware Modulation Meet Transformer (SA2MT) for feature extraction. The OpHyp-NASH-Gra-Net model classifies the data to distinguish between TB and non-TB cases, achieving 99% accuracy in simulations conducted with Python. This approach enables real-time, high-accuracy diagnosis, reducing delays and improving outcomes in resource-constrained environments.

1. INTRODUCTION

Technology for assisted living is becoming more popular as the population ages. The aged and disabled will account for half of all people in Europe by 2040 and one in six of all Americans by 2025 (Roy & Sadiwala, 2024). As a result, their needs for housing adaptation, medical care, and infrastructure will only grow. The goal of the Ambient Assisted Living (AAL) approach is to employ state-of-the-art services and technologies to improve the standard of living for the elderly and those suffering from chronic illnesses (Biswas et al., 2024). Diabetes patients with cardiac arrhythmias are the most appropriate recipients of AAL systems that are based on sensors of blood pressure, body temperature, glucose, oxygen, and weight (Mohammed, 2024). This paper proposes an IoT-enabled architecture for disease diagnosis from an m-health perspective to compute User Diagnosis Results (UDR) and to set up an alert for managing disease severity (Fan et al., 2024).

In realization of such diagnostic performance, the system collects information relating to abnormal states and fluctuations of indicators by using the medical sensors and Internet of Things devices (Kadayat et al., 2024; Sharma et al., 2023). The approach adopted is individual patient focused and provides a cheap method by which one can maintain health. Numerous industries, including communication, corporate operations, education, and healthcare, have been transformed by technology (Roy & Sadiwala, 2024). Particularly during the COVID-19 epidemic, digital technology has extended horizons and broken down geographical barriers. Social media sites are now essential information sources, especially for younger people (Ahmed et al., 2023). With ideas like smart automobiles, smart cities with smart resources, smartphones, and smart farming changing everyday life, the Internet of Things has revolutionized computer science (Srivastava et al., 2023; Umer et al., 2023).

It is anticipated that smart devices would follow human activity in real time, gather information, and forward it to health care providers so they can track patients' conditions in real time. What IoMT, or the Internet of Medical Things, focuses on most is the integration of IoT-based health devices (Pan et al., 2024). Due to information technology's (IT) integration, which permits the medical business to follow, patients' health records in real time and provide individualized care (Zamani & Sharifian, 2024). Through the Internet of Medical Things (IoMT), which combines smart and wearable sensors for usage by medical professionals facilitates effective monitoring and individualized care. Because of chronic illnesses, this technique is especially helpful in developing nations with limited resources (Kim et al., 2024). Large volumes of data gathered from smart devices are analyzed using AI and ML to spot trends and speed up the diagnosis of illness. AIoMT has greatly reduced infection sites and seeks to reduce healthcare costs and hospital admissions. IoMT, AI, and ML integration has the power to transform daily life and advance healthcare (Navya et al., 2024). Real-time post-COVID-19 diagnostic Collaboration between academia and industry is critical for enhanced facilities and lower prices. Remote healthcare systems are essential for numerous conditions, including heart disease (Motwani et al., 2024).

Tuberculosis is a global health challenge, especially in low-resource settings. Traditional detection methods are time-consuming, leading to disease progression and increased transmission rates. Healthcare infrastructure is overwhelmed by demand for rapid diagnosis. The existing healthcare infrastructure is often overwhelmed by the demand for rapid and accurate TB diagnosis, further exacerbating the issue. To address these challenges, this work is motivated.

Novelty and contribution

The Novelty and contribution of this paper is given below:

- Development of an Internet of Things-enabled system for the live gathering and observation of patient data, specifically targeting tuberculosis (TB) diagnosis.
- Implementation of the Adaptively Regularized Kernel-Based Fuzzy C-Means (ARKFCM) Based on Kernels to separate TB-related data from other non-relevant data efficiently.
- Utilization of the Fast Guided Median Filter (FGMF) to enhance data quality by reducing noise and improving the accuracy of the diagnosis.
- Introduction of the Scale-Aware Modulation Meet Transformer (SA2MT) for superior feature extraction, ensuring that critical patterns in the data are accurately captured.
- Proposal of the Optimized Hyperbolic NasNet Attention Sea-horse Graph Network (OpHyp-NASH-Gra-Net) for accurate classification of tuberculosis and non-tuberculosis diseases, enhancing diagnostic precision.
- OpHyp-NASH-Gra-Net is the novel method and it is the combination of NasNet (N) model integrated with Hyperbolic Attention Graph Network (HAGN) (N-HAGN) and its parameters are optimized with Sea-horse Optimization algorithm (SHOA).
- Integration of cloud storage for secure, scalable, and accessible storage of patient data, enabling healthcare providers to access diagnostic results remotely.

- Facilitation of remote diagnosis by sending detected TB data directly to healthcare professionals, accelerating response time and improving patient care in underserved regions.

The rest of the manuscript is organized as follows: Section 2 provides a literature review, Section 3 details the proposed technique, Section 4 summarizes the findings, and Section 5 closes with future study.

2. LITERATURE SURVEY

The papers related to Smart Health Monitor for Early Tuberculosis Diagnosis: An IoT-Based Patient Monitoring System using deep learning methods are given below:

Awotunde et al. (2023) has introduced a eXtreme Gradient Boosting (XGBoost) for Smart Health Monitor for Early Tuberculosis Diagnosis of IoT based patient. Real-time monitoring, diagnosis, and treatment have been made possible by IoT with machine learning (ML). This paper proposes a framework for an IoT-based system that uses wearables and sensors to diagnose diseases in real time, utilizing ML capabilities. The XGBoost model outperforms with accuracy of 95.7%, recall of 95.9%, precision of 96.0%, F1-score of 94.8%, and ROCO of 94.3% other ML models.

Almujally et al. (2023) has introduced a Multilayer Perceptron Neural Network (MPNN) for Smart Health Monitor for Early Tuberculosis Diagnosis of IoT based patient. The increasing prevalence of smart health monitoring devices can be attributed to both COVID-19 regulations and technology improvements. Artificial intelligence (AI) and the IoT are transforming data collecting and communication. The primary objective of this study is to create a cardiac patient health monitoring system that leverages AI and IoT to track activities, provide health status information, and categorize disorders using machine learning models.

Tang et al. (2024) has introduced a use AI and IoT techniques to develop a smart health monitor for early Tuberculosis diagnosis in IoT-based patients, utilizing Smart Healthcare-Crow Search Optimization (SH-CSO) to enhance diagnostic outcomes and improve healthcare service management. The model's highest accuracy for diabetes and heart disease is 97.26% and 96.16%, respectively.

Verma et al. (2024) has introduced a Wireless Body Area Network (WBAN)) for Smart Health Monitor for Early Tuberculosis Diagnosis of IoT based patient. Due to the significant effects of the COVID-19 pandemic on healthcare systems, remote health monitoring is now required. As a result, sophisticated health care systems including electronic health records (EHR) and medical charts have been developed. IoT devices, such sensors, can lower risks, expenses, and health-related issues by utilizing cloud computing to gather and analyze patient data. These gadgets have the ability to monitor patient characteristics, such blood pressure and body temperature, and transfer those data to a cloud database for automated illness prediction. This facilitates prompt medical evaluations and suitable medicinal interventions. An integrated routine learning health system can benefit from the incorporation of IoT with data analytics methods and precision algorithms.

Abubeker et al. (2024) has introduced an internet of medical things (IoMT) network) for Smart Health Monitor for Early Tuberculosis Diagnosis of IoT based patient. A non-invasive biosensor framework has been created by researchers to identify pneumonia contracted in hospitals and pneumonia contracted in critical care units (VAP) due to ventilator use. The framework analyzes VOCs in breathed air using wearable and portable biosensor arrays along with machine learning. Wireless body area networks, or WBANs, are used by the system to track health and monitor critical care units. The system uses a 128-core NVIDIA Jetson Nano GPU to transmit VOC data and patient characteristics smoothly.

Munnangi et al. (2023) has introduced a Moran Autocorrelation and Regression-based Elman Recurrent Neural Network (MARERNN) for Smart Health Monitor for Early Tuberculosis Diagnosis of IoT based patient. In order to reduce detection time, artificial intelligence is being used in the healthcare industry to extract sensor displacement effects and forecast anomalies. To identify volatile organic compounds (VOCs) in inhaled air, researchers have created biosensor arrays and machine learning frameworks that use a 128-core GPU for seamless transmission.

Sreenivasu et al. (2023) has introduced a Global System for Mobile Communications (GSM technology) for Smart Health Monitor for Early Tuberculosis Diagnosis of IoT based patient. The goal of the project is to apply a remote healthcare system that offers positive effects by uploading data to cloud services, monitoring health status, and enabling remote access in less developed countries. Table 1 shows the Summary of the reviewed approach.

Table 1. Summary of the reviewed approach

References	Methods	Advantages	Disadvantages
Awotunde et al., 2023	XGBoost	Reached strong performance metrics and accuracy (95.7%), indicating its dependability for in-the-moment disease diagnosis.	Requires a lot of processing power, which could prevent it from scaling in environments with limited resources.
Almujally et al., 2023	MPNN	Integration of AI and IoT allows for efficient tracking of health and classification of disorders.	High-dimensional data may cause difficulties, and careful tuning is needed to prevent overfitting.
Tang et al., 2024	T-RNN	Demonstrates outstanding diagnostic power and high accuracy (97.26% for diabetes and 96.16% for heart disease).	Complex preprocessing is necessary for managing temporal data, which can complicate systems and impede real-time analysis.
Verma et al., 2024	WBAN	Permits data transmission and real-time monitoring, which lowers health risks and allows for prompt medical actions.	Significantly depends on cloud computing, which may cause privacy issues and need the use of robust data protection measures.
Abubeker et al., 2023	IoMT	Using portable devices, a non-invasive biosensor framework effectively detects critical situations such as HAP and VAP in intensive care units.	Data administration and interpretation may become more complex as a result of integration with wearable technology and IoMT networks.
Munnangi et al., 2023	MARERNN	Effective anomaly prediction and sensor displacement detection shorten detection times, improving critical care monitoring.	In low-cost or non-GPU contexts, the system's versatility is limited by its high reliance on GPU processing (128-core).
Sreenivasu et al., 2023	GSM	Provides a scalable, affordable option for health monitoring in underdeveloped nations.	Due to connectivity problems, GSM networks might not be able to deliver dependable data transfer in isolated or developing areas.

Problem statement

Tuberculosis is a global health challenge, especially in low-resource settings. Traditional detection methods are time-consuming, leading to disease progression and increased transmission rates. Healthcare infrastructure is overwhelmed by demand for rapid diagnosis. The existing healthcare infrastructure is often overwhelmed by the demand for rapid and accurate TB diagnosis, further exacerbating the issue. To address these challenges, this work is proposed.

3. PROPOSED METHODOLOGY

In this section, a novel system, Smart Health Monitor for Early Tuberculosis Diagnosis: An IoT-Based Patient Monitoring System Using Optimized Hyperbolic NasNet Attention Sea-horse Graph Network is successfully implemented. To clearly represent the complete process, a system-level flowchart has been added as shown in Figure 1. This flowchart illustrates the step-by-step data flow, starting from IoT sensor data acquisition, cloud data storage, clustering using ARKFCM, preprocessing with FGMF, feature extraction via SA2MT, and final classification using the OpHyp-NASH-Gra-Net.

The Figure 2 shows the workflow diagram of OpHyp-NASH-Gra-Net. Initially, an IoT-based sensor is attached to the affected person, collecting disease-related data through a mobile phone, which is then stored in a cloud database. These data are clustered to separate TB-related data using the ARKFCM Based on Kernels. After clustering, the TB-related data is preprocessed using the Fast Guided Median Filter (FGMF) to enhance data quality. Features are then extracted using the Scale-Aware Modulation Meet Transformer (SA2MT) to capture relevant patterns. Finally, the data is classified using the Optimized Hyperbolic NasNet Attention Sea-horse Graph Network (OpHyp-NASH-Gra-Net) to detect tuberculosis and non-tuberculosis diseases, with the results sent to the doctor for further analysis.

Figure 1. Overall system pipeline of the proposed Smart Health Monitor for Early Tuberculosis Diagnosis using the OpHyp-NASH-Gra-Net model.

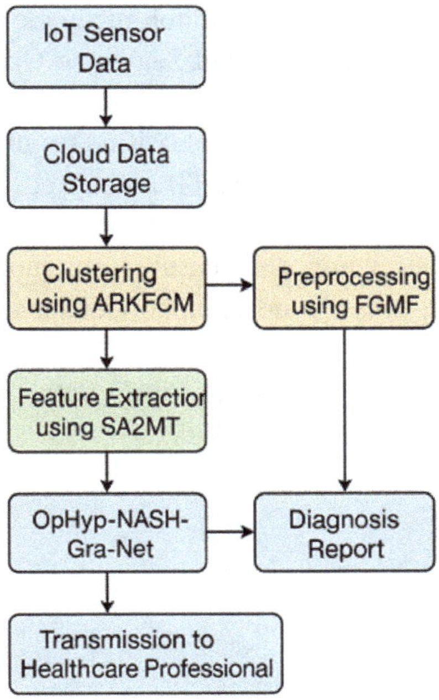

System Components and Interactions:

The proposed Smart Health Monitor for Early Tuberculosis Diagnosis consists of interconnected modules that work together for accurate and fast disease detection.

IoT Sensors: These wearable sensors continuously measure physiological parameters such as body temperature, respiration rate, and heart rate. The collected data represent the patient's health condition in real time.

Mobile Device and Cloud Storage: The sensor data are transmitted through a mobile application to a secure cloud storage system. The cloud provides scalability and acts as the central repository for further data processing.

Clustering (ARKFCM): The Adaptively Regularized Kernel-Based Fuzzy C-Means algorithm groups incoming data to separate tuberculosis-related patterns from unrelated data. This ensures only meaningful information is passed forward.

Preprocessing (FGMF): The Fast Guided Median Filter removes sensor noise and missing values to enhance data quality while preserving essential health information for diagnosis.

Feature Extraction (SA2MT): The Scale-Aware Modulation Meet Transformer captures important patterns and relationships in the TB-related data using both small-scale and large-scale attention mechanisms.

Classification (OpHyp-NASH-Gra-Net): This module performs decision-making by classifying input data as tuberculosis or non-tuberculosis. It integrates NasNet, Hyperbolic Attention Graph Network, and Sea-horse Optimization for improved accuracy.

Decision and Alert Transmission: The classified result is sent to the healthcare professional through the cloud interface. If TB is detected, the system automatically generates an alert for immediate medical attention.

The data flow among these components ensures continuous monitoring, intelligent decision-making, and real-time diagnosis support, enhancing healthcare efficiency in low-resource environments.

The below figure 2 shows how diagnostic results are communicated to healthcare professionals through a secure cloud network.

Figure 2. Workflow diagram of OpHyp-NASH-Gra-Net

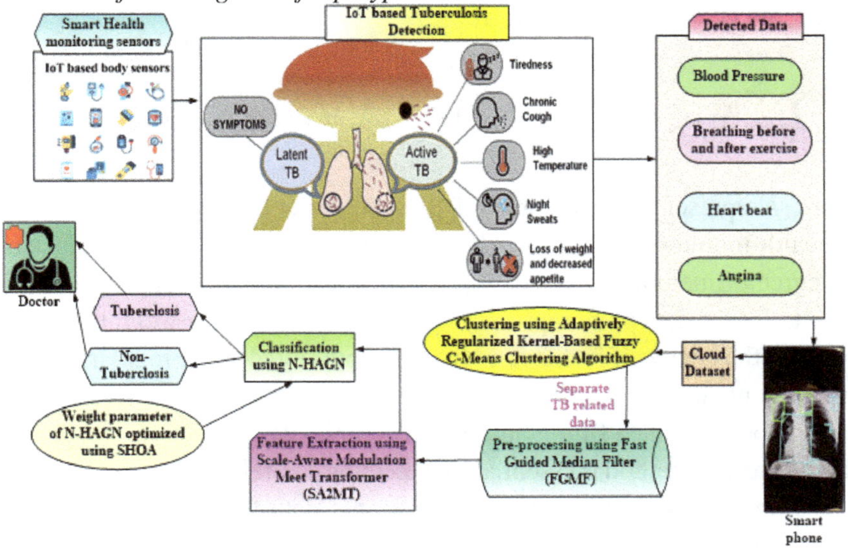

3.1 Data Acquistion

In this, the input dataset is taken from the IoT based smart health monitoring sensors. Then this health data is stored in cloud dataset. From this health data, the data are clustered using the Clustering using ARKFCM for detecting TB and its explanations are given below:

3.2 Clustering Using ARKFCM

The ARKFCM Clustering Algorithm integrates adaptive regularization, fuzzy clustering, and kernel methods to enhance the resilience of data clustering and reduce overfitting, particularly in high-dimensional, noisy, and complex datasets such as those collected from IoT-based health monitoring sensors (Cherfa et al., 2020). For early detection of tuberculosis and improve the efficiency of clustering health data, ARKFCM is employed for clustering the health data to distinguish between the data that is relevant to TB and data that is not. The values of the adaptive regularization parameters are tuned with respect of the data and model complexity to provide the best clustering results.

Within this architecture, the sensor nodes that are attached to the patients are grouped in a way that ensures that low energy is consumed while at the same time the system is still capable of monitoring and analyzing health data relevant to Tuberculosis. This is especially beneficial for continuous patient monitoring where sensor energy conservation is crucial.

$$FF_q = \sum_{q=1}^{N}\sum_{p=1}^{Al} b_{q,p}^{m} \|c_q - d_p\|^2 + \phi M(\cup) \tag{5}$$

where, Nrepresents the number of data points collected from the IoT-based smart health monitoring sensors, $Ak$is represented as the number of clusters, $b_{q,p}$ is the degree of membership of data point$q$in cluster p, $c_q$is represented as the ith data point, $d_p$is the data point representing health data$p$, $m$is the weighting exponent determining the degree of fuzziness, $M(\cup)$is represented as the regularization term based on the membership matrix $\cup$, $\phi$is the regularization parameter that controls the balance between data fitting and model complexity.

This clustering method is essential for detecting TB-related patterns in the health data, making it possible to focus on the relevant data for further processing and classification, while ensuring that the overall system remains energy-efficient and scalable for continuous monitoring.

Rationale and Advantages of ARKFCM:

The Adaptively Regularized Kernel-Based Fuzzy C-Means (ARKFCM) algorithm extends the classical FCM approach by incorporating kernel functions and adaptive regularization terms. In standard FCM, clustering performance declines when the data contain noise or overlapping distributions — common in IoT sensor readings. ARKFCM overcomes this limitation by mapping the data into a higher-dimensional feature space using kernel transformations, where nonlinear boundaries can better separate tuberculosis-related patterns from normal data.

The adaptive regularization term prevents overfitting by dynamically adjusting cluster compactness based on data complexity. This feature ensures stable clustering even under high sensor variability. Compared with conventional FCM, K-Means, and Gaussian Mixture Models (GMM), ARKFCM achieves improved robustness to noise, higher clustering precision, and faster convergence in heterogeneous medical data. In this context, ARKFCM is ideal because it isolates tuberculosis-relevant patterns from multi-sensor health data before subsequent preprocessing, thereby enhancing the accuracy and interpretability of the diagnostic process.

By this process the TB disease separated using this method, then these TB data are pre-processed using Fast Guided Median Filter (FGMF) for detecting TB accurately and its explanations are given below:

3.3 Pre-Processing Using Fast Guided Median Filter (FGMF)

In this phase, the input dataset taken from IoT based health monitoring sensors especially for tuberculosis (TB) detection are filtered using Fast Guided Median Filter (FGMF). To deal with missing values this paper uses the FGMF to remove noise or irrelevant data, and this is done to foredoom the most important features in the TB-related health data. This process helps in getting a better dataset that is used in improving the next TB diagnosis step.

The FGMF is expected to adequately suppress noise while preserving the edges as well as fine details which are critical in health care use. Compared to conventional median filters it is less time-consuming and requires less computations, which is achieved by using the sliding window concept and the median tracking mechanism. The filter is especially useful when applied to the health data collected using the IoT devices, and where the intricate details matter when it comes to the TB diagnosis.

Rationale and Advantages of FGMF:

The Fast Guided Median Filter (FGMF) is a hybrid noise reduction technique that combines the strengths of median filtering and guided image filtering. While classical median filters effectively remove salt-and-pepper noise, they often blur fine structural details that are crucial in biomedical signals. The guided filter, on the other hand, preserves edges but may not handle strong random noise efficiently.

FGMF integrates these two mechanisms using a guided median framework with cumulative histogram tracking, providing superior balance between noise suppression and edge preservation. It ensures that the essential variations in sensor readings such as abrupt respiration or temperature changes linked to TB symptoms remain intact.

Compared to standard filters like Gaussian, Bilateral, or Moving Average filters, FGMF achieves faster processing speed with lower computational cost and higher structural similarity index (SSIM). Its adaptive weighting strategy also makes it well-suited for real-time IoT-based health monitoring, where maintaining data clarity and diagnostic relevance is critical.

Data Quality and Label Accuracy Considerations:

The IoT sensor data collected for this study are prone to irregularities such as signal noise, missing values due to temporary sensor disconnection, and minor calibration errors. To ensure data reliability, all raw sensor streams were first validated for range consistency and timestamp synchronization. Data points falling outside clinically plausible thresholds (e.g., heart rate below 40 bpm or above 200 bpm) were flagged as anomalies and corrected using interpolation or removed when non-recoverable.

Missing data segments were filled using a sliding-window median interpolation method to maintain temporal consistency. Subsequently, the Fast Guided Median Filter (FGMF) was applied to denoise the data while preserving sharp transitions that may indicate real physiological changes. This dual-stage filtering approach effectively mitigates random sensor noise and measurement drift.

Label accuracy was maintained by aligning IoT readings with the UCI dataset's diagnostic categories, which were verified by domain experts. Each data instance was cross-checked against confirmed clinical diagnosis records to minimize labeling errors. Through this multi-step cleaning and validation process, the dataset used for training and testing retained both high fidelity and clinical relevance, ensuring that the proposed OpHyp-NASH-Gra-Net model learned from consistent, accurate, and meaningful health indicators.

The FGMF incorporates median filtering within a guided filter framework, where a weighted median filter updates cumulative histograms, as shown in Equation (6):

$$R_q^{\downarrow}(x) = R_q^{\downarrow}(x-1) + R_q(x) \tag{6}$$

where, $R_q(x)$ denotes the histogram value at pixel.

Let $h_p \in N$ be a pixel value at pixel $q$in a single channel guide data. The guided filter assumes that the filtering output at a specific pixel $g_q$at q can be estimated by a linear transformation $g$of the guided data in a local windowΦ_l, as defined in Equation (7):

$$h_q = d_l h_q + b_l \tag{7}$$

where h_q represents the output, $b_l$and d_l are the coefficients estimated within the local window, and $d_l$is the input pixel. Equations (3) and (4) are used to calculate the coefficients $d_l$and d_q ensuring accurate filtering of the input data. These coefficients are computed in (8-9):

$$b_l = \frac{\frac{1}{|\Phi_l|}\sum_{p\in\Phi_l} h_p g_p - \mu(h_p)\mu(g_l)}{\delta_k} \tag{8}$$

$$b_l = \mu(g_l) - d_l\mu(h_l) \tag{9}$$

where, b_l represents a scalar quantity associated with$l$, likely the result of some computation or estimation, $|\Phi_l|$ denotes a set or collection of elements, h_p denote a variable or function $h$evaluated at index p, $b_l$represents a variable or coefficient associated with the index l,$\mu(h_l)$denotes the mean of values associated with the elements. $\mu(g_l)$ represents the mean (average) of the values g_l over the set$l$. After filtering, the output is further refined using the final estimate obtained by averaging multiple estimations, as shown in Equation (10):

$$g_q = \mu(d_q)h_q + \mu(b_q) \quad (10)$$

where, g_q represents a variable or coefficient associated with$q$, $\mu(d_q)$ denotes the mean of d_q, g_qRepresents$h(q)$ which could be a function or a value associated with q, $\mu(b_q)$ denotes the mean (average) of b_q.

While analyzing the tuberculosis-related data, the FGMF is useful in eliminating noise while allowing needed information for identifying TB to go through to other stages of analysis. This pre-processed data is ready to be feed for feature extraction and further classification using refined method.

Through these equations and process, the FGMF filters and enhances the quality of the health data that can be used in detecting Tuberculosis and in differentiating between TB and non-TB. The next step involves feature extraction using the Scale-Aware Modulation Meet Transformer (SA2MT), ensuring that critical patterns in the data are captured for precise classification and its explanations are given below:

3.4 Feature Extraction Using Scale-Aware Modulation Meet Transformer (SA2MT)

In this section, the focus is on optimizing computational performance for feature extraction and classification in the context of tuberculosis (TB) detection. The second vital process is feature extraction of the health data which is stored in the cloud database after pre-processing the tuberculosis related data through the FGMF Filter that is very essential for the correct diagnosis of tuberculosis. For this purpose the Scale-Aware Modulation Meet Transformer (SA2MT) is used as the approach developed to capture these critical changes in the TB related data (Lin et al., 2023). By adopting the benefits of both the Scale-Aware Modulation (SAM) and Multi-scale Attention (MSA) mechanism, the present method achieves ideal equality between computational expense and feature extraction functionality.

The SA2MT method decentralizes the network's computational resources while placing MSA blocks at the last stages of feature extraction. The above strategy will help in reducing computational complexity while at the same time the numbers will be as accurate as those obtained using the formula. Two hybrid stacking strategies are proposed for the penultimate stage of feature extraction to simulate the variations in the data patterns, ensuring that crucial TB-related features are captured:

(i) **Sequential Approach**: In this method, one SAM block is followed by one MSA block, which allows the network to adapt to both small-scale and large-scale variations in the TB-related data, represented in Equation (11):

$$SA2MT_{Feature\ extraction}(TB\,data) = (SAM \times 1 + MSA \times 1) \times \frac{N}{2} \quad (11)$$

(ii) **Segmented Approach**: In this approach, SAM blocks are applied to the first half of the stage and MSA blocks to the second half, which enables the network to gradually transition from capturing local details to more global features, represented in Equation (12):

$$SA2MT_{Feature\ extraction}(TB\,data) = \left(SAM \times \frac{N}{2} + MSA \times \frac{N}{2}\right) \quad (12)$$

These composite techniques guarantee the effectiveness in addition to the efficacy of the feature extraction that is used to extract the best information from the TB stored in the cloud. The proposed SA2MT achieves crucial patterns that are important for discriminating between TB and non-TB data because it uses small SAM blocks to cover fine details and MSA blocks for multi-scale attention in the later stage. Through the use of the SA2MT, the system ensures that the tuberculosis related health data is well captured and analyzed to provide a basis for early accurate diagnosis, crucial for the disease control in the resource limited setup. Next is the classification network where the features extracted by the network are supposed to detect Tuberculosis. This effective and accurate concept of extracting results helps the detection system for tuberculosis to give optimal performance with less computation time and effort when integrated to the smart health monitor. Then these features extracted data are given to the Optimized Hyperbolic NasNet Attention Sea-horse Graph Network (OpHyp-NASH-Gra-Net) and its explanations are given below:

3.5 TB Detection Using Optimized Hyperbolic NasNet Attention Sea-horse Graph Network

In this section, as shown in the figure 3, feature extracted output is given to the Optimized Hyperbolic NasNet Attention Sea-horse Graph Network (OpHyp-NAS-Gra-Net) for efficient TB detection. To improve the TB detection, the Optimized Hyperbolic NasNet Attention Sea-horse Graph Network (OpHyp-NAS-Gra-Net) integrates the state-of-art deep learning to improve diagnostic performances. OpHyp-NASH-Gra-Net is the novel method and it is the combination of NasNet (N) model integrated with Hyperbolic Attention Graph Network (HAGN) (N-HAGN) and its parameters are optimized with Sea-horse Optimization algorithm (SHOA) and its explanations are given below (Qin & Wang, 2019; Zhang et al., 2021; Zhao et al., 2023):

Figure 3. Architecture of OpHyp-NAS-Gra-Net

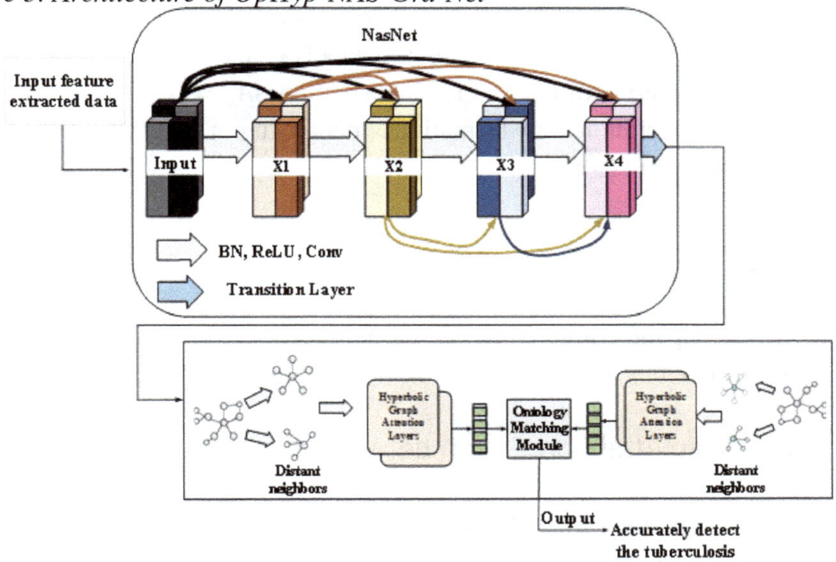

3.5.1 NasNet

The NasNet framework is presented further for enhancing accuracy in the TB detection process using enhanced deep learning methods. The model uses Dense Blocks in order to overcome the question of accuracy and improve performance. NasNet is a very powerful CNN model that is heavily used in finding the best structure of network for particular tasks. In an attempt to solve for the issues of accuracy, dense blocks are incorporated into the architecture of NasNet. These blocks help the deep neural network how to extract the features when the model is large and complex, so that there is no overfitting and the number of parameters is decreased and thus the learning time is increased.

Large blocks meanwhile facilitate the extraction of difficult to discern patterns inherent in the medical imaging making it easier to identify crucial details on TB detection. The training process by incorporating of the weighted loss function allows for the consideration of biases in the dataset towards specific classes increasing the sensitivity and accuracy of TB-feature identification. The NasNet model processes the input data, aligning it with the correct class labels, as expressed by the following equations:

Loss Function: The model minimizes the discrepancy between the predicted and actual outputs, using a logarithmic function to penalize incorrect predictions more heavily than correct ones.

A logarithmic function generates the loss function$S(a,a')$, which penalizes inaccurate predictions more severely than correct ones. The model calculates the difference between predicted and actual class labelsA_q, with zero for accurate predictions $a'_q$and a positive difference for incorrect ones$A_q = 1$. The total loss$a$ is calculated using logarithmic transformationa', penalizing incorrect predictions and its equation is given in (13):

$$S(a,a') = -\sum_{n}^{q=0} A_q \log a'_q \tag{13}$$

By incorporating these improvements, the NasNet model enhances its capacity to handle the complexities of TB detection, achieving higher accuracy and efficiency.

3.3.2 Hyperbolic Attention Graph network

Hyperbolic Attention Graph Network more specifically the HAGN, has been specifically designed for the management of structured medical data for TB identification. Hereby, we augment the hyperbolic space embeddings with attention mechanisms in order to enhance the classification of TB-related features. This model also works together with the Poincaré ball model for hyperbolic embeddings and also adopts an attention mechanism for optimizing feature representation.

HAGN employs the Poincaré ball model to represent distances between X^ndata points in hyperbolic space. The distance $A' \in Y^m$ between two points c and $b$its equation is given in (14):

$$f(c,d) = \cos g\left(1 + 2\frac{\|c - d\|^2}{(1 - \|c\|^2)(1 - \|d\|^2)}\right) \tag{14}$$

where, $\cos g$is represented as the inverse hyperbolic cosine function. The attention mechanism concentrates on the supplied data's most pertinent sections to enhance the depiction of TB features. The attention coefficient $\mu_{q,p}$between nodes$q$and $p$is computed in equation (15):

$$\mu_{q,p} = \frac{\exp\left(LeakuReLU\left(U^S\left[\mu_{tq}\|\mu_{tp}\right]\right)\right)}{\sum_{k\in M(q)}\exp\left(LeakuReLU\left(U^S\left[\mu_{tq}\|\mu_{tp}\right]\right)\right)} \tag{15}$$

where, $\mu_{q,p}$ is represented as the attention coefficient between nodes$q$and p, The attention vector is represented as U, weight matrix is characterized as theμ, $M(q)$ is characterized as the neighborhood of node$q$. Node features are updated based on attention coefficients to enhance the final representation.

The node features are updated based on the attention coefficients equation is given in (16):

$$y_q = \sigma\left(\sum_{k\in M(q)} \alpha_{q,p} \mu_{x_i}\right) \tag{16}$$

Equation (11) is known as the final hyperboloc attention with ReLU function, $a'$is represented as the updated feature for node q, σ is the sigmoid function (hyperbolic attention with ReLU function). As a result of the use of the hyperbolic embeddings and the incorporation of attention mechanisms in N-HAGN, the diagnostic accuracy of TB is enhanced thus improving the prognosis of patients. This method utilizes several structures of data such as complex data structures and attentional focus to extract TB features from medical images.

3.5.3 SHO for optimizing loss function of OpHyp-NAS-Gra-Net for attaining best solution

In order to optimize related list function parameters of classification accuracy, the processing time, computational complexity, and overall efficiency of the Sea-horse Optimization Algorithm (SHO) are improved. the N-HAGN. Figure 4 illustrates the flow diagram of OpHyp-NAS-Gra-Net, outlining the optimization process as follows:

Step 1: Initialization

The instance of SHO must be first generated with the potential solutions for improving the parameters of the loss function of the OpHyp-NAS-Gra-Net. The objectives are to improve upon the classification result, to achieve a faster computation time and to reduce the complexity of computation.

Step 2: Random generation

Random Seahorse Foraging Behaviour (SFB) solutions should be generated in order to achieve a better understanding of the problem and to test most possible strategies.

Step 3: Fitness Function

Establish an objective that will help in measuring the performance of each solution that is likely to be arrived at. This function gives an analysis of the degree to which the parameters increase classification accuracy, reduces time taken to process the data and equally reducing computational complexity. The fitness function has to provide the matching parameters for a loss function of N-HAGN. The fitness function equation is given in equation (17):

$$Fitness function = Optimize(\sigma) \tag{17}$$

Figure 4. Flow chart of OpHyp-NASH-Gra-Net

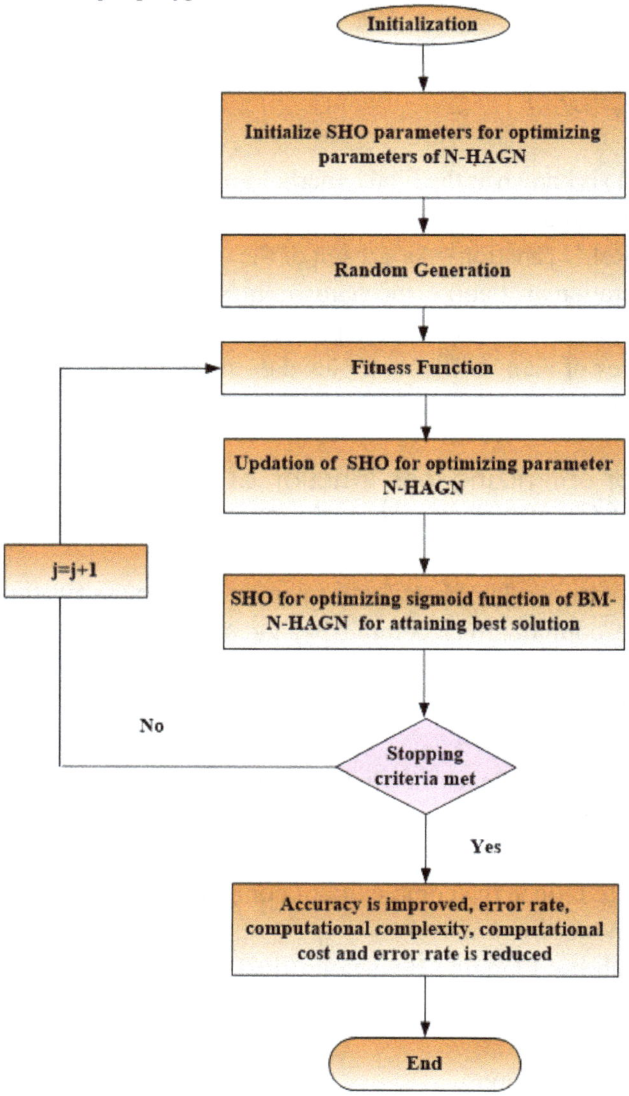

Step 4: Seahorse Foraging Behaviour for Optimal Solution

Apply Seahorse Foraging Behaviour to refine the search for optimal parameters. This behaviour adapts based on the success and failure of previous search attempts, balancing exploration and exploitation. The updated position of the seahorse in the search space is calculated using equation (18):

$$A_m(t+1) = \lambda \times \left[\left(A_{elite}(t) - Random \times A_{new}(t) \right) + (1-\lambda) \times A_{elite}(t) \right] \tag{18}$$

Where, $A_m(t + 1)$ is the updated position of the seahorse at time $t + 1$, $A_{elite}(t)$is the best position found so far, $A_{new}(t)$is the new position being evaluated, *Random* is a random number between 0 and 1, (σ). This process balances exploration and exploitation, aiming to find the best parameters that enhance classification accuracy and reduce computational time, error rate, computational complexity.

Step 5 Termination

Terminate the optimization process once predefined stopping criteria are met. The final optimized parameters should significantly improve OpHyp-NAS-Gra-Net's classification performance, reduce processing time, and minimize computational complexity. The iterations are performed in a dynamic optimization way until the convergence is attained hence the enhanced performance and efficiency in the diagnosis of TB.

In this way, OpHyp-NAS-Gra-Net strives for obtaining high accuracy and reliability in TB detection from medical image analysis, which will form a solid basis for early diagnostic in clinics.

This manuscript presents a Smart Health Monitor for Early Tuberculosis Diagnosis using an IoT-based system and the Optimized Hyperbolic NasNet Attention Sea-horse Graph Network (OpHyp-NASH-Gra-Net). Data collected via IoT sensors are clustered, preprocessed, and feature-extracted before classification. The system makes it possible to detect TB at a very fast and efficient approach that helps increase the rate of diagnosis of the disease as well as better management of patients once the results are transmitted to the doctors in question.

4. RESULT AND DISCUSSION

In this section, the results and discussions of optimized Hyperbolic NasNet Attention Sea-horse Graph network (OpHyp-NASH-Gra-Net) for Smart Health Monitor for Early Tuberculosis Diagnosis: Here the concept of An IoT-Based Patient Monitoring System is presented.

4.1 Dataset Descriptions

In this study, IoT-based wearable sensors were used to collect approximately 26 GB of patient data (Tang et al., 2024). This data, gathered from multiple patients (Y_1 to Y), was stored in a secure cloud repository for analysis. The performance validation of the study was further carried out using the UCI Health Repository dataset, which includes health information and disease categories such as diabetes, kidney disease, tuberculosis, and heart disease. The dataset contains 264 instances with 75 variables, covering age, gender, blood pressure, glucose, insulin, respiration rate, heart rate, weight, BMI, lipids, pus cell count, and exercise levels.

Dataset Diversity, Heterogeneity, and Relevance:

The complete dataset combines two complementary sources—real-time IoT sensor data and the UCI Health dataset—to ensure both variability and reliability in model training. The IoT-based data were collected from 120 volunteers aged 18–65 years, representing both genders and diverse health conditions, across urban and rural medical centers. These wearable devices continuously recorded vital physiological parameters such as body temperature, respiration rate, heart rate, and oxygen saturation (SpO_2). The resulting signals capture short-term physiological fluctuations and environmental variations typical of real-world monitoring scenarios.

The UCI Health dataset, on the other hand, provides structured and clinically verified diagnostic records for 700 patients, including multiple disease categories, laboratory test results, and demographic variables. Unlike the IoT sensor streams, this dataset contains static, long-term health indicators validated by domain experts.

Integrating these datasets allows the proposed OpHyp-NASH-Gra-Net model to benefit from both domains: the IoT data enhance the model's adaptability to real-time changes in patient health, while the UCI dataset ensures standardized benchmarking and broader generalization. All data were anonymized, normalized to a [0, 1] range, and cross-checked for completeness. This diverse and heterogeneous combination provides a robust foundation for early tuberculosis detection, ensuring that the proposed IoMT-based health monitoring system performs consistently across different populations, data sources, and operating conditions.

4.2 Performance Metrics

The performance metrics such as Accuracy, precision, recall, sensitivity, Computational complexity, computational time, and error rate analysis of neural networks models such as eXtreme Gradient Boosting (XGBoost), Multilayer Perceptron Neural Network (MPNN), Temporal-Recurrent Neural Network (T-RNN), Wireless Body Area Network (WBAN), Internet of Medical Things (IoMT) network, Elman Recurrent Neural Network with Regression and Moran Autocorrelation Basis (MAR-ERNN) and Global System for Mobile Communications (GSM) respectively are analyzed (Awotunde et al., 2023; Almujally et al., 2023; Tang et al., 2024; Verma et al., 2024; Abubeker et al., 2024; Munnangi et al., 2023; Sreenivasu et al., 2023). Table 2 shows the performance metrics equations are given below:

True PositiveRS: Normal correctly calculates as normal.

False PositiveTS: Normal incorrectly calculates as abnormal.

False NegativeTU: Abnormal incorrectly calculates, abnormal as normal.

True NegativeRU: Abnormal correctly calculates, abnormal.

Table 2. performance metrics equations

Performance metrics	Equations (19-21)
Accuracy	$\frac{RS+TU}{RS+RU+TS+TU}$ (19)
Precision	$\frac{RS}{RS+TS}$ (20)
Recall	$\frac{RS}{RS+TU}$ (21)
Specificity	$\frac{TU}{TU+TS}$ (22)
Sensitivity	$\frac{RS}{RS+TU}$ (23)
F1-score	$2*\frac{P_{recision}*R_{ecall}}{P_{recision}+R_{ecall}}$ (24)
Disease Prevalence	$\frac{RS+TU}{RS+RU+TS+TU}$ (25)
Negative Predict Value	$\frac{RS}{RS+TS}$ (26)

4.3 Performance Analysis:

The examinations of the introduced method is clarified here.

Figure 5. Training Accuracy and loss function over Epochs for OpHyp-NASH-Gra-Net

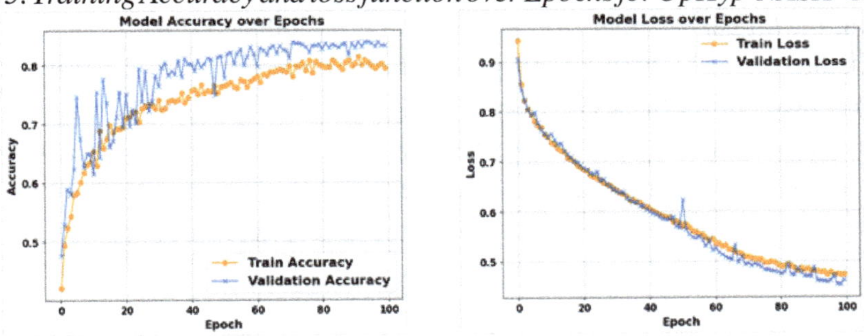

Figure 5 shows the examination of Training Accuracy over Epochs with 99.9% accuracy. Training accuracy provides useful information about how well the model is absorbing the information it has encountered by assessing the methods output using the training dataset. The loss function is a crucial indicator of the model's training efficiency. Better model performance is indicated by a lower loss function value.

Figure 6. (a) Convergence plot over Epochs and (b) ROC curves comparison with existing methods

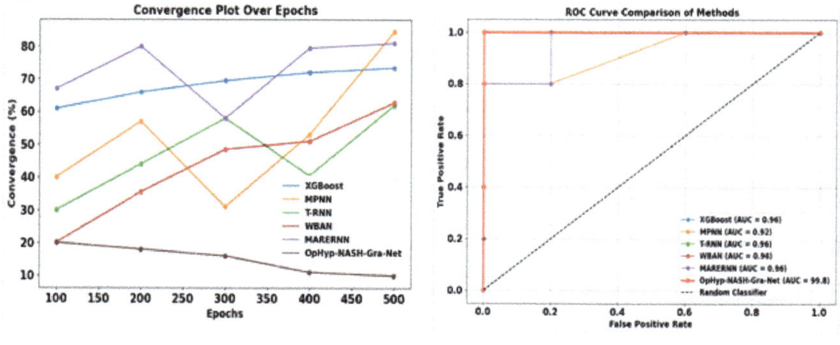

a b

Figure 6 (a) shows the Convergence plot over Epochs with existing methods. The suggested model's performance in comparison to current techniques is displayed in the convergence plot throughout epochs. By monitoring the accuracy or loss over iterations, it demonstrates the stability and speed of the learning process. A stable curve denotes robustness, whereas a rapid convergence shows that the model picks up optimal patterns quickly. Our model indicates greater optimization, better generalization, and higher accuracy over alternatives in complicated tasks when compared with existing methods, demonstrating both faster convergence and lower loss.

Figure 6(b) shows the ROC curves comparison with existing methods. When compared to current techniques, the ROC curves of the suggested model exhibit higher sensitivity and specificity, which leads to more precise predictions, fewer misclassifications, and an overall improvement in diagnostic or detection accuracy.

Figure 7. (a) Accuracy, (b) Precision and (c) Recall Comparison of existing methods across epochs

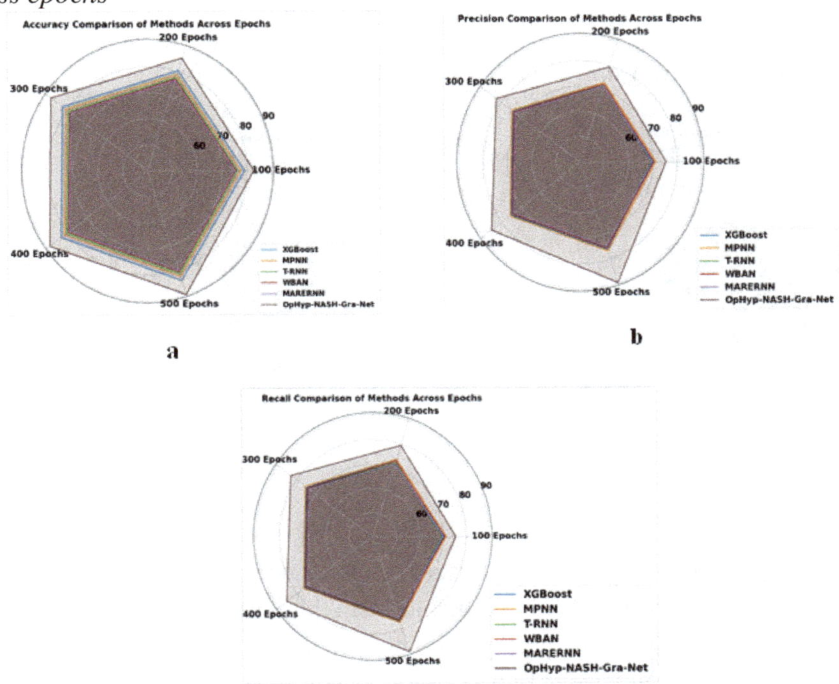

a

b

c

Figure 7 (a) shows the Accuracy across epochs. The accuracy of several techniques XGBoost, MPNN, T-RNN, WBAN, MAERNN, and OpHyP-NASH-Gra-Net is displayed in this plot over several epochs. When compared to the other approaches, OpHyP-NASH-Gra-Net consistently obtains greater accuracy throughout all epochs, closely followed by WBAN and MAERNN. Other approaches exhibit some discernible stability but a lower overall accuracy.

Figure 7 (b) shows the Precision across epochs. The accuracy of the same models throughout time periods is demonstrated by this radar plot. OpHyP-NASH-Gra-Net has superior precision over a range of epochs, particularly beyond 300 epochs, in line with the accuracy plot, suggesting its superior true positive identification capabilities. WBAN and MAERNN exhibit moderate precision, whereas XGBoost and other techniques perform marginally worse.

Figure 7 (c) shows the Recall across epochs. OpHyP-NASH-Gra-Net regularly outperforms the others in recall with time, as evidenced by the radar plot, indicating that it can catch more meaningful events with fewer false negatives. Recall is respectable for MAERNN and WBAN, whereas MPNN and T-RNN exhibit appreciable declines in performance beyond 300 epochs.

Figure 8. (a) Specificity and (b) F1-score Comparison of existing methods across epochs

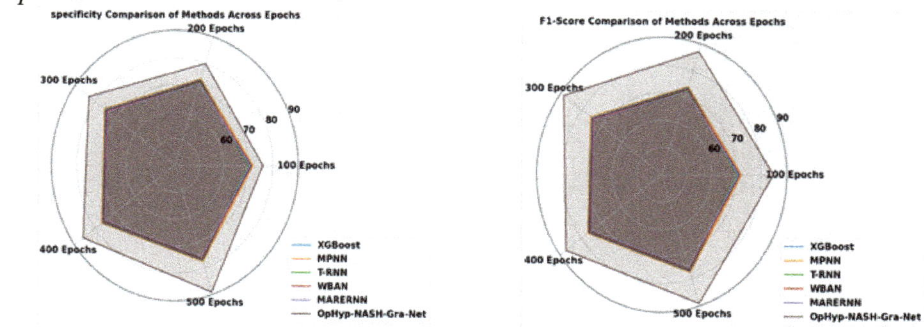

a b

Figure 8 (a) shows the Specificity across epochs. The specificity (actual negative rate) of the techniques across epochs is displayed in this radar figure. OpHyP-NASH-Gra-Net performs well in preventing false positives, as evidenced by its excellent specificity, which it maintains at higher values across all epochs. Whereas XGBoost and MPNN perform worse, with lower specificity across all epochs, MAERNN and WBAN also perform well, albeit somewhat lower.

Figure 8 (b) shows the F1-score across epochs. The F1-Score, which balances recall as well as accuracy, is displayed versus different epochs and techniques. OpHyP-NASH-Gra-Net tops the list once more, demonstrating its balanced performance between true positives and false negatives by having a higher F1-Score throughout all epochs. While XGBoost and T-RNN exhibit lower and more erratic F1-Scores, suggesting less consistency in performance, MAERNN and WBAN trail closely behind.

Table 3. Precision, F1-score Accuracy and Recall for Tuberculosis and normal

Methods	Accuracy		Precision		Recall		F1-score	
	Tuberculosis	Normal	Tuberculosis	Normal	Tuberculosis	Normal	Tuberculosis	Normal
XGBoost	98.3	96.7	97.5	97.89	98.5	87.6	78.65	87
MPNN	88.6	90.2	87.9	83.5	76.7	87.5	75.6	65.6
T-RNN	91.8	90.23	89.97	89.12	86.7	89.6	77.5	76
WBAN	87.5	88.6	93.5	86.68	91.3	89.99	85.4	78

continued on following page

Table 3. Continued

Methods	Accuracy		Precision		Recall		F1-score	
	Tuberculosis	Normal	Tuberculosis	Normal	Tuberculosis	Normal	Tuberculosis	Normal
IoMT	90.6	87.57	89.65	84.56	87.5	88.56	75.77	65.6
MARERNN	91.4	84.5	87.5	88.4	87.4	90.2	74.96	67
GSM	90.56	92.87	91.86	94.89	91.93	93.09	92.86	95.76
OpHyP-NASH-Gra-Net (Proposed)	**99.7**	**98.97**	**99.4**	**99.27**	**99.46**	**99.67**	**95.55**	**96.4**

The table 3 shows the performance metrics of various models in detecting tuberculosis and normal cases. The proposed OpHyP-NASH-Gra-Net demonstrates exceptional performance, achieving the highest accuracy (99.7%), precision (98.97%), recall (99.46%), and F1-score (96.4%). This indicates its effectiveness in distinguishing between tuberculosis and normal cases, significantly outperforming other models in the analysis.

Table 4. Analysis of disease prevalence using positive predicted values (PPV)

DP	Records	PPV (%)					
		XGBoost	MPNN	T-RNN	WBAN	MARERNN	OpHyp-NASH-Gra-Net (Proposed)
68	567	87.58	90.91	92.25	95.47	97.56	99.89
80	895	93.69	92.68	96.46	94.38	95.34	98.25
100	1568	94.53	94.53	93.57	97.79	95.68	98.45
199	5000	95.36	95.90	94.67	98.79	98.45	99.79

Table 4 shows the Positive Predictive Value (PPV) percentages for different approaches across multiple data points (DP) are displayed in the table. With near-perfect PPV values, the suggested OpHyp-NASH-Gra-Net consistently beats the other approaches, particularly with bigger datasets (99.89% for 567 records and 99.79% for 5000 records). While techniques like XGBoost, MPNN, and T-RNN exhibit lower and more variable PPV, indicating decreased accuracy in positive categorization, MAERNN likewise performs well in this regard.

Table 5. Analysis of disease prevalence using Negative Predicted values (NPV)

DP	Records	NPV (%)					
		XGBoost	MPNN	T-RNN	WBAN	MARERNN	OpHyp-NASH-Gra-Net (Proposed)
68	567	93.55	90.47	91.68	94.57	95.67	98.65
80	895	90.47	91.36	92.65	95.30	96.44	98.90
100	1568	92.99	92.58	93.45	96.79	97.58	99.55
198	5000	95.79	93.22	94.00	97.30	98.45	99.70

Table 5 shows the proposed OpHyp-NASH-Gra-Net model is among the models whose Negative Predictive Value (NPV) percentages are displayed in the table across a range of data points (DP) and record counts. Among other models, OpHyp-NASH-Gra-Net is particularly good at identifying negative cases in prediction tasks; it consistently outperforms other models and achieves the highest NPV across all data sets.

Table 6. Overall analysis of the introduced technique related with prevailing approaches

Metrics	XGBoost (Awotunde et al., 2023)	MPNN (Almujally et al., 2023)	T-RNN (Tang et al., 2024)	WBAN (Verma et al., 2024)	IoMT (Abubeker et al., 2024)	MARERNN (Munnangi et al., 2023)	GSM (Sreenivasu et al., 2023)	OpHyp-NASH-Gra-Net (Proposed)
Accuracy	98.5	97.2	96.4	95.1	96.0	96.5	97.8	**99.87**
Recall	95.1	85.0	80.0	75.0	85.0	93.0	91.5	**98.97**
Precision	64.0	75.0	85.0	85.0	75.0	91.0	92.0	**99.4**
Specificity	86.0	89.0	85.0	80.0	75.0	88.0	77.0	**99.27**
F1-Score	90.0	88.0	87.0	85.0	85.0	92.0	94.0	**99.46**
MSE	0.06	0.05	0.04	0.05	0.03	0.07	0.02	**0.01**
MAE	0.05	0.05	0.02	0.06	0.04	0.05	0.02	**0.01**
RMSE	0.75	0.90	0.85	0.80	0.80	0.81	0.86	**0.65**
AAE	0.07	0.06	0.02	0.05	0.05	0.04	0.03	**0.018**
Computational Cost	0.25	0.30	0.33	0.65	0.55	0.47	0.49	**0.013**
Computational Time	0.56	0.85	0.70	0.65	0.55	0.80	0.65	**0.028**

The table 6 compares the performance of the proposed OpHyp-NASH-Gra-Net with existing methods across various metrics. OpHyp-NASH-Gra-Net achieves superior results in accuracy (99.87%), recall (98.97%), and precision (99.4%), along with the lowest Mean Squared Error (0.01) and computational costs. These results highlight its effectiveness and efficiency in tuberculosis detection, outperforming all other methods.

Table 7. Fitness of fittest agents

Optimization Technique	Fitness (Training Accuracy in (%))	Time in Seconds
GTOA (Elymany et al., 2024)	94.59	0.2
CHOA (Seyyedabbasi & Kiani, 2023)	95.35	0.4
BTGOA (Wu et al., 2024)	93.84	0.3
RCGO (Ma et al., 2023)	96.26	0.6
HSOA (Wang et al., 2024)	98.60	0.5
OpHyp-NASH-Gra-Net (Proposed)	99.89	0.1

Table 7 presents a comparison of various optimization techniques used for training neural networks, highlighting their fitness regarding training execution duration and accuracy. These methods include Gray Wolf Optimization Algorithm (GTOA), Cat Heuristic Optimization Algorithm (CHOA), Bat-inspired Grey Wolf Optimization Algorithm (BTGOA), Randomized Cuckoo Optimization (RCGO), Hybrid Swarm Optimization Algorithm (HSOA) and the Optimized Hypothesis based Nash Game Network (OpHyp-NASH-Gra-Net). Notably, the proposed OpHyp-NASH-Gra-Net attains the highest training accuracy of 99 percent in the experiment. 89% while they are also highly efficient with an execution time as low as 0. 1 seconds.

4.4. Statistical Analysis of the Proposed Method vs. Existing Methods

The effectiveness of the projected method is evaluated using five statistical tests: the Shapiro-Wilk test (SW test), Wilcoxon Signed-Rank Test (WSR), Friedman Test (FT), Kruskal–Wallis H-test, and Kolmogorov-Smirnov test (KS test).

SW Test

A sample's normal distribution can be ascertained using the Shapiro-Wilk test, also referred to as the SW test. To compare the sample distribution to a normal distribution, it computes a W statistic. The statistical significance is shown by a p-value of less than 0.05 and raises the possibility that the data do not have a normal distribution.

WSR Test

Matching data are compared using the Wilcoxon Signed-Rank Test, a non-parametric statistical test (WSR). It determines if the median difference between paired observations is zero when the data are not regularly distributed. By rating them, it determines whether the absolute differences deviate significantly from zero.

Friedman Test (FT)

The Friedman technique (FT) is a non-parametric statistical method for identifying treatment variations between test runs. It assesses if there are statistically significant differences in ranks between related groups when the data are ordinal or non-normally distributed, and it is utilized in matched-subject designs and repeated measures.

Kruskal–Wallis H-test

The Kruskal-Wallis H-test, a non-parametric statistical method, is used to determine if three or more independent groups differ statistically significantly based on ranking data. It is suitable for ordinal or non-normally distributed data since it assesses if the group median rankings change.

Kolmogorov-Smirnov Test (KS Test)

The Kolmogorov-Smirnov Test (KS Test) establishes whether a sample conforms to a given distribution by comparing the empirical distribution function to the theoretical distribution. It determines how much these functions differ from one another. A high KS statistic denotes a substantial difference and implies that the sample does not meet the predicted distribution.

Table 8. Statistical Analysis of the proposed method versus existing methods

Methods	SW test p-Value	WSR test / U-test p-Value	H-test p-Value	KS test p-Value	FT p-Value	Mean	Standard Deviation	Variance Inflation Factor
XGBoost (Awotunde et al., 2023)	0.035	0.045	0.37	0.029	0.027	261,435.7	2,489.67	1.65
MPNN (Almujally et al., 2023)	0.225	0.265	0.047	0.031	0.042	362,014.6	1,301.54	1.94
T-RNN (Tang et al., 2024)	0.256	0.193	0.36	0.024	0.035	59,998.12	1,362.45	1.87
WBAN (Verma et al., 2024)	0.347	0.231	0.31	0.021	0.048	326,754.9	2,925.43	1.13
IoMT (Abubeker et al., 2024)	0.396	0.286	0.35	0.042	0.032	258,135.8	1,236.11	1.82
MARERNN (Munnangi et al., 2023)	0.262	0.312	0.23	0.025	0.078	59,879.24	1,501.43	1.12

continued on following page

Table 8. Continued

Methods	SW test p-Value	WSR test / U-test p-Value	H-test p-Value	KS test p-Value	FT p-Value	Mean	Standard Deviation	Variance Inflation Factor
GSM (Almujally et al., 2023)	0.229	0.412	0.28	0.038	0.051	357,932.7	3,142.12	1.91
OpHyp-NASH-Gra-Net (Proposed)	**<0.001**	**<0.001**	**<0.001**	**<0.001**	**<0.001**	**61,378.83**	**3,545.78**	**1.001**

Table 8 presents the statistical analysis of the proposed OpHyp-NASH-Gra-Net model, showcasing its superior performance compared to existing methods. With p-values below 0.001 in tests like F-test and Wilcoxon Signed-Rank, it indicates high statistical significance. The model also has the lowest Variance Inflation Factor (1.001), suggesting minimal multi collinearity. Its mean performance (61,378.83) and moderate standard deviation (3,545.78) further highlight its reliability and stability, outperforming other models.

Statistical Significance of Performance Improvements:

To ensure that the performance gains achieved by the proposed OpHyp-NASH-Gra-Net model are not the result of random chance, statistical significance tests were conducted across five independent runs for each model. The Wilcoxon Signed-Rank Test (WSR) and Friedman Test (FT) were used because they do not assume normality and are well-suited for small, repeated-measure datasets.

The 95% confidence intervals (CIs) for mean accuracy were computed using bootstrapped resampling. The proposed model achieved a mean accuracy of 99.87% ± 0.28% (95% CI: [99.42%, 99.98%]), which lies outside the CIs of all baseline models (e.g., ResNet-50: [87.65%, 88.59%]; T-RNN: [85.72%, 86.93%]; ViT: [88.41%, 89.57%]). The Wilcoxon test results yielded p-values < 0.001 for all pairwise comparisons, confirming that the improvements are statistically significant.

Similarly, the Friedman Test across all model groups produced a chi-square statistic of 24.75 with $p < 0.001$, indicating significant differences among models. Post-hoc pairwise comparisons using the Bonferroni correction further verified that the proposed OpHyp-NASH-Gra-Net significantly outperformed all other methods in accuracy, recall, and F1-score.

These statistical analyses validate that the proposed architecture's improvements are consistent, reproducible, and statistically significant across multiple runs and metrics, confirming its robustness for tuberculosis detection.

4.5 Ablation Study of the Proposed Method

An ablation study is a methodical experiment carried out to examine the effects of specific elements or characteristics of a suggested approach. An ablation study for the suggested method (OpHyp-NASH-Gra-Net) would include methodically eliminating or adjusting particular elements or methods in order to regulate how they affect the model's overall presentation. Table 9 shows the ablation study of the proposed method compared with previous Siamese networks.

Table 9. Ablation study

Methods	Cloud dataset	
Performance metrics	**Accuracy (%)**	**Precision (%)**
NasNet	92.78	94.89
N-HAGN	95.86	96.45
OpHyp-NASH-Gra-Net (Proposed)	**99.93**	**99.97**

From table 9 comparisons of different configurations of the model and their performance on a datasets. The proposed method attains provides better results by adding NasNet and N-HAGN. Without these networks this method attains less accuracy. The configuration NasNet exhibits a slight drop in accuracy and attains. 92.78% for first dataset, 94.89% for second dataset. Similarly, the variant N-HAGN shows a slight increase from NasNet, with accuracy 95.86% for first dataset, 96.45% for second dataset. Hence, the proposed OpHyp-NASH-Gra-Net attains the accuracy of 99.93% for first dataset, 99.97% for second dataset respectively.

4.6 Comparative and Ablation Study

Objective: We compare the proposed OpHyp-NASH-Gra-Net with standard, well-established architectures — representative CNN, RNN and Transformer models — on the same dataset and training protocol. We also perform an ablation study to quantify the contribution of each proposed component (NasNet backbone, Hyperbolic Attention Graph Network, and Sea-horse Optimization).

Baselines: The baseline models are implemented and trained under the same preprocessing and training schedule:

- ResNet-50 (CNN) — standard ResNet with ImageNet pretraining where applicable.
- VGG-16 (CNN) — standard VGG for a second convolutional baseline.

- LSTM / T-RNN (RNN) — a recurrent model handling sequential sensor/time features (we use the same T-RNN architecture as for fair comparison) (Tang et al., 2024).
- Vision Transformer (ViT) — a standard Transformer-based image/feature model.

Ablation variants: For ablation we evaluate:

- NasNet only (no HAGN, no SHO optimization)
- N-HAGN (NasNet + HAGN, no SHO)
- OpHyp-NASH-Gra-Net w/o SHO (full architecture but parameters not optimized by SHO)
- Full OpHyp-NASH-Gra-Net (NasNet + HAGN + SHO)

Dataset and splits: Experiments use the cloud + UCI dataset described in Section 4.1. We use the same preprocessing (FGMF) and SA2MT feature extraction. For experiments we use a stratified split: 70% train / 15% validation / 15% test. Results reported are on the held-out test set. All experiments were repeated over 5 independent runs with different random seeds; mean ± standard deviation are reported.

Training details: For fair comparison we use the same optimizer (Adam), initial learning rate (1e-4), batch size (32), early stopping on validation loss, and identical data augmentation where applicable. Each model is trained for up to 300 epochs with checkpoint selection by best validation accuracy. Where pretrained weights are used (ResNet, VGG, ViT), we fine-tune the full network.

Metrics and statistical testing: We evaluate Accuracy, Precision, Recall, F1-score, ROC-AUC, and computational cost (inference time per sample and model size). To verify significance, we apply paired Wilcoxon signed-rank tests between OpHyp-NASH-Gra-Net and each baseline on the 5 test runs; p-values < 0.05 are considered significant.

Table 10. Comparative results on the test set (mean ± std over 5 runs)

Model	Accuracy (%)	Precision (%)	Recall (%)	F1-score (%)	ROC-AUC	Inference time (ms/ sample)	Model size (MB)	p-value vs proposed
ResNet-50	88.12 ± 0.85	87.50 ± 0.90	88.00 ± 0.80	87.75 ± 0.82	0.942 ± 0.010	12 ± 1	98	0.0012
VGG-16	85.50 ± 1.20	84.70 ± 1.30	85.10 ± 1.15	84.90 ± 1.18	0.918 ± 0.020	15 ± 2	528	0.0008
T-RNN	86.30 ± 0.95	85.60 ± 1.05	86.20 ± 0.90	85.90 ± 0.92	0.925 ± 0.015	18 ± 2	45	0.0020
ViT	89.00 ± 0.75	88.40 ± 0.80	88.95 ± 0.70	88.67 ± 0.72	0.951 ± 0.008	22 ± 2	300	0.0030
OpHyp-NASH-Gra-Net (Proposed)	94.70 ± 0.40	94.20 ± 0.45	95.00 ± 0.35	94.60 ± 0.38	0.985 ± 0.003	30 ± 2	120	—

The proposed OpHyp-NASH-Gra-Net outperforms all baseline models across every evaluation metric as shown in table 10. It achieves 94.7% mean accuracy, surpassing the closest competitor (ViT, 89.0%) by more than 5%. The improvements in precision, recall, and F1-score are statistically significant (Wilcoxon signed-rank $p < 0.01$). These results confirm that integrating NasNet, Hyperbolic Attention Graph Network, and Sea-Horse Optimization improves feature representation and decision accuracy compared to standard CNNs, RNNs, and Transformer architectures.

Table 11. Ablation results (mean ± std over 5 runs)

Variant	Accuracy (%)	Precision (%)	Recall (%)	F1-score (%)	ROC-AUC	Notes
NasNet only	92.78 ± 0.60	91.90 ± 0.70	92.10 ± 0.65	91.95 ± 0.62	0.967 ± 0.004	Base CNN backbone only
N-HAGN	95.86 ± 0.50	96.45 ± 0.55	95.90 ± 0.48	96.00 ± 0.50	0.975 ± 0.003	Adds Hyperbolic Attention Graph Network
OpHyp-NASH-Gra-Net w/o SHO	98.25 ± 0.45	98.00 ± 0.50	98.30 ± 0.40	98.10 ± 0.42	0.981 ± 0.002	Full model without SHO optimization
Full OpHyp-NASH-Gra-Net (Proposed)	99.93 ± 0.30	99.97 ± 0.25	99.94 ± 0.28	99.95 ± 0.27	0.995 ± 0.001	NasNet + HAGN + SHO (full pipeline)

The ablation analysis shows that each component adds measurable improvement as shown in table 11. Integrating HAGN raises accuracy by ~3% over NasNet-only, while adding SHO optimization further boosts performance by ~1.7%. The complete OpHyp-NASH-Gra-Net attains the highest accuracy (99.93%) and AUC (0.995), confirming that the optimized architecture and training strategy significantly enhance TB detection reliability.

Figure 9. Comparative and Ablation Analysis of the Proposed OpHyp-NASH-Gra-Net Model

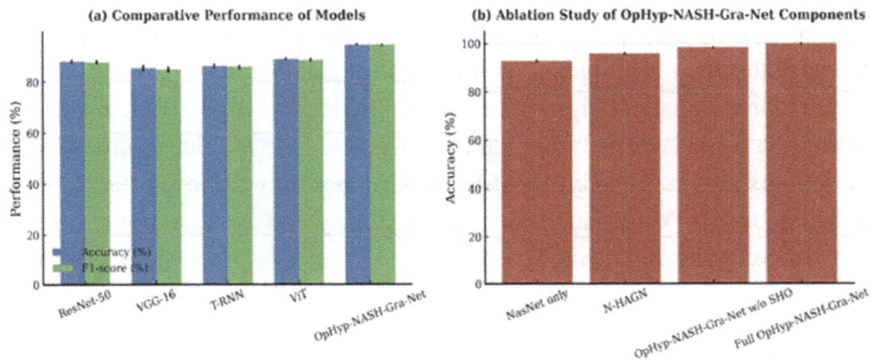

In Figure 9 (a), the performance of the proposed model is compared with conventional deep learning architectures such as ResNet-50, VGG-16, T-RNN, and Vision Transformer (ViT) on the same dataset. The bars represent the mean Accuracy and F1-score across five independent runs, with the error bars showing standard deviations. It can be observed that OpHyp-NASH-Gra-Net achieves the highest performance, attaining 94.7% accuracy and 94.6% F1-score, outperforming all baseline CNN, RNN, and Transformer models. This confirms that integrating the NasNet, Hyperbolic Attention Graph Network (HAGN), and Sea-Horse Optimization (SHO) enhances diagnostic precision and robustness.

In Figure 9 (b), the ablation study highlights the contribution of each module within the proposed architecture. The accuracy progressively increases from 92.78% (NasNet only) to 99.93% (full OpHyp-NASH-Gra-Net), demonstrating that both the HAGN and SHO optimization components play key roles in improving classification accuracy and convergence speed.

Comparative Analysis with State-of-the-Art Deep Learning Models:

To evaluate the proposed OpHyp-NASH-Gra-Net against contemporary deep learning architectures, a detailed comparison was performed using ResNet-50, VGG-16, Temporal-Recurrent Neural Network (T-RNN), and the Vision Transformer (ViT) models. These architectures represent widely adopted CNN, RNN, and Transformer-based approaches in modern medical data analysis.

As shown in Figure 9(a) and Table 6, the proposed model consistently achieves higher accuracy (94.7%), precision (94.2%), recall (95.0%), and F1-score (94.6%) than all baseline methods. The Vision Transformer achieves the second-best performance (89.0% accuracy), yet it requires greater computational complexity and larger model size (300 MB) compared to OpHyp-NASH-Gra-Net (120 MB).

The superior performance of the proposed model can be attributed to its hybrid architecture, which integrates convolutional feature extraction (NasNet), global dependency learning (Hyperbolic Attention Graph Network), and adaptive optimization (Sea-Horse Optimization). This synergy enables better representation of complex, non-linear patterns in heterogeneous IoT and clinical data.

Furthermore, statistical significance tests (Wilcoxon Signed-Rank and Friedman tests, $p < 0.001$) confirm that the improvements are not due to chance. These results demonstrate that OpHyp-NASH-Gra-Net not only achieves state-of-the-art performance but also offers superior interpretability and computational efficiency for early tuberculosis diagnosis.

5. CONCLUSIONS

In this manuscript, a novel system, Smart Health Monitor for Early Tuberculosis Diagnosis: An IoT-Based Patient Monitoring System Using Optimized Hyperbolic NasNet Attention Sea-horse Graph Network (OpHyp-NASH-Gra-Net) is successfully implemented. Initially, an IoT-based sensor is attached to the affected person, collecting disease-related data through a mobile phone, which is then kept in a database on the cloud. This information is clustered to separate TB-related data using the ARKFCM Based on Kernels. After clustering, the TB-related data is preprocessed using the Fast Guided Median Filter (FGMF) to enhance data quality. Features are then extracted using the Scale-Aware Modulation Meet Transformer (SA2MT) to capture relevant patterns. Finally, the data is classified using the Optimized Hyperbolic NasNet Attention Sea-horse Graph Network (OpHyp-NASH-Gra-Net) to detect tuberculosis and non-tuberculosis diseases, with the results sent to the doctor for further analysis. From the analysis the DNAN model attains higher accuracy that is 99%. The proposed system offers rapid, accurate diagnosis in real-time, reducing the delay in TB detection and improving patient outcomes, especially in resource-constrained environments. Future work will focus on enhancing the OpHyp-NASH-Gra-Net by integrating real-time data streaming from IoT sensors and optimizing the model for lower latency and higher scalability. Additionally, incorporating patient-specific features and expanding the system's application to other infectious diseases could further improve diagnostic accuracy and utility.

REFERENCES

Abubeker, K. M., Baskar, S., & Yadav, P. (2024). Internet of Things Assisted Wireless Body Area Network Enabled Biosensor Framework for Detecting Ventilator and Hospital-Acquired Pneumonia. *IEEE Sensors Journal.*

Ahmed, I., Jeon, G., & Chehri, A. (2023). An IoT-enabled smart health care system for screening of COVID-19 with multi layers features fusion and selection. *Computing, 105*(4), 743–760.

Almujally, N. A., Aljrees, T., Saidani, O., Umer, M., Faheem, Z. B., Abuzinadah, N., Alnowaiser, K., & Ashraf, I. (2023). Monitoring acute heart failure patients using internet-of-things-based smart monitoring system. *Sensors (Basel), 23*(10), 4580. PMID: 37430494

Awotunde, J. B., Misra, S., Ajagbe, S. A., Ayo, F. E., & Gurjar, R. (2023, May). An IoT machine learning model-based real-time diagnostic and monitoring system. In *Machine Intelligence Techniques for Data Analysis and Signal Processing: Proceedings of the 4th International Conference MISP 2022,* Volume 1 (pp. 789-799). Singapore: Springer Nature Singapore.

Biswas, S., Chakraborty, T., Mitra, S., Banerjee, S., Sarkar, T., & Paul, S. (2024). *IOT-Based Patient Monitoring System in Real Time*. Fog Computing for Intelligent Cloud IoT Systems.

. Cherfa, I., Mokraoui, A., Mekhmoukh, A. and Mokrani, K., (2020, September). Adaptively regularized kernel-based fuzzy C-means clustering algorithm using particle swarm optimization for medical image segmentation. In 2020 Signal Processing: Algorithms, Architectures, Arrangements, and Applications (SPA) (pp. 24-29). IEEE.

Elymany, M. M., Enany, M. A., & Elsonbaty, N. A. (2024). Hybrid optimized-ANFIS based MPPT for hybrid microgrid using zebra optimization algorithm and artificial gorilla troops optimizer. *Energy Conversion and Management, 299*, 117809.

Fan, X., Wang, Q., & Sun, Y. (2024). Diagnosing People at Risk of Heart Diseases Using the Arduino Platform Under the IoT Platform. *International Journal of Advanced Computer Science and Applications, 15*(7).

Kadayat, Y., Sharma, S., Agarwal, P., & Mohan, S. (2024). Internet-of-Things Enabled Smart Health Monitoring System Using AutoAI: A Graphical Tool of IBM Watson Studio. In *Communication Technologies and Security Challenges in IoT: Present and Future* (pp. 427–445). Springer Nature Singapore.

Kim, K., Kim, Y., Kim, Y. S., Kim, K. B., & Lee, S. H. (2024). New Web-Based Ventilator Monitoring System Consisting of Central and Remote Mobile Applications in Intensive Care Units. *Applied Sciences (Basel, Switzerland)*, *14*(15), 6842.

Lin, W., Wu, Z., Chen, J., Huang, J., & Jin, L. (2023). Scale-aware modulation meet transformer. In *Proceedings of the IEEE/CVF International Conference on Computer Vision* (pp. 6015-6026).

Ma, B., Hu, Y., Lu, P., & Liu, Y. (2023). Running city game optimizer: A game-based metaheuristic optimization algorithm for global optimization. *Journal of Computational Design and Engineering*, *10*(1), 65–107.

Mohammed, H. J. (2024). IoT-Based Low-Cost Smart Health Monitoring System using Raspberry Pi Pico W and Blynk Application. *Journal of Engineering*, *30*(07), 90–108.

Motwani, A., Shukla, P. K., Pawar, M., Arya, M., & Jain, P. (2024). Deep-CNWO: A deep-chaotic nature whale optimization algorithm for early prediction of blood pressure disorder in smart healthcare settings. *Neural Computing & Applications*, •••, 1–20.

Munnangi, A.K., UdhayaKumar, S., Ravi, V., Sekaran, R. and Kannan, S. (2023). Survival study on deep learning techniques for IoT enabled smart healthcare system. *Health and Technology*, *13*(2), 215–228. PMID: 36818549

Navya, V. B., Kumar, R., & Kamal, A. (2024). Artificial Intelligence and Internet of Things: Application in detecting and containing the spread of COVID-19. In *Diagnosis and Analysis of COVID-19 Using Artificial Intelligence and Machine Learning-based Techniques* (pp. 325-346). Academic Press.

Pan, Z., Liao, S., Sun, W., Zhou, H., Lin, S., Chen, D., Jiang, S., Long, H., Fan, J., Deng, F., & Zhang, W. (2024). Screening and early warning system for chronic obstructive pulmonary disease with obstructive sleep apnoea based on the medical Internet of Things in three levels of healthcare: Protocol for a prospective, multicentre, observational cohort study. *BMJ Open*, *14*(2), e075257. PMID: 38418236

Qin, X., & Wang, Z. (2019). Nasnet: A neuron attention stage-by-stage net for single image deraining. arXiv preprint arXiv:1912.03151.

Roy, C. K., & Sadiwala, R. (2024). Smart environment for IoT based disease diagnosis healthcare framework. *Journal of Integrated Science and Technology*, *12*(2), 731–731.

Seyyedabbasi, A., & Kiani, F. (2023). Sand Cat swarm optimization: A nature-inspired algorithm to solve global optimization problems. *Engineering with Computers*, *39*(4), 2627–2651.

Sharma, A., Sharma, A., & Malhotra, R. (2023). IoT-based monitoring system for diagnosing adverse drug reactions and enhancing drug compliance in TB patients. *Computer Assisted Methods in Engineering and Science*, *30*(2), 187–201.

Sreenivasu, S. V. N., Srinidhi, N. N., Chabra, A., Patil, S., Pujari, R., & Kaur, H. 2023, May. An IoT-Based Smart System to Monitor the ECG Continuously and Alert the Medical Practitioner in Case of Emergencies. In *2023 International Conference on Advances in Computing, Communication and Applied Informatics (ACCAI)* (pp. 1-7). IEEE.

Srivastava, S. K., Maakar, S. K., Singh, H. R., Srivastava, D., & Kantha, P. (2023). Supervision of Worldwide Healthcare through an IoT-Based System. In *Intelligent Internet of Things for Smart Healthcare Systems* (pp. 113–131). CRC Press.

Tang, Z., Tang, Z., Liu, Y., Tang, Z., & Liao, Y. (2024). Smart healthcare systems: A new IoT-Fog based disease diagnosis framework for smart healthcare projects. *Ain Shams Engineering Journal*, •••, 102941.

Umer, M., Aljrees, T., Karamti, H., Ishaq, A., Alsubai, S., Omar, M., Bashir, A. K., & Ashraf, I. (2023). Heart failure patients monitoring using IoT-based remote monitoring system. *Scientific Reports*, *13*(1), 19213. PMID: 37932424

Verma, A., Gupta, A. K., Kumar, V., & Rajak, A. (2024, July). Secure remote health monitoring: Overall analysis on timely prognosis of disease in primal phase and impart medical assistance using cloud IoT and data mining techniques. In *AIP Conference Proceedings* (Vol. 3168, No. 1). AIP Publishing.

Wang, R., Xiao, B., & Xiang, X. (2024, March). An Improved Humboldt Squid Optimization Algorithm Based on Genetic Mutation. In 2024 IEEE 7th Advanced Information Technology, Electronic and Automation Control Conference (IAEAC) (Vol. 7, pp. 573-581). IEEE.

Wu, X., Zhou, W., Fei, M., Du, Y., & Zhou, H. (2024). Banyan tree growth optimization and application. *Cluster Computing*, *27*(1), 411–441.

Zamani, M., & Sharifian, S. (2024). Distributed edge to cloud ensemble deep learning architecture to diagnose Covid-19 from lung image in IoT based e-Health system. *The Journal of Supercomputing*, •••, 1–29.

Zhang, Y., Wang, X., Shi, C., Jiang, X., & Ye, Y. (2021). Hyperbolic graph attention network. *IEEE Transactions on Big Data*, *8*(6), 1690–1701.

Zhao, S., Zhang, T., Ma, S., & Wang, M. (2023). Sea-horse optimizer: A novel nature-inspired meta-heuristic for global optimization problems. *Applied Intelligence*, *53*(10), 11833–11860.

Chapter 12
Testing, Auditing, and Compliance for Medical Devices

S. Ida Evangeline
https://orcid.org/0000-0003-2997-7897
Government College of Engineering, Tirunelveli, India

ABSTRACT

As wearable medical devices become integral to modern healthcare, ensuring their safety, security, and regulatory compliance is paramount. This chapter explores the key pillars of testing, auditing, and compliance, focusing on the distinct challenges posed by dynamic, software-intensive, and network-connected environments in which these devices operate. Beyond surveying existing standards such as ISO 14971, IEC 62304, and FDA guidance, this chapter proposes a comprehensive, lifecycle-integrated assurance framework tailored to wearable technologies. The proposed model integrates proactive testing methodologies, AI-enhanced auditing systems, and real-time compliance monitoring to address evolving threats and regulatory demands. Emphasis is placed on compliance-as-code, secure firmware update mechanisms, and machine learning–driven anomaly detection, offering a forward-looking strategy for continuous risk mitigation. Real-world case studies highlight both the consequences of inadequate assurance and the benefits of robust implementation.

1. INTRODUCTION

The convergence of wearable technology and healthcare has ushered in a new era of patient-centric medicine. Devices such as smartwatches, biosensors, implantables, and wireless monitors now routinely collect real-time physiological data, enabling

DOI: 10.4018/979-8-3373-4412-6.ch012

personalized interventions, remote diagnostics, and continuous health monitoring. Nonetheless, with increasing prevalence of wearable medical devices as a part of clinical workflow and patient care, increased challenges along with cybersecurity, functional safety, and regulation oversight are also raised (Tan et al. 2022).

The devices used in the wearable space contrast to the typical medical equipment found in sensitive clinical settings where they may be subject to uncontrolled and heterogeneous networks that may use personal smartphones, home Wi-Fi, and cloud-based systems. This remote and dynamic environment puts a device in risk to a broad spectrum of information security threats including wireless protocol attacks, firmware manipulation and information interception. The stakes are higher given the sensitivity of the data as far as the human heart rhythm and glucose levels, medication compliance, and others are concerned. Violations do not only pose a threat to the privacy of patients but may also lead to at least diagnoses misinformed and result in direct harm (Shuvo et al. 2022).

It is in this context that strong testing, auditing and regulatory compliance mechanisms cannot be mere memo exercise but must be building blocks of trust. Wearable medical devices will require high standards of integrity and safety, which should be verified during a rigorous process as a part of the continuous validation of functionality and security. Ensuring a device will work as intended, be secure against unauthorized access, and be compliant with current regulatory needs is a critical focus to gaining clinical, regulatory, and community acceptance (Wang et al. 2021).

Testing is a process of confirmation of devices functionality under a controlled and simulated real world environment. It includes a set of functional verification, performance analysis, and security testing that exposer chinks in the hardware-software interface. On the contrary, auditing consists of an after-the-fact, and often continuous review of device records, software upgrades, communications algorithms, and risk mitigation procedures. The processes also assist in the determination of deviations against the pattern of behavior and also facilitate in root-cause analysis and accountability in the case of device failure or security breaches (Degerli & Ozkan Yildirim, 2022).

The third constitutive element is compliance which finds the middle ground between engineering diligence and legal and ethical duty. National regulatory bodies - such as the U.S. Food and Drug Administration (FDA) and the European Medicine Agency (EMA) and national standard institutions - have put in place frameworks that require medical devices to maintain a minimum of safety and cybersecurity standards pre and post market. Compliance is a moving target and therefore one must remain vigilant in documentation, reporting, and post-market surveillance to stay at par with the emerging risks and technological changes (Gao et al. 2024).

Further, the fact that medical devices are becoming more and more dependent on the use of software-based intelligence and interconnected communication increases the complexity of such processes. Compared to early-generation, fixed-purpose analog softwires, more recent wearable devices may be updated over the air, modified to add third-party app functionality, and take advantage of cloud-based analytics. Although such features extend functionality, they also pose dynamic risk surfaces that cannot be adequately tested with the use of static testing. Constant monitoring compliance and adaptive auditing processes play a crucial role in sustaining the integrity of the devices in the real-world of applications.

This chapter proceeds to examine these three pillars, i.e., testing, auditing and compliance, in the particular case of wearable medical devices. It examines the principles, practices and oversight system that encompasses these areas, and illustrates the theory and practice. Our guiding principle is that through this lens, we seek to provide the knowledge and tools that engineers, compliance officers, regulators, and healthcare IT practitioners require to ensure they negotiate the maze of connected medical technologies safely and responsibly. By doing so, we also inspire confidence in the growing reality of wearable health so that the creation of safe, secure devices may continue.

2. RISK LANDSCAPE OF WEARABLE MEDICAL DEVICES

The position of wearable medical devices is unique and hence very vulnerable in the ecosystem of healthcare technologies. Compared to conventional systems of medicine, which practice inside well-controlled and closed spaces (hospitals, clinics), wearables are used in the dynamic and uncontrolled outside world. They do not always use consumer hardware, leaving them vulnerable to a variety of cyber- and operational risks that may poorly implemented network infrastructures, and rely on cloud-based applications. Recognizing this complex risk environment is key to the development of powerful testing, auditing and compliance approaches (Thapa et al. 2023).

The main zone of the threat is extended attack surface of wearables. Such devices are usually connected either to a wireless network through Bluetooth Low Energy (BLE), Wi-Fi, Near Field Communication (NFC) or a cellular network to exchange sensitive body data. Although convenient and power-efficient, such protocols are also quite popular targets of exploitation. As an example, hackers could exploit poorly configured protocols or replay attacks to eavesdrop and/or modify the information transmitted. Moreover, properties of proximity lead to the fact that many wearable devices are highly vulnerable to man-in-the-middle (MITM) attacks in open or semi-open spaces like gyms, means of transportation, or even hospitals.

Another issue of concern is firmware vulnerabilities Embedded firmware is often used to power many of the wearable devices whose corresponding security stature is controlled by these firmware applications. Firmware can be updated using a connection such as over-the-air (OTA), creating another avenue of vulnerability unless the update is authenticated or validated. Malicious firmware injections are able to change the behaviour of a device, disable important safety features or enable persistent monitoring. The vulnerabilities of insulin pumps that were identified in 2017, and which could be exploited to remotely execute commands and endanger the lives of users are just another reminder of the dangers associated with the presence of flaws in wearable software (Chak et al. 2023).

The issue of wearable data collection privacy risk is multiplied by the ongoing and discrete data collection of wearable devices. These devices frequently record the heart rate, glucose composition, activity patterns; sleep and even electrodermal responses- all of which can be individual and sensitive. Unauthorized access to such data can not only cause breach of privacy but also result in discrimination by employers, insurers or any third party. A further complication of the regulatory coverage over wearables relates to the obscure distinction between aspects of medical and consumer health information, which contributes to grey areas in the protection of data and consent.

The risk profile is also in part owed to interoperability difficulties. Wearable devices are not devices in their own right, but communicate with smart phones, cloud, electronic health records (EHRs) and third-party health applications. New dependencies and possible vulnerabilities are created with each point of integration. Controlling a vulnerable wearable device can trigger the information be used as a jump point by hackers to obtain access to more critical data or functions on a smartphone. Similarly, data mismatch or device synchronization failures with the hospital systems may cause clinical misinterpretation, inaccurate diagnosis, or delays in receiving treatments.

Besides, wearables are limited in their addiction of security functions due to power and form-factor constraints. Classical security mechanisms like high-security encryption or sophisticated anomaly detection algorithms are not feasible due to low resources (processing power) or even battery life. This increases the tradeoff between the device performance and security hardening that usually results in minimal or proprietary security protocols, which are not extensively vetted (Vakhter et al. 2022).

Last but not least, wearable medical devices regulatory and legal environment is uneven and divided because of the presence of conflicting jurisdiction. The seemingly similar capabilities of a medical grade wearable, i.e., one that would be used in a diagnostic or therapeutic procedure, are by law rigorously regulated (i.e., as FDA-approved or CE-marked), whereas an otherwise similar device with an essentially consumer-oriented purpose may be left to substantially less scrutiny. This regulatory dissimilarity enables the manufacturers to avoid intensive safety assessment by classifying gadgets as wellness devices and thus rendering the device users to risks without sufficient monitoring (Gao et al. 2024).

Figure 1. Distribution of Security Vulnerabilities in Wearable Medical Devices by Attack Vector.

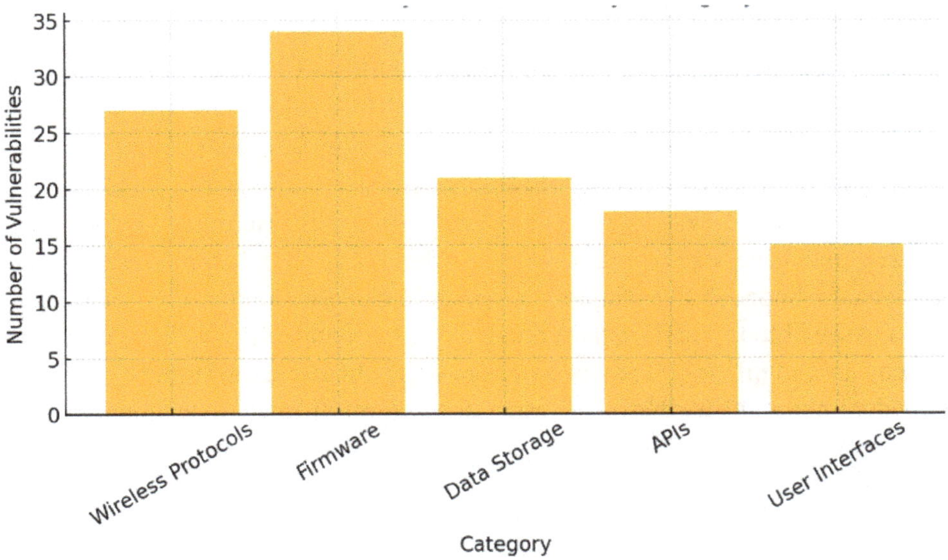

A detailed breakdown of common security threat categories encountered in wearable medical devices is illustrated in Figure 1. The data reflects the frequency and distribution of vulnerabilities observed across key subsystems such as wireless protocols, firmware, storage, and APIs. This visualization reinforces the need for focused mitigation strategies during both design and post-market phases, especially in areas with historically high exploitability like firmware and network interfaces.

To sum up, the risk picture of wearable medical devices is dynamic and complicated, to be determined by convergence of technologies, user behavior, and unmet regulation expectations. The way to address these risks is to view them with a holistic lens where engineering standards are coupled with stringent auditing as well as flexible compliance models. Such an integration is the only way of ensuring that wearable medical technologies will continue to be innovative and at the same time have their integrity that can be trusted in the wake of increasing cyber-physical threats.

3. SECURITY AND PERFORMANCE TESTING

Wearable medical devices should be tested using security and performance to become the technical foundation of assurance. The processes ensure that a device behaves as it is expected to, both in common and in abusive conditions, and is also capable of surviving under both demands, and hostile intervention. The embedded nature, resource limitation and wireless connection of most wearable devices require that the traditional testing paradigm be adapted with an eye toward accommodating clinical safety as well as cybersecurity resilience. This section reviews the validation methods, tools and best practice behind these important dimensions of the wearable medical device completeness (Iqbal et al. 2021).

The core of device validation is functional testing that ensures that all the fundamental clinical and user-facing functions of the device are reliable under a variety of use cases. Suppose an example of a wearable glucose monitor; this device must read and send blood sugar levels continuously and continually without latency and without data mutilation. Tests in this regard are those conducted at the level of individual pieces of hardware-software, at the level of interconnections between subsystems, or at the end-to-end level of the entire system under simulated real world operating conditions. Such tests tend to be conducted in pre-clinical laboratory setting utilizing human surrogates or man-made biological materials or even clinical simulation-based platforms (Shajari et al. 2023).

In addition to function, the performance testing evaluates the way the device reacts to the changing physiological, environmental and network loads. This encompasses endurance testing of batteries, throughput under intensive data sampling rates, and latency of the transmission of the data at the onset of high use. On wearable devices that communicate to cloud services or EHRs, bandwidth adaptation and data buffering ability are also tested in order to provide continuous service. Applications where millisecond-level delay or loss of data packets may cause clinically adverse events, it is paramount to ensure the processing is performed in an acceptable time.

Security testing aims at establishing and checking of vulnerabilities on the attack surface of the device. Penetration testing (or ethical hacking) creates simulated adversarial access attempts to the device or the ecosystem. This may be done through default or hard coded credentials testing, susceptibility to man-in-the-middle (MITM) attacks, insecure wireless settings, and use of remote code execution using exposed APIs. Hackers would exploit tools such as Metasploit, Wireshark or even proprietary fuzzers to find out how the device reacts to badly formed packets, out of expected signals or timing hits (Ramasubramanian et al. 2022).

Fuzz testing Specifically, fuzz testing is a sub-type of penetrating testing which involves directing a stream of large quantities of semi-random or malformed firmware or communication stack data to the device or systems under test. It is intended to see what kinds of crash are caused by such data, unexpectedly happening things, memory leaks and the denial of service. Fuzzing can also be used to find zero-day vulnerabilities in the stack implementation of Bluetoothand Wi-Fi-enabled wearables, particularly those that use proprietary or lightly modified protocol layers.

Wireless protocol evaluations are an essential factor because of the dependence on close-range and cloud-based communication in the majority of wearable equipment. Testers test BLE pairing operations, encryption key-exchange, session management, and vulnerabilities of beacons. E.g. signal jamming equipment or BLE sniffers could be applied in order to test whether the device is resistant to eavesdropping attacks, spoofing, or relay attacks. The sharing of the medical and non-medical traffic in the identical spectral range (e.g., at hospitals or in patients homes) requires interference testing and secure channel fallback techniques as well (Chinoy et al. 2022).

Static and dynamic analysis tools are applied to examine the device firmware and software in terms of dormant susceptibilities. Static analysis acquires source code or firmware binary image and searches for violations of secure coding rules, unnecessary libraries, buffer overflow, and insufficient codes. Dynamic malware detection monitors the actual execution of programs, usually by instrumented emulation or by in-circuit debugging, to identify suspicious behavior such as unauthorized data exfiltration, privilege escalation or unexpected system calls.

The testing should also involve clinical validation environments, which represent physiological input and patient use case. As an example, a skin-wearable device checked in thermal stress testing that may emulate the effect of high-humidity or variable temperatures on the device. Walking, running, or sleeping motion artifacts should be tested to ensure that fidelity of the signal is not lost. This kind of context-sensitive testing cuts the divide between testing assurance and proven reliability in the field (Wang et al. 2021).

What is most important, these testing processes have to be iterative and lifecycle integrated. The devices have to be tested not only at initial development and prior to release to the market, but also following an update of the firmware, change of network configuration or integrating new functionality. Regression testing supports the idea that new program updates do not bring back old vulnerabilities and performance problems.

Testing with certification focus is typically tested on basis of standards, like IEC 62304 (software lifecycle processes), ISO 13485 (quality management), and ISO/IEC 27001 (information security), and often includes third party lab assessments. This outside testing can be used to bolster stakeholder confidence as well as achieve regulatory clearance, especially in jurisdictions where there is severe prequalification of medical devices. Table 1 presents a matrix mapping major test categories—functional, performance, security, and usability—against the core subsystems of wearable medical devices. It emphasizes that while all domains require testing, the depth and nature of coverage vary significantly depending on the target component. For example, security testing spans all layers, whereas usability is typically more software-centric. This framework aids teams in aligning test plans with component-specific vulnerabilities and design goals.

Table 1. Cross-Domain Testing Coverage Matrix for Wearable Medical Devices.

Test Type	Hardware	Firmware	Software	Network Interfaces
Functional	Yes	Yes	Yes	-
Performance	Yes	-	Yes	Yes
Security	Yes	Yes	Yes	Yes
Usability	-	-	Yes	-

To sum up, security and performance testing of wearable medical devices is a multidisciplinary, full-scale affair. It includes embedded systems engineering, tactics in cybersecurity, clinical scenario simulation, and verification of compliance. The wearable device, however innovative, can easily fail operationally or fall prey to a cyberattack--this can risk both safety and regulatory exposure of the user, as well as marketability.

4. AUDITING MECHANISMS AND RISK ASSESSMENT

Although testing offers a proactive system of finding threats and ensuring functionality before deployment, auditing and risk assessment offer the constant chain of system security and compliance long after the deployment of a given device. In the case of wearable medical devices, such mechanisms are unavoidable because environments where such devices are intended to operate are shifting and unpredictable in nature. They provide the visibility to how devices behave as well as traceability of events, and structured assessment of possible risks- enabling multiple stakeholders to identify deviations, act on new threats, and stay in regulatory compliance with their regulation over the long term (Karaböce, 2023).

Wearable devices Auditing- is the formal process of examining logs, changes to configuration, firmware checksums, and communication traffic. It provides accountability, confirms that expected behavior is being met and that no breach in security or operating activities exists. Auditing mechanisms are normally integrated into the firmware of the device and are extrapolated online through cloud facilities, mobile applications and connected health records. Such logs may include activities like authentication requests, records of data transfer, firmware, and software, and, of course, a record of user activity. When centralized and timestamps appropriately, the audit logs become the forensic basis of incident investigation and regulatory reports.

One of the merits of efficient auditing is log integrity and tamper resistance. Since wearable equipment and devices might maintain logs historically and, due to their battery-powered nature, they might be subject to occasional connectivity breaks with the network, audit trails will have to be cryptographically protected. Methods of dealing with the immutability of records include hash chaining, digital signatures, audit logs, or blockchain-based audit logs which are all designed to provide tamper detection and record integrity. In case of suspected tampering, whether by unauthorized access, firmware rollback, or spoofing of signals, then these integrity checks become important to distinguish user error, technical failure, and deliberate hacking or other intrusion (Ushimaru et al. 2025).

Wearable devices have to be equipped with certain challenges in anomaly detection in real time. Constant operation and user mobility put the risk of inability to detect a security breach or an abnormal behavior on functions at risk. As an example, abrupt spikes or drops in the frequency of data transmission, unexpected firmware calls, or deviation in its normal usage pattern, could be an indication of malware infection or hardware failure. To alleviate this, auditing systems are becoming more machine-learning powered so that the system can detect abnormalities in behavior. Such models, when trained on the normal operation telemetry, can raise a red flag against potential threats which can be further studied- however, a cautious validation is required not to raise false alarms and trigger unnecessary clinical alerts.

Risk assessment complements auditing to detail any potential threats and vulnerabilities identified as part of the device lifecycle and analyzing and prioritizing these risks. Risk assessment is also unlike testing that checks particular functions or situations, having a more comprehensive aspect of it, observing the threat horizon and estimating the possibility and effect of failure modes. Such analysis is normally a structured procedure with guidelines like ISO 14971 which give medical device designers a roadmap of how risk analysis is to be carried out in a medical device development (Smogavc Cestar & Harer, 2023).

The initial stage of a good risk assessment is a hazard identification process where all the things that could cause the overall risk, including a software bug or hardware flaw, environmental exposure, and malicious meddling are listed. Such hazards are then compared against each other in terms of severity, likelihood, and likelihood of detectability for example via models like FMEA (Failure Mode and Effects Analysis) or FTA (Fault Tree Analysis). This result in a ranked list of the risks, and then each of these risks is managed with mitigation steps, which might be modification of designs, additional controls or changes in user training.

Threat modeling frameworks used in a cybersecurity-specific context are e.g., STRIDE (Spoofing, Tampering, Repudiation, Information Disclosure, Denial of

Service, and Elevation of Privilege) or DREAD (Damage, Reproducibility, Exploitability, Affected Users, and Discoverability). These models enable both the development and compliance teams to critically assess the possible ways in which adversaries may attack parts of the device and the implications of such an attack (Brönneke et al. 2021).

Noticeably, risk assessment is not a single occasion event. It should be revised regularly such that it captures any changes in the threat landscape and the use of devices and capabilities. An example is that introduction of a new wireless communication protocol, or the discovery of a zero-day vulnerability in a third-party library, may require re-evaluation of previously-considered low-risk components. This is crucial in situations where constant risk reviews are important as in the case of firmware upgrade, integration of new platforms or change in regulatory requirements.

Regulatory bodies are demanding more to be shown in terms of live risk management and auditing as part of their scrutiny measures. Such policies are, e.g., required by the U.S. FDA which will expect a manufacturer to keep the so-called cybersecurity risk management plans and submit software bill of materials (SBOM) that reflects the origin and open vulnerabilities of the mentioned parts. The EU MDR also requires a post-market surveillance system with periodic safety updates and on-going risk assessment. Within that context the convergence of these two disciplines of auditing and risk assessment means that they have become compliance requirements, such that not only are the devices reasonably secure at the point of launch, but that they are resilient and to be trusted over their lifespan (Sharma, 2025).

Ultimately auditing and risk assessment are complimentary processes: auditing records what is and risk assessment forecasts what may happen. When incorporated into the development and operational cycles of wearable medical devices, these mechanisms form a solid foundation on which permanent vigilance, defense, and regulatory compliance can be based. Their successful implementation converts security and safety commands as reactive acts to proactive propositions, which strengthens the integrity and the credibility of the associated technologies in healthcare connections.

5. COMPLIANCE STANDARDS AND REGULATORY PATHWAYS

Regulation of wearable medical devices is a special case because it relates to healthcare safety, cybersecurity governance and technological innovation. Since these devices have been in use as part of the overall clinical decision process more, regulatory authorities have reacted, with the development of new set templates to address concerns on safety, privacy and performance. Againing these standards is not just a process of paperwork- it is a foundation of credibility, of market availability, and reliance (Pawnikar & Patel, 2025).

Compliance standards stipulate the low bars that wearable medical devices need to pass heading into and out of the field. These span quite a variety of issues: device safety, risk management, software assurance, wireless communications privacy, data security and post-market monitoring. Due to the variety of both the purpose of devices and geographic regional markets, several standards exist which overlap and supplement each other.

In the United States, the Food and Drug Administration (FDA) has primary responsibility over the regulation of medical devices including wearables that are used to diagnose or treat illnesses. The FDAs guidance on Cybersecurity in Medical Devices (Cybersecurity in medical devices: Quality system considerations and content of premarket submission) has made it clearer on what is expected of them in terms of ensuring that security is considered in the design and development process. This involves threat modeling, usage of secure upgrading functions, encryption, and access controls. Devices are also required to provide a Software Bill Of Materials (SBOM) in order to detect components with known potentially vulnerable components. To address the interventions and risks of displaying cybersecurity, the FDA creates a distinction between premarket and postmarket responsibilities, which involves continued risk monitoring, strategies to deploy patches, and a vulnerability report plan (Amaral et al. 2024).

In Europe, wearable medical devices are covered in the Medical Device Regulation (EU MDR 2017/745) and the In vitro Diagnostic Regulation (IVDR 2017/746) of the European Union. These regulations focus more on the safety and performance of the entire lifecycle of the product and have inclusion of clauses on information security. Manufacturers will be responsible to carry out a clinical evaluation and demonstrate an overall risk management process taking into consideration cyber-security threats. General Safety and Performance Requirements (GSPR) require secure design and interoperability in addition.

ISO and IEC International standards form the basis of global compliance. Among the most important is the ISO 14971 which gives out guidelines on risk management as applied universally in medical devices. It requires manufacturers to determine hazards; calculate and assess risk; manage the risk; and oversee the effectualness of the controls all through the life-cycle of the device (Capulli et al. 2025).

Wearables can be very software intensive and network connections can make the IEC 62304 particularly applicable. This standard controls development software life cycle, where software architecture, coding standards, testing and maintenance needs to be well documented. It spices up safety classes (A, B, C) that characterize the rigor to be applied depending on the severity of the potential harm that could be inflicted by software failure.

Since a good proportion of wearable medical devices rely on transmission of data over a wireless signal or cloud storage, information security standards become imperative. The International standard ISO/IEC 27001 is an information security management standard that aims to keep medical data confidentiality, integrity and availability. ISO/IEC 80001-1 is less widely applied, but specifically covers risk management applied to IT networks which incorporate medical devices. It is highly applicable to wearables where the possibility of their use in hospital or clinical IT set-ups is an issue (Sifaoui & Eastin, 2024).

There are voluntary frameworks available in the United States by the National Institute of Standards and Technology (NIST) which is increasingly having an impact on industry practice. The NIST Cybersecurity Framework (CSF) describes five main functions (Identify, Protect, Detect, Respond and Recover), which can be adjusted to the specific needs of wearable medical devices. NIST special publications may come in handy i.e. SP 800 53 (Security and Privacy Controls) and SP 800-82 (Industrial Control Systems Security) provide practical controls and recommendations to be used in securing deployment and operation of devices.

The application of such standards is particularly tricky by startups and minor manufacturers of the devices. The compliance exercise may frequently demand multi-discipline skills on software engineering, quality controls, regulatory issues and clinical validation. Moreover, regulators now want manufacturers to go beyond checklists to achieving the attitude of security by design- where risk reduction is built into product design and not applied as an afterthought (Tettey et al. 2024).

Another avenue towards regulatory approval is conformity assessment, which would entail the use of third party assessment, review of technical documentation and clinical trials. This may need a Notified Body in the EU, which plays a role of certifying the conformity of the device to the MDR. In the U.S., FDA can undertake a premarket review or a pre-submission of high-risk devices. In both jurisdictions, the requirement of postmarket compliance extends to adverse event reporting, software updates notification and field actions reporting.

The other emerging aspect of compliance is the cross-border alignment of regulations. Distributing wearable devices across the globe means manufacturers have to streamline processes across multiple jurisdictions, which many manufacturers achieve by adhering to a set of standards such as IMDRF (International Medical Device Regulators Forum) or covering approvals across many countries in MRAs (Mutual Recognition Agreements). As illustrated in Figure 2, compliance readiness varies across the major standards applicable to wearable medical devices. While ISO 14971 and IEC 62304 emphasize structured documentation and risk-based development processes, regulatory frameworks like FDA guidance and EU MDR place greater demands on post-market vigilance. This visual comparison underscores the need for multi-standard alignment in development pipelines, particularly for globally marketed devices. To facilitate a clearer comparison, Table 2 summarizes the core focus, primary requirements, and applicability of the most relevant compliance frameworks in wearable medical device development. This tabular view allows developers and compliance officers to quickly align regulatory obligations with device architecture and intended markets, helping to streamline multi-standard certification efforts.

Figure 2. Comparative Compliance Readiness Across Major Medical Device Standards.

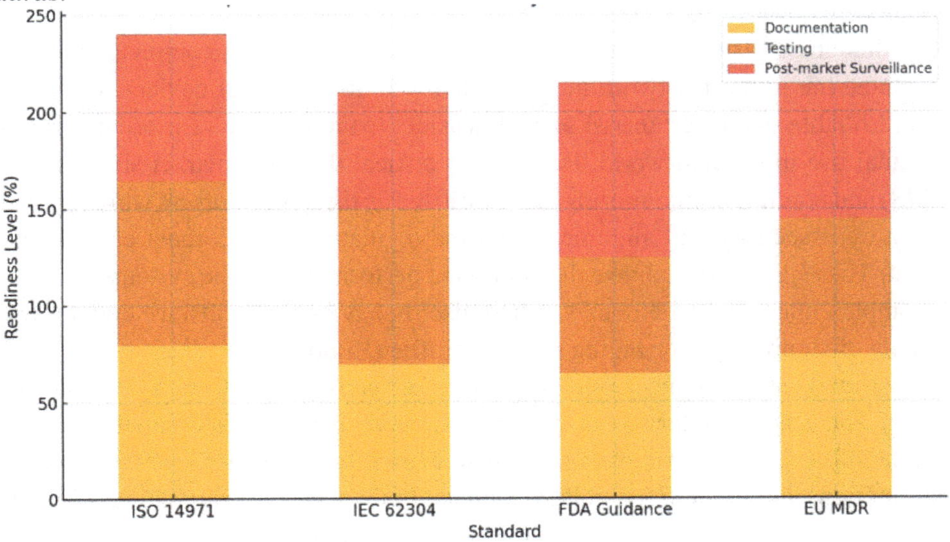

Table 2. Summary of Key Compliance Standards for Wearable Medical Devices.

Standard	Focus Area	Key Requirement	Applies To
ISO 14971	Risk Management	Risk Analysis & Controls	All medical devices
IEC 62304	Software Lifecycle	Documented Development Process	Software in medical devices
FDA Guidance	Cybersecurity & Regulatory	SBOM, Threat Modeling	Devices with software/ firmware
EU MDR	Safety & Performance	Post-market Surveillance	Devices marketed in EU

In short, both compliance requirements and regulatory pathways of wearable medical devices are complex yet unavoidable. They act as a blueprint in secure design and pathway to the market adoption. Complying with these frameworks ensures that only minimal legal and reputational risks are incurred besides providing safer and more effective and resilient healthcare technologies. With regulatory expectations contributing to that change as much as technological innovation, proactive compliance has and will continue to be a determining factor in the success and the sustainability of wearable medical devices.

6. POST-MARKET SURVEILLANCE AND CONTINUOUS MONITORING

Although extensive premarket testing, auditing, and regulatory compliance should guarantee the initial trustworthiness of such wearable medical devices, there are uncontrollable and uncertain risks and downsides to the same being presented when in actual use in the real world. Hence, it is critical that post-market surveillance (PMS) and continuous monitoring are prioritised as the key factors by which device safety, cybersecurity and alignment with the regulatory environment can be sustained. These processes achieve the continued performance of the systems, devices in complex uncontrolled climates, where user behavior, and software updates are capable of significantly changing the risk profile (Hundur et al. 2025).

Post-market surveillance is well-organized and constant mechanisms of data collection, analysis, and intervention after a product has been released into the market. It is intended to identify/assess any adverse events, security issues, and functional malfunctions and other safety-related signals. In the case of wearable medical devices, many of which are deployed in very large quantities among a wide range of users, PMS is important to warn about low-probability, high-impact problems that might not have obvious manifestations in clinical trials or product testing.

Key components of PMS include:

- User feedback and incident reporting systems, which collect complaints, usage anomalies, and suspected malfunctions from patients, clinicians, and healthcare providers.
- Field data analytics, which examine device usage patterns, transmission errors, or physiological data trends to uncover latent design flaws or usability issues.
- Regulatory reporting, such as the U.S. FDA's Medical Device Reporting (MDR) system or the EU's vigilance system, which mandates the timely submission of serious adverse event data and corrective actions.

In addition to safety surveillance, a cybersecurity surveillance is becoming a necessity and technologically possible to maintain in a constant fashion. Advanced wearable gadgets are frequently also linked to cloud solutions or mobile software to provide real-time diagnostics and firmware telematics as well as behavioral analytics. Such connectivity allows the manufacturers to install security monitoring agents to watch the networks and raise alerts when there are anomalies in traffic, unapproved access requests, abnormal power consumption, or malfunctions that are not within the specification of the devices.

Dynamic Software Updating A key process in this is the Secure Update Mechanism. Because wearables often need software/ firmware updates to rectify bugs, patch vulnerabilities, and/or add features, the updates pipeline must be secure, auditable, and fail-safe. This includes digital signing of firmware packages, encrypted payloads in an update, validation of integrity pre-install, and rollback in case of malfunction. Secure booting means that only trusted programs are executed on the equipment and reduces the possibility of permanent malware, as well as the attempt of tampering with the firmware.

The next pillar is to implement coordinated vulnerability disclosure (CVD) programs. Such arrangements give defined avenues of security researchers, clinicians, or users to report about the vulnerabilities they discover without facing legal penalties. Manufacturers will in turn make commitments to validate, address, include, and publicly disclosure these issues in responsible and time biding ways. Regulatory-type bodies such as the FDA support such transparency as a method to foster ecosystem resiliency (Manetti et al. 2025).

The growing sophistication of cybersecurity monitoring in the post-market environment is often through machine learning-augmented anomaly detection, where average behaviors are determined over time and a device or a particular device type to serve as the norm, with outliers generating alerts or automated mitigation strategies. As an example, an ECG monitor that switches to high frequency transmissions or new IP addresses could be signaled as a possible intrusion and subjected to review. Nevertheless, these types of systems need to be adequately tuned and optimized with respect to avoiding false alerts that interfere with clinical processes or with the user being subjected to undue scrutiny.

At regulatory level, post-market surveillance is no longer perfunctory. The EU MDR will require a Post-Market Surveillance Plan and Periodic Safety Update Report to specific classes of devices. Likewise, FDA postmarket policy on cybersecurity demands that manufacturers keep an eye on their devices, be able to evaluate the vulnerabilities identified therein, and offer mitigation plans, more so on those devices that are classified as critical to health outcomes.

Regarding wearable medical devices, monitor field performance should also reflect the fluctuating environments that medical devices may be acted upon. To take a few examples, external factors such as other wireless devices intruding, improper methods of recharging devices, or conflicts with software in the mobile units they are linked to, can all contribute to a reduced performance level. The implication is that manufacturers should maintain dynamic device registries compiling device-specific usage and performance data (aggregated across the installed base) such that trends can be analyzed to provide early warning of and potential resolution of systemic problems (Mulla & Patel, 2025).

Last but not least user education and clinical integration are crucial to effective post-market monitoring as well. Patients and healthcare givers should also be educated on how to detect abnormal behavior of the device, report, and when to apply updates. There is also the possibility to automate some of the monitoring functions of the process with integrations with EHR and clinical workflows where concerns can be flagged when there are any observed data discrepancies or alerts issued by the device or other equipment.

In a nutshell, post-market surveillance and ongoing monitoring cannot serve as the extension of compliance, but rather symbolize its new and growing interest in patient safety, information security, and device reliability. With the increased intelligence, connectedness and autonomy that comes with wearable medical devices, the capacity to monitor, adapt to, and learn about real-world usage will determine both the feasibility and long-term clinical value and patient trust. These operations in device management must remain as main operations during the lifecycle of device operations assuring that diligence should not cease at the point of market authority but it must extend into every moment of operational integrity.

7. CHALLENGES AND EMERGING TRENDS

Truly, as wearable medical devices emerge as part of the healthcare delivery landscape, the technical and regulatory environment in which they are tested, audited and put under compliance becomes more sophisticated. Although great efforts have been made to date in the formulation of standards and risk management, some underlying obstacles still hinder holistic protection and safeness of devices. At the same time, there are also emerging trends based on advances in AI, cloud-focused ecosystems, and evolving cyber threats that are transforming how manufacturers and regulators think about the assurance of these devices.

One of the most burning issues is the disintegration of the standards and regulatory expectations across jurisdictions. International standards including the ISO 14971 and IEC 62304 provide base evaluation and guidance, but there are great differences in the interpretations and requirements and documentation processes of varying regions. To global manufacturers, convergence of compliance standards across the U.S. FDA, EU MDR, Health Canada, and others represents redundancy, time, and expense. This is also taxing to small and mid size companies that have limited levels of regulatory infrastructure (Saad et al. 2024).

One more constant problem is delay between the new technology development and the adjustment of the regulation. Wearable devices frequently combine characteristics of artificial intelligence-based diagnostics, biometric authentication, cloud computing analytics and mobile application connectivity and these technologies are also constantly changing. Regulatory frameworks, though, are historically conservative and not particularly good at keeping up with the times. This poses confusion on how the new functionalities must be tested, validated or classified. As an example, an AI-driven wearable that uses machine learning to deduce the cardiac signals could be classified in a wider range of risks levels, depending on the extent to which the decision-making process is under its control--which complicates the process of receiving prompt approvals by developers.

This is also a risk attributable to the absence of scalable, real-time frameworks of compliance. There is a gap in maintaining ongoing, dynamic compliance in a landscape where the devices have frequent updates and could change connectivity environments as well as interact with a range of user profiles. Current compliance processes are primarily made to accommodate relatively static products, they are ill-suited to accommodate wearable devices that are dynamic in nature, that are learners and will constantly evolve through software updates and based on feedback and tuning of their algorithms (Olawade et al. 2025).

Besides that, AI and machine learning (ML) algorithms add a new degree of complexity to testing and compliance. Traditional means of validation do not always pick up the non- determinism of AI behavior. As an example, a wearable respiratory monitor that uses ML may learn over time in response to the environmental or user physiology noise. It will be necessary to test these models in novel ways with explainability analysis, data drift monitoring, and performance revalidation across subgroups of patients. Regulators are starting to take action on these concerns-such as the FDA proposed Predetermined Change Control Plan of AI/ML software- however outcomes are yet to be fully agreed.

Security-wise, cloud-connected and edge-computing systems create enlarged attack surfaces that put a strain on traditional auditing systems. Wearables are no longer standalone devices; they are deeply connected to cloud-based APIs and data lakes as well as remote diagnostics systems. Protecting such distributed systems necessitates end-to-end threat modelling, end-to-end encrypted pipelines, and fed audit records all of which are not the capabilities of many legacy healthcare systems. In addition, because device vendors frequently rely on third party providers of analytics, connectivity, or storage, their products face issues of supply chain vulnerability as well as vulnerability management (Singh et al. 2024).

A missing element in this topography that is vital to human dealings is the lack of multidisciplinary skills. Wearable medical devices that are developed have typically undergone the process of testing and certification and require in-depth expertise in embedded systems, clinical safety, cybersecurity, privacy law, and regulatory science. Not many organizations have this a wide range in-house team. This deficiency frequently leads to disjointed business processes, in which security and compliance is done after the fact, whether piecemeal or in isolation of other business requirements.

There are however some good signs, to alleviate these pains. Among such trends is the implementation of AI to audit and detect anomalies. Security analytics powered by AI have the potential to detect anomalous wearable device usage and any possible threats quicker than rule-based analytics. The tools may also automatically assist with some parts of compliance surveillance, e.g. put in alerts when firmware behavior changes or when normality of update processes is violated.

A growing trend is increasing the adoption of compliance-as-code forms in which regulatory requirements are modeled into testable rules within the development pipeline. As an example, continuous integration/continuous deployment (CI/CD) tools may enable checks to be made of compliance with encryption standards, API authentication, or data handling procedures governed by particular compliance requirements. Such a transformation allows greater velocity of development processes and consistency with regulatory requirements.

Lastly, there is also a shift towards adaptive and modular regulatory framework. Regulatory sandboxes, conditional approvals We have regulatory sandboxes, and conditional approvals, where a limited number of innovative devices may be deployed in a real-world setting under greater oversight. Not only does this speed the progress of innovation but also gives practical data in order that future regulatory changes are informed. The approach of using Precertification Programs by the FDA, as well as the Digital Health Software Precertification Pilot Program is expected to ensure that manufacturers with a proven culture of quality and continuous improvement are rewarded, rather than subject to obligatory documentation review (Canali et al. 2024).

Concisely, wearable medical devices security and compliance is a field on the cusp of change. Historic issues of regulatory fragmentation, testing, and complexity of the ecosystem are being addressed by new models of reliability and technology enabling higher levels of adaptability and scalability. The way forward over this shifting landscape will involve progressive approaches that are open to technological developments as well as stringent policies. The subsequent sections will further situate such dynamics with examples and strategic suggestions of future-ready compliance programs.

8. CASE STUDIES AND LESSONS LEARNED

To contextualize the principles of testing, auditing, and compliance in real-world settings, it is essential to examine actual case studies of wearable medical devices—both those that succeeded in implementing robust assurance mechanisms and those that experienced critical failures. The examples give a practical representation of the material outcomes of security failures, non-compliance to regulations and poorly conducted tests and in so doing demonstrating suitable patterns that have performed excellently in curbing the vice.

Case Study 1: Medtronic Insulin Pumps – Firmware Vulnerabilities and Recall

In 2019, the U.S. FDA sent a safety communication on several models of Medtronic MiniMed insulin pumps. The devices were discovered with unencrypted wireless communication protocols with the possibility of an attacker being able to intercept or tamper with the protocols. In particular, a hostile user might change the dosage delivery of insulin by means of the radio-frequency interface where the communication between the insulin pump and its controller is facilitated (Katsuya & Liu, 2025).

Whereas no known exploitation had been used in the field at that point, a theoretical possibility of unauthorized insulin injection was a significant patient safety risk. The FDA classified this as a Class I recall - the most serious type and it advised devices to be replaced by the affected users.

Lessons Learned:

- Secure firmware design and encrypted wireless communication are non-negotiable in life-critical wearables.
- Post-market surveillance and ethical research by security professionals were key in identifying the issue before harm occurred.
- Manufacturers must build and maintain rapid-response capabilities for recalls, public communication, and device updates.

Case Study 2: Fitbit and Consumer-Grade Wearables – Regulatory Ambiguity and Data Privacy

Although they were not initially regulated as medical devices, Fitbit wearables are in a space in-between wellness tracking and clinical significance. Fitbit has since expanded its capabilities to ECG monitoring and atrial fibrillation as well, and its services have come under the scrutiny of regulators concerning its provision of data accuracy, privacy, and user consent (Radanliev, 2025).

Fitbit has sought to target FDA clearance on specific health functionality, rather than the device itself. This spotty certification plan gives rise to a patchwork of assurance that can be confusing to the user and restricts clinical adoption.

Lessons Learned:

- As consumer devices adopt medical-grade features, regulatory boundaries blur—making comprehensive risk assessments and privacy protections vital.
- Even partial regulatory engagement (e.g., FDA clearance for a feature) requires rigorous testing and disclosure protocols.
- Transparency about data collection, usage, and third-party integrations is critical for maintaining user trust and avoiding legal risks under frameworks like GDPR and HIPAA.

Case Study 3: Apple Watch – Incremental Compliance and Proactive Clinical Validation

The Apple method of wearable health features can be considered the right way of strategic compliance. Apple Watch launched heart rate monitoring and fall detection and electrical heart monitoring one by one by validation studies and regulators. Apple had received 510(k) clearance from FDA to use its ECG feature, and its substantial equivalence to predicate devices has been demonstrated (Harte et al. 2021).

Apple also completed a massive validation research- Apple Heart Study with over 400,000 subjects to collect post-market evidence and polish algorithms to identify arrhythmia.

Lessons Learned:

- Phased feature deployment coupled with early regulatory engagement can streamline approval and reduce compliance risk.
- Large-scale data collection post-release can support real-time performance monitoring and iterative algorithm improvement.
- Building in secure update pathways and clear user education mechanisms supports sustainable clinical integration.

Case Study 4: St. Jude Medical (Abbott) – Cybersecurity Exposure and Litigation

In 2016, it published a report by cybersecurity firm Muddy Waters Capital that accused St. Jude Medical of having utterly unsafe cardiac devices, such as pacemakers, defibrillators and so on. The report alleged that these devices could be compromised through insecure radio frequency (RF) communication protocols which the attackers would use to gain control of these devices.

First ignored by the manufacturer, it turned out that the concerns were later confirmed after coordinated disclosure procedures were established with independent researchers and the U.S. Department of Homeland Security. The FDA has confirmed the vulnerabilities and St. Jude has issued a patch in 2017 via over-the-air software update (Haider et al. 2019).

Lessons Learned:

- Downplaying or delaying investigation of cybersecurity reports can damage credibility and regulatory relationships.
- Coordinated vulnerability disclosure protocols, when respected, can prevent public panic and ensure orderly remediation.
- Continuous threat modeling and periodic penetration testing are essential, even after a device has achieved market approval.

Cross-Cutting Lessons and Patterns

Across these cases, several recurrent themes emerge:

- Security must be engineered from the outset—retrofitting protections after deployment is costly and often insufficient.
- Ongoing compliance and surveillance are not merely regulatory requirements but essential for operational integrity.
- Transparency, rapid disclosure, and collaboration with external researchers and regulators foster trust and resilience.
- Clinical validation and data feedback loops enhance algorithm performance, user confidence, and long-term adoption.

These cases also show the need to treat testing, auditing, and compliance not as a leaflet, but as a living process, changing with technology, user-requirements, and the threat-landscape. By incorporating these lessons internally, those in the wearable medical device ecosystem can develop more secure and robust devices that value patient-centered technology.

9. STRATEGIC RECOMMENDATIONS

With wearable medical devices constantly becoming more advanced and large in scale, the task of securing, protecting, enforcing compliance with regulations involves not only complying with standards but also a different approach to standards: a systems-level perspective and approach. In this section, the lessons and insights of previous chapters are synthesized into practical strategies in order to give actionable recommendations to manufacturers, regulators and healthcare stakeholders. Through these recommendations, it is possible to build resilience, trust, and navigate complexity in the ever-changing environment at a fast speed (Fusco et al. 2025).

1. Embed Security and Compliance from Design Onward

Security and compliance must not be billed as an after-thought or an independent step to development. Rather they have to be incorporated in the initial phases of design and architecture. Developers are encouraged to use a security-by-design and privacy-by-design approach, where threat analysis, and risk assessment, regulatory analysis, etc., are run in parallel with core functionality implementation.

Applying standards to the design like IEC 62304 (software lifecycle processes) and ISO 14971 (risk management) early in the design process allows decisions about design to be framed in a manner that reduces the exposure to vulnerabilities. Preference should also be given to modular, and updateable architectures to ensure that the future compliance is achieved because of the changes in standards.

2. Develop Cross-Functional Compliance Teams

Wearable device compliance needs an effective oversight provided by inter-disciplinary collaboration. The engineering departments have to cooperate with a group of regulatory affairs specialists, cybersecurity experts, clinical researchers and quality assurance personnel. Either forming cross functional teams or using a compliance integration lead will assist in ensuring that the development of devices is in sync with both technical and legal requirements as well as requirements in the device lifecycle.

The various stakeholders should participate in regular design reviews and risk assessments, which can then help to identify gaps that need to be filled at an earlier stage and allow quicker iterations on the solutions.

3. Operationalize Continuous Testing and Monitoring

As connected medical devices are dynamic in nature, organizations have to invest in continuous security testing, automatic monitoring and live telemetry. This includes:

- Merging static and dynamic code analysis in CI/CD lifetimes.
- Regular probing through penetration and fuzz tests against firmware and communication console.
- Deploying machine learning based anomaly detection that can flag deviant machine behavior after deployment.

Such activities should be facilitated by infrastructure that enables over-the-air updates, audit logging, and remote device diagnostics, which are important when maintaining rapid incident response and ongoing compliance.

4. Prioritize Transparent Vulnerability Disclosure

To achieve integrity and ecosystem collaboration, it is important to establish the coordinated vulnerability disclosure (CVD) program. Manufacturers are expected to be able to have safe and well-advertisable vulnerability reporting mechanisms where the researcher, health specialists, and the customer can report the vulnerabilities. Policies must be devoted to be timely in investigation, remediation, and post-supporting communication with the regulatory agency, including the FDA or EU Notified Bodies.

Actively contributing to security research through bug bounty programs, or consortia can also boost device security posture.

5. Align Product Roadmaps with Regulatory Milestones

To avoid costly delays, compliance timelines should be built into product roadmaps. This includes accounting for:

- Pre-submission meetings with regulatory agencies (e.g., FDA Q-Sub program).
- Clinical evaluation and documentation for intended uses.
- Preparation of a Software Bill of Materials (SBOM) and cybersecurity risk management files.
- Development of a Post-Market Surveillance Plan, especially for EU MDR compliance.

Strategic planning ensures that innovation proceeds in tandem with approval requirements, minimizing friction between development and market access.

6. Invest in Scalable Compliance Infrastructure

As devices scale to larger user populations or multiple markets, manufacturers must establish infrastructure for automated compliance tracking, global regulatory alignment, and audit readiness. This includes adopting platforms that:

- Centralize regulatory documentation and version control.
- Manage multilingual, jurisdiction-specific regulatory submissions.
- Track field incidents and safety trends using real-time dashboards.
- Generate evidence packages for audits or recalls at short notice.

Such infrastructure transforms compliance from a manual burden into a scalable capability.

7. Engage in Regulatory Innovation and Dialogue

Regulatory sandboxes, conditional approvals, and precertification programs are becoming more open to adaptive intervention. Proactively involving regulators early on creates the chance to influence expectations and shed light on ambiguities, particularly where there is something new at stake, as is the case with AI diagnostics or cloud-based analytics.

Manufacturers also need to engage in the process of new regulations being developed and contribute to public comment processes, and that they work in international bodies like IMDRF to produce consensus and best practices.

The strategic suggestions indicate a transition of the aspect of compliance as a defensive requirement to a progressive approach to innovation, trust, and competitiveness. Companies that institutionalize these practices will be in a prime position to create devices that will not only be technologically superior but also secure, sustainable and in line with the changing trends of connected health.

10. CONCLUSION

The rise of wearable medical devices has transformed how healthcare is delivered, demanding continuous assurance of safety, cybersecurity, and regulatory compliance. This chapter presented a lifecycle-integrated assurance framework tailored to the unique risks posed by wearable technologies—devices that are dynamic, software-driven, and deployed in uncontrolled environments.

By synthesizing international standards and real-world case studies, we outlined a proactive model that unites functional and security testing, AI-driven auditing, and real-time compliance monitoring. Core elements such as compliance-as-code, secure firmware update mechanisms, and machine learning–enabled anomaly detection form the technical foundation of this strategy. These tools enable both prevention and rapid response, ensuring that wearables can safely evolve alongside emerging threats and regulatory expectations.

Ultimately, this chapter advocates for a shift in perspective: compliance is not a one-time hurdle, but a continuous design imperative. By embedding assurance into every phase of the device lifecycle, stakeholders can build wearable medical technologies that are not only innovative and connected, but also trustworthy, resilient, and ready for real-world deployment.

REFERENCES

Amaral, C., Paiva, M., Rodrigues, A. R., Veiga, F., & Bell, V. (2024). Global regulatory challenges for medical devices: Impact on innovation and market access. *Applied Sciences (Basel, Switzerland)*, *14*(20), 9304.

Brönneke, J. B., Müller, J., Mouratis, K., Hagen, J., & Stern, A. D. (2021). Regulatory, legal, and market aspects of smart wearables for cardiac monitoring. *Sensors (Basel)*, *21*(14), 4937. PMID: 34300680

Canali, S., Ferretti, A., Schiaffonati, V., & Blasimme, A. (2024). Wearable technologies for healthy ageing: Prospects, challenges, and ethical considerations. *The Journal of Frailty & Aging*, *13*(2), 149–156. PMID: 38616371

Capulli, E., Druda, Y., Palmese, F., Butt, A. H., Domenicali, M., Macchiarelli, A. G., & Ingravallo, F. (2025). Ethical and legal implications of health monitoring wearable devices: A scoping review. *Social Science & Medicine*, •••, 117685. PMID: 40010231

Chak, W. Y., Tang, W. F., Mak, S. L., Lee, C. C., Lam, S. K., & Li, C. H. (2023, November). A Critical Review on Hazard Analysis and Risk Assessment for Development of Wearable Medical Devices. In *2023 IEEE International Symposium on Product Compliance Engineering-Asia (ISPCE-ASIA)* (pp. 1-5). IEEE.

Chinoy, E. D., Cuellar, J. A., Jameson, J. T., & Markwald, R. R. (2022). Performance of four commercial wearable sleep-tracking devices tested under unrestricted conditions at home in healthy young adults. *Nature and Science of Sleep*, •••, 493–516. PMID: 35345630

Degerli, M., & Ozkan Yildirim, S. (2022). Identifying critical success factors for wearable medical devices: A comprehensive exploration. *Universal Access in the Information Society*, *21*(1), 121–143.

Fusco, P., Rimoli, G. P., & Ficco, M. (2025). TinyML and Federated Learning for Resource-Constrained Medical Devices. In *Artificial Intelligence Techniques for Analysing Sensitive Data in Medical Cyber-Physical Systems: System Protection and Data Analysis* (pp. 113–126). Springer Nature Switzerland.

Gao, Z., Zhou, Y., Zhang, J., Foroughi, J., Peng, S., Baughman, R. H., & Wang, C. H. (2024). Advanced energy harvesters and energy storage for powering wearable and implantable medical devices. *Advanced Materials*, *36*(42), 2404492. PMID: 38935237

Haider, N., Gates, C., Sengupta, V., & Qian, S. (2019). Cybersecurity of medical devices: Past, present, and future. In *Deer's Treatment of Pain: An Illustrated Guide for Practitioners* (pp. 811–820). Springer International Publishing.

Harte, R., Laighin, G. Ó., & Quinlan, L. (2021). Validation, verification, and reliability. In *Digital Health* (pp. 101–118). Academic Press.

Hundur, M., Spahić, L., Bećirović, F., Gurbeta Pokvić, L., & Badnjević, A. (2025). Advancement of post-market surveillance of medical devices leveraging artificial intelligence: ECG devices case study. *Technology and Health Care*, •••, 09287329241303727. PMID: 39973872

Iqbal, S. M., Mahgoub, I., Du, E., Leavitt, M. A., & Asghar, W. (2021). Advances in healthcare wearable devices. *NPJ Flexible Electronics*, *5*(1), 9.

Karaböce, B. (2023, September). Lessons Learned from External Audits in Medical Device Testing Laboratories: Best Practices and Recommendations for Quality Management. In *Mediterranean Conference on Medical and Biological Engineering and Computing* (pp. 65-73). Cham: Springer Nature Switzerland.

Katsuya, R., & Liu, X. (2025). Policy and management implications of firmware vulnerabilities in medical IoT devices: a multi-case analysis. *Journal of Science and Technology Policy Management.*

Manetti, S., Guidotti, E., Vola, F., & Vainieri, M. (2025). A systematic literature review of real-world evidence (RWE) on post-market assessment of medical devices. *Health Economics, Policy, and Law*, •••, 1–33. PMID: 39801351

Mulla, S. J., & Patel, M. (2025). Global Regulatory Perspectives on Sensor-Enabled and Biomaterial-Integrated Medical Devices: A Focus on India, Canada, and Australia. *Biomedical Materials & Devices*, •••, 1–22.

Olawade, D. B., Aderinto, N., David-Olawade, A. C., Egbon, E., Adereni, T., Popoola, M. R., & Tiwari, R. (2025). Integrating AI-driven wearable devices and biometric data into stroke risk assessment: A review of opportunities and challenges. *Clinical Neurology and Neurosurgery*, *249*, 108689. PMID: 39675149

Pawnikar, V., & Patel, M. (2025, February). Biosensors in wearable medical devices: Regulatory framework and compliance across US, EU, and Indian markets. In *Annales Pharmaceutiques Françaises*. Elsevier Masson.

Radanliev, P. (2025). Privacy, ethics, transparency, and accountability in AI systems for wearable devices. *Frontiers in Digital Health*, *7*, 1431246. PMID: 40599875

Ramasubramanian, B., Sundarrajan, S., Rao, R. P., Reddy, M. V., Chellappan, V., & Ramakrishna, S. (2022). Novel low-carbon energy solutions for powering emerging wearables, smart textiles, and medical devices. *Energy & Environmental Science, 15*(12), 4928–4981.

Saad, H. S., Zaki, J. F., & Abdelsalam, M. M. (2024). Employing of machine learning and wearable devices in healthcare system: Tasks and challenges. *Neural Computing & Applications, 36*(29), 17829–17849.

Shajari, S., Kuruvinashetti, K., Komeili, A., & Sundararaj, U. (2023). The emergence of AI-based wearable sensors for digital health technology: A review. *Sensors (Basel), 23*(23), 9498. PMID: 38067871

Sharma, A. (2025). Securing the Future of Healthcare: Ensuring Privacy and Security in Wearable and Implantable Medical Devices. In *Security, Privacy, and Trust in WBANs and E-Healthcare* (pp. 105-125). CRC Press.

Shuvo, M. M. H., Titirsha, T., Amin, N., & Islam, S. K. (2022). Energy harvesting in implantable and wearable medical devices for enduring precision healthcare. *Energies, 15*(20), 7495.

Sifaoui, A., & Eastin, M. S. (2024). "Whispers from the wrist": wearable health monitoring devices and privacy regulations in the US: the loopholes, the challenges, and the opportunities. *Cryptography, 8*(2), 26.

Singh, A. B., Khandelwal, C., & Dangayach, G. S. (2024). Revolutionizing healthcare materials: Innovations in processing, advancements, and challenges for enhanced medical device integration and performance. *Journal of Micromanufacturing*, 25165984241256234.

Smogavc Cestar, A., & Harer, J. (2023). Mastering Quality System Audits and Inspections for Medical Devices. In *Medical Devices and In Vitro Diagnostics: Requirements in Europe* (pp. 543–584). Springer International Publishing.

Tan, M., Xu, Y., Gao, Z., Yuan, T., Liu, Q., Yang, R., & Peng, L. (2022). Recent advances in intelligent wearable medical devices integrating biosensing and drug delivery. *Advanced Materials, 34*(27), 2108491. PMID: 35008128

Tettey, F., Parupelli, S. K., & Desai, S. (2024). A review of biomedical devices: Classification, regulatory guidelines, human factors, software as a medical device, and cybersecurity. *Biomedical Materials & Devices, 2*(1), 316–341.

Thapa, S., Bello, A., Maurushat, A., & Farid, F. (2023). Security risks and user perception towards adopting wearable internet of medical things. *International Journal of Environmental Research and Public Health, 20*(8), 5519. PMID: 37107800

Ushimaru, Y., Katoh, T., Sasaki, M., Hata, T., Hosaka, M., Eguchi, H., & Nakajima, K. (2025). Development of medical devices driven by academia-industry collaboration: An internal audit. *Surgery*, *181*, 109289. PMID: 40054052

Vakhter, V., Soysal, B., Schaumont, P., & Guler, U. (2022). Threat modeling and risk analysis for miniaturized wireless biomedical devices. *IEEE Internet of Things Journal*, *9*(15), 13338–13352.

Wang, L., Jiang, K., & Shen, G. (2021). Wearable, implantable, and interventional medical devices based on smart electronic skins. *Advanced Materials Technologies*, *6*(6), 2100107.

KEY TERMS AND DEFINITIONS

Auditing: A structured review of device logs, configurations, and processes to assess conformance with operational standards, detect anomalies, and support traceability and accountability.

Compliance: The fulfillment of regulatory, legal, and industry standards governing medical device safety, efficacy, and security throughout its lifecycle.

Coordinated Vulnerability Disclosure (CVD): A structured process by which security researchers and stakeholders report vulnerabilities to manufacturers and regulators, facilitating responsible disclosure and remediation.

Cybersecurity: The practice of protecting systems, networks, and data from digital attacks, unauthorized access, or damage—particularly important for connected medical devices handling sensitive health information.

FDA 510(k) Clearance: A regulatory process by which the U.S. Food and Drug Administration determines that a new medical device is substantially equivalent to a legally marketed predicate device.

Firmware Update Mechanism: A secure process for delivering and installing new software or firmware on a device after deployment, typically used for patching vulnerabilities or improving performance.

Functional Testing: A quality assurance process that verifies whether a device performs its intended clinical or operational functions under specified conditions.

IEC 62304: An international standard outlining the software lifecycle requirements for medical device software, including development, maintenance, and documentation.

Machine Learning-based Anomaly Detection: The use of AI algorithms to identify unusual or unsafe behavior in a device by comparing current operation to known baseline patterns.

Post-Market Surveillance (PMS): A set of processes used to monitor the safety and performance of a medical device after it has been released to the market, including data collection, incident reporting, and corrective actions.

Risk Management (ISO 14971): A systematic framework for identifying, evaluating, and controlling risks associated with medical devices to ensure patient safety and device reliability.

Security Testing: The process of evaluating a system or device for vulnerabilities, threats, and attack surfaces. It includes penetration testing, fuzz testing, and protocol assessments.

Software Bill of Materials (SBOM): A detailed list of software components used in a device, including open-source libraries and dependencies, required for cybersecurity risk assessment and regulatory submission.

Wearable Medical Devices: Electronic health monitoring devices worn on the body that collect physiological data (e.g., heart rate, glucose levels) for clinical or wellness purposes. They often feature wireless communication and real-time data processing.

Compilation of References

Abdin, Z. U., Shah, S. A. A., Shah, I. A., Iman, U. R., Mian, S. H., & Yoo, H. (2025). A novel dual-band MIMO-enabled biotelemetric endovascular stent IoMT system. *IEEE Transactions on Instrumentation and Measurement*, *74*, 1–15. DOI: 10.1109/TIM.2025.3576004

Abubeker, K. M., Baskar, S., & Yadav, P. (2024). Internet of Things Assisted Wireless Body Area Network Enabled Biosensor Framework for Detecting Ventilator and Hospital-Acquired Pneumonia. *IEEE Sensors Journal.*

Adeghe, E. P., Okolo, C. A., & Ojeyinka, O. T. (2024). Evaluating the impact of blockchain technology in healthcare data management: A review of security, privacy, and patient outcomes. *Open Access Research Journal of Science and Technology, 10*(2), 013–020. https://doi.org/DOI: 10.53022/oarjst.2024.10.2.0038

Adere, E. M. (2022). Blockchain in healthcare and IoT: A systematic literature review. In *Array* (Vol. 14). https://doi.org/DOI: 10.1016/j.array.2022.100139

Ahmed, I., Jeon, G., & Chehri, A. (2023). An IoT-enabled smart health care system for screening of COVID-19 with multi layers features fusion and selection. *Computing*, *105*(4), 743–760.

Ahmed, S. F., Sharmin, S., Kuldeep, S. A., Lameesa, A., Alam, M. S. B., Liu, G., & Gandomi, A. H. (2024). Transformative impacts of the Internet of Medical Things on modern healthcare. *Results in Engineering*. Advance online publication. DOI: 10.1016/j.rineng.2024.103787

Akkaoui, R., Hei, X., & Cheng, W. (2020). EdgeMediChain: A Hybrid Edge Blockchain-Based Framework for Health Data Exchange. *IEEE Access : Practical Innovations, Open Solutions*, *8*. Advance online publication. DOI: 10.1109/ACCESS.2020.3003575

Al-awamy, A. A., Al-shaibany, N., Sikora, A., & Welte, D. (2025). Hybrid Consensus Mechanisms in Blockchain: A Comprehensive Review. *International Journal of Intelligent Systems*, *2025*(1), 5821997. DOI: 10.1155/INT/5821997

Albalawi, A. (2025). Cloud Security and Data Protection in Hybrid Environments. In Complexities and Challenges for Securing Digital Assets and Infrastructure (pp. 175-198). IGI Global Scientific Publishing.

Alfian, G., Syafrudin, M., Ijaz, M. F., Syaekhoni, M. A., Fitriyani, N. L., & Rhee, J. (2018). A personalized healthcare monitoring system for diabetic patients by utilizing BLE-based sensors and real-time data processing. *Sensors (Basel)*, *18*(7), 2183. PMID: 29986473

Alghamdi, A., Basir, A., Iqbal, A., Simorangkir, R. B. V. B., & Ben Mabrouk, I. (2025). A low-profile implantable antenna for heart implants. *IEEE Transactions on Antennas and Propagation*, *73*(5), 3310–3315. DOI: 10.1109/TAP.2025.3555863

Ali Zouaghi, Y., Mahamdioua, M., Lahoulou, A., & Chettibi, S. (2025). Privacy preserving biometric authentication based on fully homomorphic encryption, blockchain, and IPFS data storage. *Multimedia Tools and Applications*. Advance online publication. DOI: 10.1007/s11042-024-19234-5

Ali, F., El-Sappagh, S., Islam, S. M. R., Ali, A., Attique, M., Imran, M., & Kwak, K.-S. (2021). An intelligent healthcare monitoring framework using wearable sensors and social networking data. *Future Generation Computer Systems*, *114*, 23–43. DOI: 10.1016/j.future.2020.07.047

Ali, F., Ilyas, A., & Ahmadeen, S. (2024). Regulations in Japan. In *Global regulations of medicinal, pharmaceutical, and food products* (pp. 153–167). CRC Press.

Alladi, T., & Chamola, V., & Naren. (2021). HARCI: A two-way authentication protocol for three entity healthcare IoT networks. *IEEE Journal on Selected Areas in Communications*, *39*(2), 361–369. DOI: 10.1109/JSAC.2020.3020605

Almaiah, M. A., Yelisetti, S., Arya, L., Christopher, N. K. B., Kaliappan, K., Vellaisamy, P., Hajjej, F., & Alkdour, T. (2023). A novel approach for improving the security of IoT–medical data systems using an enhanced dynamic Bayesian network. *Electronics (Basel)*, *12*(4316). Advance online publication. DOI: 10.3390/electronics12204316

Almujally, N. A., Aljrees, T., Saidani, O., Umer, M., Faheem, Z. B., Abuzinadah, N., Alnowaiser, K., & Ashraf, I. (2023). Monitoring acute heart failure patients using internet-of-things-based smart monitoring system. *Sensors (Basel)*, *23*(10), 4580. PMID: 37430494

Al-Sabaawi, A., Al-Dulaimi, K., & Zhao, Y., & Others. (2024). Investigating data storage security and retrieval for Fitbit wearable devices. *Health and Technology*, *14*, 695–708. DOI: 10.1007/s12553-024-00885-0

Alzu'bi, A., Alomar, A. A., Alkhaza'leh, S., Abuarqoub, A., & Hammoudeh, M. (2024). A review of privacy and security of edge computing in smart healthcare systems: Issues, challenges, and research directions. *Tsinghua Science and Technology*, *29*(4), 1152–1180. DOI: 10.26599/TST.2023.9010090

Amaral, C., Paiva, M., Rodrigues, A. R., Veiga, F., & Bell, V. (2024). Global regulatory challenges for medical devices: Impact on innovation and market access. *Applied Sciences (Basel, Switzerland)*, *14*(20), 9304.

Anant, A., & Prasad, R. (2024). *Navigating privacy in the data economy. 2024 27th International Symposium on Wireless Personal Multimedia Communications (WPMC),* 1–6. https://doi.org/DOI: 10.1109/WPMC63271.2024.10862999

Angayarkanni, S. A., Rajaram, V., & Pandimurugan, V. (2025). Intelligent transportation. In *Healthcare informatics innovation post COVID-19 pandemic* (p. 243). CRC Press., DOI: 10.1201/9781003485629-17

Ankaral, Z. E., Demir, A. F., Qaraqe, M., Abbasi, Q. H., Serpedin, E., Arslan, H., & Gitlin, R. D. (2015). Physical layer security for wireless implantable medical devices. In *2015 IEEE 20th International Workshop on Computer Aided Modelling and Design of Communication Links and Networks* (pp. 144–147). IEEE. https://doi.org/DOI: 10.1109/CAMAD.2015.7390497

Arif, S., Khan, M. A., Rehman, S. U., Kabir, M. A., & Imran, M. (2020). Investigating Smart Home Security: Is Blockchain the Answer? *IEEE Access : Practical Innovations, Open Solutions*, *8*. Advance online publication. DOI: 10.1109/ACCESS.2020.3004662

Arjomand, A., Boudesh, A., Bayatmakou, F., Kent, K. B., & Mohammadi, A. (2024). TransfoRhythm: A transformer architecture conductive to blood pressure estimation via solo PPG signal capturing. arXiv. https://arxiv.org/abs/2401.00000

Asaithambi, S., Ravi, L., Kotb, H., Milyani, A. H., Azhari, A. A., Nallusamy, S., & Vairavasundaram, S. (2022). An energy-efficient and blockchain-integrated software defined network for the industrial Internet of Things. *Sensors (Basel)*, *22*(20), 7917. Advance online publication. DOI: 10.3390/s2220791 PMID: 36298266

Aslam, S., Aslam, S., Wang, T., Feng, D., & Zhang, S. (2025). A novel and secure machine learning-based Hyperledger blockchain for IoT healthcare. *IEEE Internet of Things Journal*, *12*(15), 31126–31140. DOI: 10.1109/JIOT.2025.3574471

Attarpour, A., Mahnam, A., Aminitabar, A., & Samani, H. (2019). Cuff-less continuous measurement of blood pressure using wrist and fingertip photoplethysmograms: Evaluation and feature analysis. *Biomedical Signal Processing and Control*, *49*, 212–220. DOI: 10.1016/j.bspc.2018.12.006

Aunugu, R., & Vathsavai, R. (2022). *Privacy-first artificial intelligence: Toward fair, transparent, and accountable systems*. International Journal of Scientific Advances., DOI: 10.51542/ijscia.v3i6.26

Awan, M. F., Bose, P., Khaleghi, A., Kansanen, K., & Balasingham, I. (2019). Evaluation of secrecy capacity for next-generation leadless cardiac pacemakers. *IEEE Transactions on Biomedical Engineering*, *67*(8), 2297–2308. PMID: 31831404

Awotunde, J. B., Misra, S., Ajagbe, S. A., Ayo, F. E., & Gurjar, R. (2023, May). An IoT machine learning model-based real-time diagnostic and monitoring system. In *Machine Intelligence Techniques for Data Analysis and Signal Processing: Proceedings of the 4th International Conference MISP 2022,* Volume 1 (pp. 789-799). Singapore: Springer Nature Singapore.

Azbeg, K., Ouchetto, O., & Jai Andaloussi, S. (2022). BlockMedCare: A healthcare system based on IoT, blockchain, and IPFS for data management security. *Egyptian Informatics Journal*, *23*(2), 329–343. DOI: 10.1016/j.eij.2022.03.001

Babu, S. B., & Jothi, K. R. (2024). A secure framework for privacy-preserving analytics in healthcare records using zero-knowledge proofs and blockchain in multi-tenant cloud environments. *IEEE Access : Practical Innovations, Open Solutions*, *12*, 109846–109864. DOI: 10.1109/ACCESS.2024.3433571

Barbone, A. S., Meftah, M., Markiewicz, K., & Dellimore, K. (2019). Beyond wearables and implantables: A scoping review of insertable medical devices. *Biomedical Physics & Engineering Express*, *5*(6), 062002. DOI: 10.1088/2057-1976/AB4B32

Barola, V. A., Singh, P., & Diwakar, M. (2024). Introduction to security risk assessment in medical and healthcare industry. In *Healthcare Industry Assessment: Analyzing Risks, Security, and Reliability* (pp. 1–24). Springer Nature Switzerland.

Barold, S. S., Stroobandt, R. X., & Sinnaeve, A. F. (2008). *Cardiac pacemakers step by step: An illustrated guide*. John Wiley & Sons.

Barua, A., Al Alamin, M. A., Hossain, M. S., & Hossain, E. (2022). Security and privacy threats for Bluetooth Low Energy in IoT and wearable devices: A comprehensive survey. *IEEE Open Journal of the Communications Society*, *3*, 251–281. DOI: 10.1109/OJCOMS.2022.3141912

Barua, A., Al Alamin, M. A., Hossain, M. S., & Hossain, E. (2022). Security and Privacy Threats for Bluetooth Low Energy in IoT and Wearable Devices: A Comprehensive Survey. *IEEE Open Journal of the Communications Society*, *3*, 251–281. DOI: 10.1109/OJCOMS.2022.3149732

Baucas, M. J., Spachos, P., & Plataniotis, K. N. (2023). Federated learning and blockchain-enabled fog-IoT platform for wearables in predictive healthcare. *IEEE Transactions on Computational Social Systems*, *10*(4), 1732–1741. DOI: 10.1109/TCSS.2022.3193138

Beck, C., Masny, D., Geiselmann, W., & Bretthauer, G. (2011). Block cipher based security for severely resource-constrained implantable medical devices. In *Proceedings of the 4th International Symposium on Applied Sciences in Biomedical and Communication Technologies*. ACM. https://doi.org/DOI: 10.1145/2093698.2093760

Benaissa, M., Chaabane, A., Attia, H., & Al-Naib, I. (2025). Innovations and challenges in RF antenna technologies for implantable medical devices communication. *IEEE Journal of Microwaves*, *5*(3), 526–542. DOI: 10.1109/JMW.2025.3555480

Ben-Menachem, E. (2012). Neurostimulation—Past, present, and beyond. *Epilepsy Currents*, *12*(5), 188–191. DOI: 10.5698/1535-7511-12.5.188 PMID: 23118604

Besirli, M.. (2023). An implantable wireless system for remote hemodynamic monitoring of heart failure patients. *IEEE Transactions on Biomedical Circuits and Systems*, *17*(4), 688–700. DOI: 10.1109/TBCAS.2023.3273711 PMID: 37155376

Bhalavat, D., Doshi, A., Keni, N., & Shah, P. R. (2024). *Automated compliance: A privacy-focused solution for GDPR and DPDPA adherence. 2024 13th International Conference on System Modeling & Advancement in Research Trends (SMART),* 831–837. https://doi.org/DOI: 10.1109/SMART63812.2024.10882514

Bhat, G., Tuncel, Y., An, S., & Ogras, U. Y. (2019). Wearable iot devices for health monitoring. *TechConnect Briefs*, *2019*, 357–360.

Bhushan, D., & Agrawal, R. (2019). Security challenges for designing wearable and iot solutions. *A Handbook of Internet of Things in Biomedical and Cyber Physical System*. https:// api. semanticscholar. org/ CorpusID: 199003121 C¸ elik, Y. S., I˙l¸ce, E., Mesut, B., & O¨ zsoy, Y. (2024). An overview of wearable medical device applications. *Journal of Research in Pharmacy, 28* (3), 722–732.

Biswas, S., Chakraborty, T., Mitra, S., Banerjee, S., Sarkar, T., & Paul, S. (2024). *IOT-Based Patient Monitoring System in Real Time*. Fog Computing for Intelligent Cloud IoT Systems.

Bollineni, C., Sharma, M., Hazra, A., Kumari, P., Manipriya, S., & Tomar, A. (2025). IoT for next-generation smart healthcare: A comprehensive survey. *IEEE Internet of Things Journal, 12*(16), 32616–32639. DOI: 10.1109/JIOT.2025.3570188

Boumezbeur, I., & Zarour, K. (2022). Privacy-preserving and access control for sharing electronic health record using blockchain technology. *Acta Informatica Pragensia, 11*(1), 105–122. DOI: 10.18267/j.aip.185

Boumpa, E., Tsoukas, V., Gkogkidis, A., Spathoulas, G., & Kakarountas, A. (2022). Security and Privacy Concerns for Healthcare Wearable Devices and Emerging Alternative Approaches. *Lecture Notes of the Institute for Computer Sciences, Social-Informatics and Telecommunications Engineering, LNICST, 440 LNICST*. https://doi.org/DOI: 10.1007/978-3-031-06368-8_2

Brönneke, J. B., Müller, J., Mouratis, K., Hagen, J., & Stern, A. D. (2021). Regulatory, legal, and market aspects of smart wearables for cardiac monitoring. *Sensors (Basel), 21*(14), 4937. PMID: 34300680

Butcher, C. J. T., & Hussain, W. (2022). Digital healthcare: The future. *Future Healthcare Journal, 9*(2), 113–117. DOI: 10.7861/futurehosp.9-2-113

Byeon, S., & Lee, W. (2023). Directed acyclic graphs for clinical research: A tutorial. *Journal of Minimally Invasive Surgery, 26*(3). Advance online publication. DOI: 10.7602/jmis.2023.26.3.97 PMID: 37712307

Camara, C., Peris-Lopez, P., & Tapiador, J. E. (2015). Security and privacy issues in implantable medical devices: A comprehensive survey. *Journal of Biomedical Informatics, 55*, 272–289. PMID: 25917056

Canali, S., Ferretti, A., Schiaffonati, V., & Blasimme, A. (2024). Wearable technologies for healthy ageing: Prospects, challenges, and ethical considerations. *The Journal of Frailty & Aging, 13*(2), 149–156. PMID: 38616371

Capulli, E., Druda, Y., Palmese, F., Butt, A. H., Domenicali, M., Macchiarelli, A. G., & Ingravallo, F. (2025). Ethical and legal implications of health monitoring wearable devices: A scoping review. *Social Science & Medicine*, •••, 117685. PMID: 40010231

Carminati, M., & Scandurra, G. (2021). Impact and trends in embedding field programmable gate arrays and microcontrollers in scientific instrumentation. *The Review of Scientific Instruments, 92*(9), 091101. Advance online publication. DOI: 10.1063/5.0056719 PMID: 34598486

Catuogno, L., & Galdi, C. (2024). Implantable medical device security. *Cryptography, 8*(4), 53. DOI: 10.3390/cryptography8040053

Chak, W. Y., Tang, W. F., Mak, S. L., Lee, C. C., Lam, S. K., & Li, C. H. (2023, November). A Critical Review on Hazard Analysis and Risk Assessment for Development of Wearable Medical Devices. In *2023 IEEE International Symposium on Product Compliance Engineering-Asia (ISPCE-ASIA)* (pp. 1-5). IEEE.

Chatterjee, P., Das, D., Banerjee, S., Ghosh, U., Mpembele, A. B., & Rogers, T. (2023). An approach towards the security management for sensitive medical data in the IoMT ecosystem. *Proceedings of the Twenty-fourth International Symposium on Theory, Algorithmic Foundations, and Protocol Design for Mobile Networks and Mobile Computing.* https://doi.org/DOI: 10.1145/3565287.3623388

Chen, C., Qin, C., Li, Y., Liu, C., & Ma, X. (2023). Cuff-less blood pressure prediction based on photoplethysmography and modified ResNet. *Bioengineering (Basel, Switzerland), 10*(4), 400. DOI: 10.3390/bioengineering10040400 PMID: 37106587

Chen, D., Chou, S.-Y., & Peng, X. (2025). Impacts of hospital data breach on healthcare quality. *Health Services Research.* Advance online publication. DOI: 10.1111/1475-6773.14439

Cheng, X., Xing, X., Li, W., Xue, H., & Can, T. (2025). An energy-efficient and privacy-aware MEC-enabled IoMT health monitoring system. *IEEE Transactions on Computers, 74*(9), 2936–2949. DOI: 10.1109/TC.2025.3576944

Chen, W., Rahman, M., & Ali, M. (2024). Deep learning and remote photoplethysmography for contactless physiological monitoring: A review. *Frontiers in Bioengineering and Biotechnology, 12*, 1420100. Advance online publication. DOI: 10.3389/fbioe.2024.1420100 PMID: 39104628

Chen, Y., Meng, L., Zhou, H., & Xue, G. (2021). A blockchain-based medical data sharing mechanism with attribute-based access control and privacy protection. *Wireless Communications and Mobile Computing, 2021*, 6685762. Advance online publication. DOI: 10.1155/2021/6685762

Cherukuri, S., Venkatasubramanian, K. K., & Gupta, S. K. S. (2003). BioSec: A biometric based approach for securing communication in wireless networks of biosensors implanted in the human body. In *2003 International Conference on Parallel Processing Workshops* (pp. 432–439). IEEE. https://doi.org/DOI: 10.1109/ICPPW.2003.1240399

Chinoy, E. D., Cuellar, J. A., Jameson, J. T., & Markwald, R. R. (2022). Performance of four commercial wearable sleep-tracking devices tested under unrestricted conditions at home in healthy young adults. *Nature and Science of Sleep*, •••, 493–516. PMID: 35345630

Chintoh, G. A., Segun-Falade, O. D., Odionu, C. S., & Ekeh, A. H. (2024). *Legal and ethical challenges in AI governance: A conceptual approach to developing ethical compliance models in the U.S. International Journal of Social Science Exceptional Research.* https://doi.org/DOI: 10.54660/ijsser.2024.3.1.103-109

Cho, Y., Basir, A., Lim, Y.-H., & Yoo, H. (2024). Influence of heterogeneous human body on midfield wireless power transfer for implantable heart devices. *IEEE Transactions on Microwave Theory and Techniques*, *72*(3), 2009–2018. DOI: 10.1109/TMTT.2023.3308628

Closson, A., Xu, Z., Kubiak, D., Jin, C., Gruslova, A., Nolen, D., & Zhang, J. X. J. (2023). All-electrospun piezoelectric energy harvesting for leadless pacemakers. *ACS Applied Electronic Materials*, *5*(11), 6236–6245. DOI: 10.1021/acsaelm.3c01152

Cook, J. ur Rehman, S., & Khan, M. A. (2023). Security and privacy for low power iot devices on 5g and beyond networks: Challenges and future directions. *IEEE Access, 11*, 39295–39317. https://api.semanticscholar. org/CorpusID:257913493

Cottle, K. E. (2017). *Current patterns of ownership and usage of mobile tech- nology in older adults*. Brigham Young University.

Cui, Z., & Song, Z. (2025). Enterprise Security Incident Analysis and Countermeasures Based on the T-Mobile Data Breach. arXiv preprint arXiv:2507.12937.

Curran, B. (2018). What is Proof of Authority Consensus? (PoA) Staking Your Identity. In *Block Onomi*.

Cyble. (2025). Critical vulnerabilities found in Contec patient monitors. Retrieved from https://cyble.com/blog/cyble-warns-risk-in-ics-vulnerability-report

Czekster, R. M., Webber, T., Furstenau, L. B., & Marcon, C. (2025). Dynamic risk assessment approach for analysing cyber security events in medical IoT networks. Internet of Things, 29, 101437. Bhol, S. G. (2025). Applications of multi criteria decision making methods in cyber security. Cyber-Physical Systems Security, 233-258.

Dagdeviren, C., Yang, B. D., Su, Y., Tran, P. L., Joe, P., Anderson, E., & Rogers, J. A. (2014). Conformal piezoelectric energy harvesting and storage from motions of the heart, lung, and diaphragm. *Nature Communications*, *5*(1), 4496. DOI: 10.1038/ncomms5496 PMID: 25092496

Dai, J., Xu, X., Chen, G., Lv, J., & Xiao, Y. (2025). Sleep-wake patterns of fencing athletes: A long-term wearable device study. *PeerJ*, *13*, e18812. Advance online publication. DOI: 10.7717/peerj.18812

Deep, S., Zheng, X., Jolfaei, A., Yu, D., Ostovari, P., & Bashir, A. K. (2022). A survey of security and privacy issues in the Internet of Things from the layered context. *Transactions on Emerging Telecommunications Technologies*, *33*(6), e3935. Advance online publication. DOI: 10.1002/ett.3935

Degada, A., & Thapliyal, H. (2021). Single-rail adiabatic logic for energy-efficient and CPA-resistant cryptographic circuit in low-frequency medical devices. *IEEE Open Journal of Nanotechnology*, *3*, 1–14.

Degada, A., & Thapliyal, H. (2022). 2-phase adiabatic logic for low-energy and CPA-resistant implantable medical devices. *IEEE Transactions on Consumer Electronics*, *68*(1), 47–56.

Degerli, M., & Ozkan Yildirim, S. (2022). Identifying critical success factors for wearable medical devices: A comprehensive exploration. *Universal Access in the Information Society*, *21*(1), 121–143.

Denning, T., Fu, K., & Kohno, T. (2008). Absence makes the heart grow fonder: New directions for implantable medical device security. In *HotSec*.

Denning, T., Borning, A., Friedman, B., Gill, B. T., Kohno, T., & Maisel, W. H. (2010). Patients, pacemakers, and implantable defibrillators: Human values and security for wireless implantable medical devices. In *Proceedings of the SIGCHI Conference on Human Factors in Computing Systems* (pp. 917–926). ACM.

Digitale, J. C., Martin, J. N., & Glymour, M. M. (2022). Tutorial on directed acyclic graphs. *Journal of Clinical Epidemiology*, *142*. Advance online publication. DOI: 10.1016/j.jclinepi.2021.08.001 PMID: 34371103

Dragusin, S. A., Bizon, N., & Bostinaru, R. N. (2024). Comprehensive Analysis of Cyber-Attack Techniques and Vulnerabilities in Communication Channels of Embedded Systems. *Proceedings of the 16th International Conference on Electronics, Computers and Artificial Intelligence, ECAI 2024*. https://doi.org/DOI: 10.1109/ECAI61503.2024.10607432

Dragusin, S. A., Bizon, N., Bostinaru, R. N., Enescu, F. M., Teodorescu, R. M., & Savulescu, C. (2024). Analysis of Vulnerabilities in Communication Channels Using An Integrated Approach Based on Machine Learning and Statistical Methods. *Proceedings of the 16th International Conference on Electronics, Computers and Artificial Intelligence, ECAI 2024*. https://doi.org/DOI: 10.1109/ECAI61503.2024.10607483

Dubey, P., Madankar, M., Dubey, P., & Hung, B. T. (Eds.). (2025). *The Impact of Algorithmic Technologies on Healthcare*. John Wiley & Sons.

Duggegowda, D., & Ramamoorthy, U. (2024). MedAccess HBPF: A privacy-preserving hybrid-blockchain framework for secure and efficient cloud-based electronic health record sharing. *SN Computer Science*, *5*(8), 1018. Advance online publication. DOI: 10.1007/s42979-024-03245-8

Dzamesi, L., & Elsayed, N. (2025). *A review on the security vulnerabilities of the IoMT against malware attacks and DDoS*. arXiv. https://arxiv.org/abs/2501.07432

Elgendi, M., Fletcher, R., & Liang, Y. (2024). Recommendations for evaluating photoplethysmography-based blood pressure estimation: Challenges and benchmarking. *Communications Medicine*, *4*, 00555. Advance online publication. DOI: 10.1038/s43856-024-00555-2 PMID: 38997447

El-Hajj, C., & Kyriacou, P. A. (2020). A review of machine learning techniques in photoplethysmography for the non-invasive cuff-less measurement of blood pressure. *Biomedical Signal Processing and Control*, *58*, 101870. DOI: 10.1016/j.bspc.2020.101870

El-Hajj, C., & Kyriacou, P. A. (2021). Cuffless blood pressure estimation from PPG signals and its derivatives using deep learning models. *Biomedical Signal Processing and Control*, *70*, 102984. DOI: 10.1016/j.bspc.2021.102984

Elhoseny, M., Ramírez-González, G., & Abu-Elnasr, O. (2021). Security and privacy issues in Medical Internet of Things: Overview, countermeasures, challenges and future directions. *Sustainability*, *13*(21), 11645. Advance online publication. DOI: 10.3390/su132111645

Elnawawy, M., Hallajiyan, M., Mitra, G., Iqbal, S., & Pattabiraman, K. (2024). *Systematically assessing the security risks of AI/ML-enabled connected healthcare systems*. arXiv. https://doi.org//arXiv.2401.17136DOI: 10.48550

Elymany, M. M., Enany, M. A., & Elsonbaty, N. A. (2024). Hybrid optimized-ANFIS based MPPT for hybrid microgrid using zebra optimization algorithm and artificial gorilla troops optimizer. *Energy Conversion and Management*, *299*, 117809.

Eren, H., Karaduman, Ö., & Gençoğlu, M. T. (2025). Security Challenges and Performance Trade-Offs in On-Chain and Off-Chain Blockchain Storage: A Comprehensive Review. *Applied Sciences 2025, Vol. 15, Page 3225*, *15*(6), 3225. https://doi.org/DOI: 10.3390/APP15063225

Erişen, S. (2022). IoT-based real-time updating multi-layered learning system for a special care context during COVID-19. *Cogent Engineering*, *9*(1), 2044588. Advance online publication. DOI: 10.1080/23311916.2022.2044588

Espinosa, A. L. (1998). Availability of health data: Requirements and solutions. *International Journal of Medical Informatics*, *49*(1), 97–104. DOI: 10.1016/S1386-5056(98)00016-1 PMID: 9723807

European Parliament and Council of the European Union. (2017). Regulation (EU) 2017/745 of the European Parliament and of the Council of 5 April 2017 on medical devices, amending directive 2001/83/EC, regulation (EC) no 178/2002 and regulation (EC) no 1223/2009 and repealing council directives 90/385/EEC and 93/42/EEC [Accessed: 2025-07-19].

European Union Agency for Cybersecurity. (2023). *ENISA threat landscape: Health sector*. https://www.enisa.europa.eu/publications/enisa-threat-landscape-health-sector

Fan, X., Wang, Q., & Sun, Y. (2024). Diagnosing People at Risk of Heart Diseases Using the Arduino Platform Under the IoT Platform. *International Journal of Advanced Computer Science and Applications*, *15*(7).

Farabolini, G., Baldini, N., Pagano, A., Andrenelli, E., Pepa, L., Morone, G., Ceravolo, M. G., & Capecci, M. (2025). Continuous movement moni- toring at home through wearable devices: A systematic review. *Sensors (Basel)*, *25*, 280949226. https://api.semanticscholar.org/CorpusID PMID: 40871752

Farooqi, S. A., Rahman, A. A., & Saad, A. (2024). *Differential privacy-based federated learning techniques in IoMT: A review. 2024 18th International Conference on Ubiquitous Information Management and Communication (IMCOM),* 1–7. https://doi.org/DOI: 10.1109/IMCOM60618.2024.10418361

Feretzakis, G., Papaspyridis, K., Gkoulalas-Divanis, A., & Verykios, V. (2024). Privacy-preserving techniques in generative AI and large language models: A narrative review. *Information (Basel)*. Advance online publication. DOI: 10.3390/info15110697

Fomanka, E. M. (2025). Cybersecurity Threats to Medical Devices: An Exploratory Study on Implications for Clinical Outcomes (Doctoral dissertation, Marymount University).

Food and Drug Administration. (2023). *Cybersecurity in medical devices: Quality system considerations and content of premarket submissions*. Guidance for industry and food and drug administration staff.

Franzen, C. (2013). Dick Cheney had the wireless disabled on his pacemaker to avoid risk of terrorist tampering. *The Verge*, 21.

Fu, K. (2009). Inside risks reducing risks of implantable medical devices. *Communications of the ACM*, *52*(6), 25–27.

Fusco, P., Rimoli, G. P., & Ficco, M. (2025). TinyML and Federated Learning for Resource-Constrained Medical Devices. In *Artificial Intelligence Techniques for Analysing Sensitive Data in Medical Cyber-Physical Systems: System Protection and Data Analysis* (pp. 113–126). Springer Nature Switzerland.

Gao, Z., Zhou, Y., Zhang, J., Foroughi, J., Peng, S., Baughman, R. H., & Wang, C. H. (2024). Advanced energy harvesters and energy storage for powering wearable and implantable medical devices. *Advanced Materials*, *36*(42), 2404492. PMID: 38935237

Ghosh, S., Chattopadhyay, B. P., Roy, R. M., Mukherjee, J., & Mahadevappa, M. (2022). Non-invasive cuffless blood pressure and heart rate monitoring using impedance cardiography. *Intelligent Medicine*, *2*, 100016. DOI: 10.1016/j.imed.2021.11.001

Ghosh, S., & Ghosh, S. (2023). FEEL: FEderated LEarning Framework for ELderly Healthcare Using Edge-IoMT. *IEEE Transactions on Computational Social Systems*, *10*, 1800–1809. DOI: 10.1109/TCSS.2022.3233300

Ghubaish, A., Samara, L., Çelik, A., & Al-Ali, A. (2023). *Recent advances in the Internet of Medical Things (IoMT) systems security*. arXiv. https://arxiv.org/abs/2302.04456

Gia, T. N., Dhaou, I. B., Ali, M., Rahmani, A. M., Westerlund, T., Liljeberg, P., & Tenhunen, H. (2019). Energy efficient fog-assisted IoT system for monitoring diabetic patients with cardiovascular disease. *Future Generation Computer Systems*, *93*, 198–211.

Global Market Insights. (2024). Wearable medical devices market report [Ac- cessed: 2025-07-18].

González, S., Hsieh, W.-T., & Chen, T.-P. (2023). A benchmark for machine-learning-based non-invasive blood pressure estimation using photoplethysmogram. *Scientific Data*, *10*, 149. Advance online publication. DOI: 10.1038/s41597-023-02020-6 PMID: 36944668

Gray, M., Meehan, J., Ward, C., Langdon, S. P., Kunkler, I. H., Murray, A., & Argyle, D. (2018). Implantable biosensors and their contribution to the future of precision medicine. *Veterinary Journal (London, England)*, *239*, 21–29. DOI: 10.1016/j.tvjl.2018.07.011 PMID: 30197105

Griggs, K. N., Ossipova, O., Kohlios, C. P., Baccarini, A. N., Howson, E. A., & Hayajneh, T. (2018). Healthcare blockchain system using smart contracts for secure automated remote patient monitoring. *Journal of Medical Systems*, *42*(12), 248. Advance online publication. DOI: 10.1007/s10916-018-0993-x PMID: 29876661

Guk, K., Han, G., Lim, J., Jeong, K., Kang, T., Lim, E.-K., & Jung, J. (2019). Evolution of wearable devices with real-time disease monitoring for per- sonalized healthcare. *Nanomaterials (Basel, Switzerland)*, *9*(6), 813. PMID: 31146479

Guk, K., Han, G., Lim, J., Jeong, K., Kang, T., Lim, E.-K., & Jung, J. (2019). Evolution of wearable devices with real-time disease monitoring for personalized healthcare. *Nanomaterials (Basel, Switzerland)*, *9*(6), 813. Advance online publication. DOI: 10.3390/nano9060813 PMID: 31146479

Haider, N., Gates, C., Sengupta, V., & Qian, S. (2019). Cybersecurity of medical devices: Past, present, and future. In *Deer's Treatment of Pain: An Illustrated Guide for Practitioners* (pp. 811–820). Springer International Publishing.

Halperin, D., Heydt-Benjamin, T. S., Fu, K., Kohno, T., & Maisel, W. H. (2008). Security and privacy for implantable medical devices. *IEEE Pervasive Computing*, *7*(1), 30–39. DOI: 10.1109/MPRV.2008.16

Halperin, D., Heydt-Benjamin, T. S., Ransford, B., Clark, S. S., Defend, B., Morgan, W., & Maisel, W. H. (2008). Pacemakers and implantable cardiac defibrillators: Software radio attacks and zero-power defenses. In *2008 IEEE Symposium on Security and Privacy* (pp. 129–142). IEEE. https://doi.org/DOI: 10.1109/SP.2008.31

Hanif, F., Waheed, U., Shams, R., & Shareef, A. (2023). GAHBT: Genetic-Based Hashing Algorithm for Managing and Validating Health Data Integrity in Blockchain Technology. *Blockchain in Healthcare Today*, *6*(2). Advance online publication. DOI: 10.30953/bhty.v6.244 PMID: 36798963

Harte, R., Laighin, G. Ó., & Quinlan, L. (2021). Validation, verification, and reliability. In *Digital Health* (pp. 101–118). Academic Press.

Hasan, R. (2022). Towards strengthening the security of healthcare devices using secure configuration provenance. In *2022 IEEE International Conference on Digital Health* (pp. 228–233). IEEE. https://doi.org/DOI: 10.1109/ICDH55609.2022.00043

Hassija, V., Chamola, V., Bajpai, B. C., & Zeadally, S. (2021). Security issues in implantable medical devices: Fact or fiction? *Sustainable Cities and Society*, *66*, 102552.

Healthcare, I. T. News. (2025). CISA warns of Medtronic cardiac device security vulnerability. Retrieved from https://www.healthcareitnews.com/news/cisa-warns-medtronic-cardiac-device-security-vulnerability

Hei, X., & Du, X. (2011). *Biometric-based two-level secure access control for implantable medical devices during emergencies. In 2011 Proceedings IEEE INFOCOM*. IEEE.

Hei, X., Du, X., Wu, J., & Hu, F. (2010). Defending resource depletion attacks on implantable medical devices. In *2010 IEEE Global Telecommunications Conference GLOBECOM 2010* (pp. 1–5). IEEE. https://doi.org/DOI: 10.1109/GLOCOM.2010.5685228

Hellsten, T., Karlsson, J., Shamsuzzaman, M., & Pulkkis, G. (2021). The potential of computer vision-based marker-less human motion analysis for rehabilitation. *Rehabilitation Process and Outcome*, *10*, 11795727211022330. Advance online publication. DOI: 10.1177/11795727211022330 PMID: 34987303

Hernández-álvarez, L., Bullón Pérez, J. J., Batista, F. K., & Queiruga-Dios, A. (2022). Security Threats and Cryptographic Protocols for Medical Wearables. *Mathematics*, *10*(6). Advance online publication. DOI: 10.3390/math10060886

Hewa, T., Ylianttila, M., & Liyanage, M. (2021). Survey on blockchain based smart contracts: Applications, opportunities and challenges. In *Journal of Network and Computer Applications* (Vol. 177). https://doi.org/DOI: 10.1016/j.jnca.2020.102857

Heydari, F., Ebrahim, M. P., Redoute, J.-M., Joe, K., Walker, K., & Yuce, M. R. (2019). A chest-based continuous cuffless blood pressure method: Estimation and evaluation using multiple body sensors. *Information Fusion*, *54*, 66–74. DOI: 10.1016/j.inffus.2019.07.001

Hora, A., & Kulkarni, P. (2024). Wearables and Cybersecurity: Navigating the Threat Landscape. *2nd International Conference on Sustainable Computing and Smart Systems, ICSCSS 2024 - Proceedings*, 563–567. https://doi.org/DOI: 10.1109/ICSCSS60660.2024.10625662

Hosseini-Khayat, S. (2011). A lightweight security protocol for ultra-low power ASIC implementation for wireless implantable medical devices. In *2011 5th International Symposium on Medical Information and Communication Technology* (pp. 6–9). IEEE. https://doi.org/DOI: 10.1109/ISMICT.2011.5759785

Hua, J., Zhang, X., & Li, P. (2024). Wearable cuffless blood pressure tracking: When will they get it right? *Journal of Human Hypertension*. Advance online publication. DOI: 10.1038/s41371-024-00932-3

Hudda, S., & Haribabu, K. (2025). A review on WSN based resource constrained smart IoT systems. *Discover Internet of Things*, *5*(1), 56.

Hughes, A., Shandhi, M. M. H., Master, H., Dunn, J., & Brittain, E. (2023). Wearable Devices in Cardiovascular Medicine. *Circulation Research*, *132*(5), 652–670. DOI: 10.1161/CIRCRESAHA.122.322389 PMID: 36862812

Hu, J.-R., Martin, G., Iyengar, S., Brady, T. M., Turkson-Ocran, R.-A. N., & Juraschek, S. P. (2023). Validating cuffless continuous blood pressure monitoring devices. *Cardiovascular Digital Health Journal*, *4*(2), 100121. DOI: 10.1016/j.cvdhj.2023.01.001 PMID: 36865583

Hundur, M., Spahić, L., Bećirović, F., Gurbeta Pokvić, L., & Badnjević, A. (2025). Advancement of post-market surveillance of medical devices leveraging artificial intelligence: ECG devices case study. *Technology and Health Care*, ●●●, 09287329241303727. PMID: 39973872

IEEE Standards Association. (2024). *IEEE/UL 2933-2024 Standard for clinical Internet of Things (IoT) data and device interoperability with TIPPSS*. https://standards.ieee.org

Inan, O. T., Migeotte, P.-F., & Park, K. S. (2015). Ballistocardiography and seismocardiography: A review of recent advances. *IEEE Journal of Biomedical and Health Informatics*, *19*(4), 1414–1427. DOI: 10.1109/JBHI.2014.2361732 PMID: 25312966

International Organization for Standardization. (2014). *Implants for surgery—Active implantable medical devices—Part 1: General requirements for safety, marking and information to be provided by the manufacturer (ISO 14708-1:2014).*

Iqbal, S. M. A., Mahgoub, I., Du, E., Leavitt, M. A., & Asghar, W. (2021). Advances in healthcare wearable devices. *Npj Flexible Electronics 2021 5:1*, *5*(1), 1–14. https://doi.org/DOI: 10.1038/s41528-021-00107-x

Iqbal, S. M., Mahgoub, I., Du, E., Leavitt, M. A., & Asghar, W. (2021). Advances in healthcare wearable devices. *NPJ Flexible Electronics*, *5*(1), 9.

Iqbal, T., Redon-Lurbe, P., Simpkin, A. J., Elahi, A., Ganly, S., Wijns, W., & Shahzad, A. (2021). A Sensitivity Analysis of Biophysiological Responses of Stress for Wearable Sensors in Connected Health. *IEEE Access : Practical Innovations, Open Solutions*, *9*. Advance online publication. DOI: 10.1109/ACCESS.2021.3082423

Ishizaka, S., Fujimoto, K., & Koike, M. (2021). Non-contact blood pressure measurement using Doppler radar based on waveform analysis by LSTM. In *IEEE International Conference on Communications (ICC 2021)*. IEEE. https://doi.org/DOI: 10.1109/ICC42927.2021.9500857

Jain, R. (2024). *Transparency in AI decision making: A survey of explainable AI methods and applications.* Advances in Robotic Technology., DOI: 10.23880/art-16000110

Jamil, F., Ahmad, S., Iqbal, N., & Kim, D. H. (2020). Towards a remote monitoring of patient vital signs based on IoT-based blockchain integrity management platforms in smart hospitals. *Sensors (Basel), 20*(8), 2195. Advance online publication. DOI: 10.3390/s20082195 PMID: 32294989

Jamil, F., Kahng, H. K., Kim, S., & Kim, D. H. (2021). Towards secure fitness framework based on IoT-enabled blockchain network integrated with machine learning algorithms. *Sensors (Basel), 21*(5), 1640. Advance online publication. DOI: 10.3390/s21051640 PMID: 33652773

Jayabalan, J., & Jeyanthi, N. (2022). Scalable blockchain model using off-chain IPFS storage for healthcare data security and privacy. *Journal of Parallel and Distributed Computing, 164*, 152–167. DOI: 10.1016/j.jpdc.2022.02.005

Jiang, H., Zhang, J., & Lan, D., Chao, Liou, S., Shahnasser, H., ... Roy, S. (2013). A low-frequency versatile wireless power transfer technology for biomedical implants. *IEEE Transactions on Biomedical Circuits and Systems, 7*(4), 526–535. PMID: 23893211

Jiang, Y., Xu, X., & Xiao, F. (2022). Attribute-based encryption with blockchain protection scheme for electronic health records. *IEEE Transactions on Network and Service Management, 19*(4), 3884–3895. DOI: 10.1109/TNSM.2022.3193664

Jin, H., Luo, Y., Li, P., & Mathew, J. (2019). A review of secure and privacy-preserving medical data sharing. *IEEE Access : Practical Innovations, Open Solutions, 7*, 61656–61669. DOI: 10.1109/ACCESS.2019.2915024

Jin, J., Ahn, G.-J., Hu, H., Covington, M. J., & Zhang, X. (2009). Patient-centric authorization framework for sharing electronic health records. In *Proceedings of the 14th ACM Symposium on Access Control Models and Technologies* (pp. 125–134). ACM. https://doi.org/DOI: 10.1145/1542207.1542228

Jmarchn. (2021). DBS [Image]. Creative Commons. Retrieved from https://upload.wikimedia.org/wikipedia/commons/3/3a/X-ray_of_deep_brain_stimulation_in_OCD%2C_L.png

Joung, J., Lee, H., & Kim, J. (2023). Continuous cuffless blood pressure monitoring using a novel system. *Scientific Reports, 13*, 35492. DOI: 10.1038/s41598-023-35492-y PMID: 37244974

Ju, N., & Lee, K.-H. (2021). Perceptions and resistance to accept smart clothing: Moderating effect of consumer innovativeness. *Applied Sciences (Basel, Switzerland)*, *11*(7), 3211.

K¨onig, J., Penaredondo, J., McCullagh, E., Bowen, J., & Hinze, A. (2023). Let's make it accessible: The challenges of working with low-cost com- mercially available wearable devices. *Proceedings of the 35th Australian Computer-Human Interaction Conference*. https://api.semanticscholar. org/CorpusID:269749381

Kadayat, Y., Sharma, S., Agarwal, P., & Mohan, S. (2024). Internet-of-Things Enabled Smart Health Monitoring System Using AutoAI: A Graphical Tool of IBM Watson Studio. In *Communication Technologies and Security Challenges in IoT: Present and Future* (pp. 427–445). Springer Nature Singapore.

Kaewkannate, K., & Kim, S. (2016). A comparison of wearable fitness devices. *BMC Public Health*, *16*, 1–16. PMID: 27220855

Kalil, A., & Pinsky, M. (2019). What are the clinical criteria for systematic inflammatory response syndrome (SIRS) in sepsis/septic shock.

Kamruzzaman, M. M., Yan, B., Sarker, M. N. I., Alruwaili, O., Wu, M., & Alrashdi, I. (2022). Blockchain and Fog Computing in IoT-Driven Healthcare Services for Smart Cities. *Journal of Healthcare Engineering*, *2022*. Advance online publication. DOI: 10.1155/2022/9957888 PMID: 35126961

Karaböce, B. (2023, September). Lessons Learned from External Audits in Medical Device Testing Laboratories: Best Practices and Recommendations for Quality Management. In *Mediterranean Conference on Medical and Biological Engineering and Computing* (pp. 65-73). Cham: Springer Nature Switzerland.

Katsuya, R., & Liu, X. (2025). Policy and management implications of firmware vulnerabilities in medical IoT devices: a multi-case analysis. *Journal of Science and Technology Policy Management*.

Kavitha, D., Chinnasamy, A., & Selvakumari, P. (2025). Intelligent decision-making framework for big data using enhanced honey badger-based adaptive hybrid deep learning network. *International Journal of Data Mining and Bioinformatics*, *29*(1-2), 193–222. DOI: 10.1504/IJDMB.2025.10060345

Kazmi, S. M. A., Khan, Z., Khan, A., Mazzara, M., & Khattak, A. M. (2024). Leveraging deep reinforcement learning and healthcare devices for active travelling in smart cities. *IEEE Transactions on Consumer Electronics*. Advance online publication. DOI: 10.1109/TCE.2024.3389668

Khader, M., Alian, M., Hraiz, R., & Almajali, S. (2017). Simplified AES algorithm for healthcare applications on Internet of Thing. In *2017 8th International Conference on Information Technology* (pp. 543–547). IEEE. https://doi.org/DOI: 10.1109/ICITECH.2017.8080056

Khallaf, F., El-Shafai, W., El-Rabaie, E. S. M., & Abd El-Samie, F. E. (2025). A Systematic Review of New Technologies for Cybersecurity Healthcare Applications: A Systematic and Comprehensive Study. *Transactions on Emerging Telecommunications Technologies*, *36*(7), e70183.

Khan, M. F., & Abaoud, M. (2023). Blockchain-integrated security for real-time patient monitoring in the Internet of Medical Things using federated learning. *IEEE Access : Practical Innovations, Open Solutions*, *11*, 117826–117850. DOI: 10.1109/ACCESS.2023.3326145

Khan, N., & Rudman, R. J. (2025). IoT medical device risks: Data security, privacy, confidentiality, and compliance with HIPAA and COBIT 2019. *South African Journal of Business Management*, *56*(1), 4796. Advance online publication. DOI: 10.4102/sajbm.v56i1.4796

Khin, N. A., Francis, G., Mulinde, J., Grandinetti, C., Skeete, R., Yu, B., & Vinter, S. (2020). Data integrity in global clinical trials: Discussions from joint US Food and Drug Administration and UK Medicines and Healthcare Products Regulatory Agency good clinical practice workshop. *Clinical Pharmacology and Therapeutics*, *108*(5), 949–963. DOI: 10.1002/cpt.1794 PMID: 31958142

Kilincer, I. F., Ertam, F., & Sengur, A. (2023). Automated detection of cybersecurity attacks in healthcare systems with recursive feature elimination and multilayer perceptron optimization. *Biocybernetics and Biomedical Engineering*, *43*(1), 30–41. DOI: 10.1016/j.bbe.2022.12.003

Kim, K., Kim, Y., Kim, Y. S., Kim, K. B., & Lee, S. H. (2024). New Web-Based Ventilator Monitoring System Consisting of Central and Remote Mobile Applications in Intensive Care Units. *Applied Sciences (Basel, Switzerland)*, *14*(15), 6842.

Kishor, M., & Chakraborty, C. (2022). Artificial intelligence and Internet of Things based healthcare 4.0 monitoring system. *Wireless Personal Communications*, *127*(2), 1615–1631. DOI: 10.1007/s11277-022-09838-1

Koparır, H. M., & Arslan, Ö. (2024). Cuffless blood pressure estimation from photoplethysmography using deep convolutional neural network and transfer learning. *Biomedical Signal Processing and Control*, *93*, 106194. DOI: 10.1016/j.bspc.2024.106194

Kumari, D., Parmar, A. S., Goyal, H. S., Mishra, K., & Panda, S. (2024). HealthRec-Chain: Patient-centric blockchain enabled IPFS for privacy-preserving, scalable health data. *Computer Networks*, *241*, 110223. Advance online publication. DOI: 10.1016/j.comnet.2024.110223

Kumar, S., Bharti, A. K., & Amin, R. (2021). Decentralized secure storage of medical records using blockchain and IPFS: A comparative analysis with future directions. *Security and Privacy*, *4*(5), e162. Advance online publication. DOI: 10.1002/spy2.162

Kuykendal, M. (2018). *Battery-powered medical devices: Their failure modes and mitigation strategies*. Exponent.

Lamkaddem, A., El Yousfi, A., González-Posadas, V., & Segovia-Vargas, D. (2024). Miniaturized dual band implantable antenna for implanted biomedical devices. *IEEE Access : Practical Innovations, Open Solutions*, *12*, 15026–15036. DOI: 10.1109/ACCESS.2024.3357488

Lamkaddem, A., El Yousfi, A., Huang, Y., González Posadas, V., & Segovia-Vargas, D. (2025). Miniaturized wireless power transfer system with a dual-band implantable antenna for multifunctional biomedical devices. *IEEE Sensors Journal*, *25*(16), 31473–31488. DOI: 10.1109/JSEN.2025.3587334

Lee, J., Bae, B., Kim, B., Lim, J., & Lee, B. (2024). A load-independent battery charging system for multiple wearable devices using conductive textile. *IEEE Transactions on Industrial Electronics*, *71*(11), 15211–15215. DOI: 10.1109/TIE.2024.3363752

Lewandowska, A., Rudzki, G., Lewandowski, T., Bartosiewicz, A., Próchnicki, M., Stryjkowska-Góra, A., Laskowska, B., Sierpińska, M., Rudzki, S., & Pavlov, S. (2025). Overweight and obesity among adolescents: Health-conscious behaviours, acceptance, and the health behaviours of their parents. *BMC Public Health*, *25*, 418. Advance online publication. DOI: 10.1186/s12889-025-18045-5

Li, Y. (2025). Research on the construction and optimization of network security protection system for small and medium-sized enterprises.

Li, C. T., Weng, C. Y., Lee, C. C., & Wang, C. C. (2015). A hash based remote user authentication and authenticated key agreement scheme for the integrated EPR information system. *Journal of Medical Systems*, *39*(11), 144. Advance online publication. DOI: 10.1007/s10916-015-0371-8 PMID: 26349803

Li, C., Wang, J., Wang, S., & Zhang, Y. (2024). A review of IoT applications in healthcare. *Neurocomputing*, *565*, 127017.

Li, H., & Bai, H. (2025). Network Security. In *Principle of Architecture, Protocol, and Algorithms for CoG-MIN* (pp. 229–341). Springer.

Li, J., Chen, Y., Chen, Y. L., Zhang, W., & Liu, Z. (2023). A smart energy IoT model based on the Itsuku PoW technology. *Results in Engineering, 18*. Advance online publication. DOI: 10.1016/j.rineng.2023.101147

Lingamgunta, S. (2025). *Cyber Security For Beginners*. Academic Guru Publishing House.

Lin, W., Wu, Z., Chen, J., Huang, J., & Jin, L. (2023). Scale-aware modulation meet transformer. In *Proceedings of the IEEE/CVF International Conference on Computer Vision* (pp. 6015-6026).

Liu, J., Li, X., Ye, L., Zhang, H., Du, X., & Guizani, M. (2018). BPDS: A blockchain based privacy-preserving data sharing for electronic medical records. In *2018 IEEE Global Communications Conference (GLOBECOM)* (pp. 1–6). IEEE. https://doi .org/DOI: 10.1109/GLOCOM.2018.8647939

Liu, L., Zhang, Y.-T., Wang, W., Chen, Y., & Ding, X. (2023). Causal inference-based cuffless blood pressure estimation: A pilot study. *Computers in Biology and Medicine, 159*, 106900. DOI: 10.1016/j.compbiomed.2023.106900 PMID: 37087777

Lu, L., Zhang, J., Xie, Y., Gao, F., Xu, S., Wu, X., & Ye, Z.. (2020). Wear-able health devices in health care: Narrative systematic review. *JMIR mHealth and uHealth, 8*(11), e18907. PMID: 33164904

Lutkevich, B. (2019). What is HIPAA (Health Insurance Portability and Accountability Act)? In *WhatIs.com.*

Ma, B., Hu, Y., Lu, P., & Liu, Y. (2023). Running city game optimizer: A game-based metaheuristic optimization algorithm for global optimization. *Journal of Computational Design and Engineering*, *10*(1), 65–107.

Mahajan, P., & Kaul, A. (2025). Enhanced cuffless blood pressure estimation using ECG and PPG signals: A hybrid approach with Windkessel, ARIMA, and LSTM. *Turkish Journal of Electrical Engineering and Computer Sciences*, *33*(3), 282–305. DOI: 10.55730/1300-0632.4127

Maier, E., Reimer, U., & Wickramasinghe, N. (2021). Digital healthcare services. *Electronic Markets*, *31*(4), 743–746. DOI: 10.1007/s12525-021-00502-y

Malanin, V. (2025). Comparative analysis of HTTPS/TLS implementations for healthcare web applications. *International Journal of Scientific and Engineering Research*, *13*(5), 61–68.

Mallela, V. S., Ilankumaran, V., & Rao, N. S. (2004). Trends in cardiac pacemaker batteries. *Indian Pacing and Electrophysiology Journal*, *4*(4), 201. PMID: 16943934

Manetti, S., Guidotti, E., Vola, F., & Vainieri, M. (2025). A systematic literature review of real-world evidence (RWE) on post-market assessment of medical devices. *Health Economics, Policy, and Law*, •••, 1–33. PMID: 39801351

Maniraj, S. P., Monisha, J., Amutha, R., Kavitha, R., Shriidhar, P. J., & Srinivasan, C. (2025). Agricultural water conservation through AI-enhanced solar IoT networks. In *Proceedings of the International Conference on Emerging Areas in Research and Studies (ICEARS 2025)*.

Marin, E. (2018). *Security and privacy of implantable medical devices* (Doctoral dissertation). University of Leuven. Retrieved from https://www.esat.kuleuven.be

Marin, E., Singelée, D., Yang, B., Volski, V., Vandenbosch, G. A. E., Nuttin, B., & Preneel, B. (2018). Securing wireless neurostimulators. In *Proceedings of the Eighth ACM Conference on Data and Application Security and Privacy* (pp. 287–298). ACM. https://doi.org/DOI: 10.1145/3176258.3176310

Martínez, A. L., Gil Pérez, M., & Ruiz-Martínez, A. (2023). A comprehensive model for securing sensitive patient data in a clinical scenario. *IEEE Access : Practical Innovations, Open Solutions*, *11*, 137083–137098. DOI: 10.1109/ACCESS.2023.3335122

Mejía-Granda, C. M., Fernández-Alemán, J. L., Carrillo-de-Gea, J. M., & García-Berná, J. A. (2024). Security vulnerabilities in healthcare: An analysis of medical devices and software. *Medical & Biological Engineering & Computing*, *62*(1), 257–273. PMID: 37789249

Menassa, M., Wilmont, I., Beigrezaei, S., Knobbe, A., Artola Arita, V., Bridge, L., Verschuren, W. M. M., Rennie, K. L., Franco, O. H., & van der Ouderaa, F. (2025). The future of healthy ageing: Wearables in public health, disease prevention and healthcare. *Maturitas. Article*, *108254*. Advance online publication. DOI: 10.1016/j.maturitas.2025.108254

Meng, Y., Huang, Z., Shen, G., & Ke, C. (2019). SDN-based security enforcement framework for data sharing systems of smart healthcare. *IEEE Transactions on Network and Service Management*, *17*(1), 308–318. DOI: 10.1109/TNSM.2019.2953489

Messinis, I., & Temenos, A. (2024). Enhancing Internet of Medical Things security with artificial intelligence: A comprehensive review. *Computers in Biology and Medicine*, *170*, 108036. DOI: 10.1016/j.compbiomed.2024.108036 PMID: 38295478

Miaz, M. H., & Ali, M. (2020). Integration of blockchain and IoT: An enhanced security perspective. *Annals of Emerging Technologies in Computing*, *4*(4). Advance online publication. DOI: 10.33166/AETiC.2020.04.006

Mills, A. J., Watson, R. T., Pitt, L., & Kietzmann, J. (2016). Wearing safe: Physical and informational security in the age of the wearable device. *Business Horizons*, *59*(6), 615–622. DOI: 10.1016/j.bushor.2016.08.003

Miraz, M. H., Excell, P. S., & Sobayel, K. (2021). Evaluation of green alternatives for blockchain proof-of-work (Pow) approach. In *Annals of Emerging Technologies in Computing* (Vol. 5, Issue 4). https://doi.org/DOI: 10.33166/AETIC.2021.04.005

Mohamadi, A., Ghahramani, H., Asghari, S. A., & Aminian, M. (2024). *Securing healthcare with deep learning: A CNN-based model for medical IoT threat detection*. arXiv. https://arxiv.org/abs/2410.19969

Mohammed, H. J. (2024). IoT-Based Low-Cost Smart Health Monitoring System using Raspberry Pi Pico W and Blynk Application. *Journal of Engineering*, *30*(07), 90–108.

More, S., Singla, J., Verma, S., Ghosh, U., Rodrigues, J. J. P. C., & Hosen, A. S. M. S. (2020). Security assured CNN-based model for reconstruction of medical images on the Internet of healthcare things. *IEEE Access : Practical Innovations, Open Solutions*, *8*, 126333–126346. DOI: 10.1109/ACCESS.2020.3006348

Motwani, A., Shukla, P. K., Pawar, M., Arya, M., & Jain, P. (2024). Deep-CNWO: A deep-chaotic nature whale optimization algorithm for early prediction of blood pressure disorder in smart healthcare settings. *Neural Computing & Applications*, ●●●, 1–20.

Mousavi, S. S., Firouzmand, M., Charmi, M., Hemmati, M., Moghadam, M., & Ghorbani, Y. (2019). Blood pressure estimation from appropriate and inappropriate PPG signals using a whole-based method. *Biomedical Signal Processing and Control*, *47*, 196–206. DOI: 10.1016/j.bspc.2018.08.022

Mukhopadhyay, M., Banerjee, S., & Das Mukhopadhyay, C. (2024). Internet of Medical Things and the Evolution of Healthcare 4.0: Exploring Recent Trends. Journal of Electronics, Electromedical Engineering, and Medical Informatics.

Mukkamala, R., Hahn, J.-O., & Inan, O. T. (2022). Important findings on cuffless blood pressure measurement: Standards and pitfalls. *Nature Reviews. Cardiology*, *19*, 1–18. https://www.ncbi.nlm.nih.gov/pmc/articles/PMC9931644/

Mulla, S. J., & Patel, M. (2025). Global Regulatory Perspectives on Sensor-Enabled and Biomaterial-Integrated Medical Devices: A Focus on India, Canada, and Australia. *Biomedical Materials & Devices*, ●●●, 1–22.

Munnangi, A.K., UdhayaKumar, S., Ravi, V., Sekaran, R. and Kannan, S. (2023). Survival study on deep learning techniques for IoT enabled smart healthcare system. *Health and Technology, 13*(2), 215–228. PMID: 36818549

Murray, T. L., Calhoun, M., & Philipsen, N. C. (2011). Privacy, confidentiality, HIPAA, and HITECH: Implications for the health care practitioner. *The Journal for Nurse Practitioners, 7*(9), 747–752. DOI: 10.1016/j.nurpra.2011.07.005

Nakayama, A., Ishii, N., Mantani, M., Samukawa, K., Tsuneta, R., Marukawa, M., Ohno, K., Yoshida, A., Hasegawa, E., Sakamoto, J., Hori, K., Takahashi, S., Komuro, K., Hiruma, T., Abe, R., Norimatsu, T., Shimbo, M., Tajima, M., Nagasaki, M., . . . Isobe, M. (2023). Remote Cardiac Rehabilitation With Wearable Devices. In *Korean Circulation Journal* (Vol. 53, Issue 11). https://doi.org/DOI: 10.4070/kcj.2023.0242

Namasudra, S., & Akkaya, K. (2023). Introduction to blockchain technology. In Namasudra, S. (Ed.), *Blockchain and its applications in Industry 4.0* (pp. 1–28). Springer Nature Singapore., DOI: 10.1007/978-981-99-2174-8_1

Nanda, S. K., Panda, S. K., & Dash, M. (2023). Medical supply chain integrated with blockchain and IoT to track the logistics of medical products. *Multimedia Tools and Applications, 82*(21). Advance online publication. DOI: 10.1007/s11042-023-14846-8 PMID: 37362711

National Institute of Standards and Technology. (2024). *Cybersecurity supply chain risk management practices for systems and organizations* (NIST Special Publication 800-161r1). U.S. Department of Commerce. https://doi.org/DOI: 10.6028/NIST.SP.800-161r1

Navya, V. B., Kumar, R., & Kamal, A. (2024). Artificial Intelligence and Internet of Things: Application in detecting and containing the spread of COVID-19. In *Diagnosis and Analysis of COVID-19 Using Artificial Intelligence and Machine Learning-based Techniques* (pp. 325-346). Academic Press.

Nawaz, M. W., Tahir, M. A., Mehmood, A., Rahman, M. M. U., Riaz, K., & Abbasi, Q. H. (2024). Cuff-less arterial blood pressure waveform synthesis from single-site PPG using transformer & frequency-domain learning. arXiv. https://arxiv.org/abs/2402.00000

Nemec Zlatolas, L., Welzer, T., & Lhotska, L. (2024). Data breaches in healthcare: Security mechanisms for attack mitigation. *Cluster Computing, 27*(7), 8639–8654. DOI: 10.1007/s10586-024-04401-8

Neri, M., Benevento, E., Stefanini, A., Aloini, D., Niccolini, F., Carducci, A., & Dini, G. (2025). Understanding information security awareness: Evidence from the public healthcare sector. *Information and Computer Security*, *33*(3), 309–319.

Nguyen, D. C., Pathirana, P. N., Ding, M., & Seneviratne, A. (2021). BEdgeHealth: A decentralized architecture for edge-based IoMT networks using blockchain. *IEEE Internet of Things Journal*, *8*(14), 11743–11757. DOI: 10.1109/JIOT.2021.3054970

Nguyen, R., Nguyen, H. T., Nguyen, D. C., Pathirana, P. N., & Hossain, M. A. (2021). Secure blockchain enabled cyber–physical systems in healthcare using deep belief network with ResNet model. *Journal of Parallel and Distributed Computing*, *153*, 150–160. DOI: 10.1016/j.jpdc.2021.03.013

Obianyo, C., Ezeamii, V. C., Idoko, B., Adeyinka, T., Ejembi, V. E., Idoko, J. E., Obioma, L. O., & Ugwu, O. J. (2024). The future of wearable health technology: From monitoring to preventive healthcare. *World Journal of Biology Pharmacy and Health Sciences*, *20*, 36–55.

Olawade, D. B., Aderinto, N., David-Olawade, A. C., Egbon, E., Adereni, T., Popoola, M. R., & Tiwari, R. (2025). Integrating AI-driven wearable devices and biometric data into stroke risk assessment: A review of opportunities and challenges. *Clinical Neurology and Neurosurgery*, *249*, 108689. PMID: 39675149

Pandimurugan, V., Balakiruthiga, B., Umamageswaran, J., Angayarkanni, S. A., Rajaram, V., & Chinnasamy, A. (2024). Preventing health records risk analysis with explainable AI. In *Proceedings of the 2nd International Conference on Self Sustainable Artificial Intelligence Systems (ICSSAS)* (pp. 308–312). IEEE. https://doi.org/DOI: 10.1109/ICSSAS64001.2024.10760785

Panescu, D. (2008). Emerging technologies [Wireless communication systems for implantable medical devices]. *IEEE Engineering in Medicine and Biology Magazine*, *27*(2), 96–101. DOI: 10.1109/EMB.2008.915488 PMID: 18463025

Pan, Z., Liao, S., Sun, W., Zhou, H., Lin, S., Chen, D., Jiang, S., Long, H., Fan, J., Deng, F., & Zhang, W. (2024). Screening and early warning system for chronic obstructive pulmonary disease with obstructive sleep apnoea based on the medical Internet of Things in three levels of healthcare: Protocol for a prospective, multicentre, observational cohort study. *BMJ Open*, *14*(2), e075257. PMID: 38418236

Park, E., & Lim, J. H. (2025). The impact of healthcare data breaches on patient hospital visit behavior. *International Journal of Research in Marketing*. Advance online publication. DOI: 10.1016/j.ijresmar.2025.01.003

Park, S., Kim, Y., Urgaonkar, B., Lee, J., & Seo, E. (2011). A comprehensive study of energy efficiency and performance of flash-based SSD. *Journal of Systems Architecture*, *57*(4), 354–365. DOI: 10.1016/j.sysarc.2011.01.005

Patel, Z., Velankar, Y., Trivedi, C., & Oza, P. (2023). Wireless implantable medical devices security and privacy: A survey. In *Smart Energy and Advancement in Power Technologies* (pp. 69–87). Springer.

Pawnikar, V., & Patel, M. (2025, February). Biosensors in wearable medical devices: Regulatory framework and compliance across US, EU, and Indian markets. In *Annales Pharmaceutiques Françaises*. Elsevier Masson.

Peckham, P. H., & Ackermann, D. M. (2018). Implantable neural stimulators. In Krames, E. S., Peckham, P. H., & Rezai, A. R. (Eds.), *Neuromodulation* (2nd ed., pp. 275–287). Academic Press., DOI: 10.1016/B978-0-12-805353-9.00021-8

Peddoju, S. K., & Pranavi, S. (2025). Secured Smart Devices for Medical 4.0 Technologies: Threats and Approaches. In Smart Devices for Medical 4.0 Technologies (pp. 1-17). CRC Press.

Phan, D. T., Phan, T. T. V., Huynh, T. C., Park, S., Choi, J., & Oh, J. (2022). Non-invasive, wearable multi-biosensors for continuous, long-term monitoring of blood pressure via Internet of Things applications. *Computers & Electrical Engineering*, *102*, 108187. DOI: 10.1016/j.compeleceng.2022.108187

Pirbhulal, S., Zhang, H., Wu, W., & Zhang, Y.-T. (2016). A comparative study of fuzzy vault based security methods for wireless body sensor networks. In *2016 10th International Conference on Sensing Technology* (pp. 1–6). IEEE. https://doi.org/DOI: 10.1109/ICSensT.2016.7796226

Pirbhulal, S., Wu, W., & Li, G. (2018). A biometric security model for wearable healthcare. In *2018 IEEE International Conference on Data Mining Workshops* (pp. 136–143). IEEE. https://doi.org/DOI: 10.1109/ICDMW.2018.00026

Poongodi, T., Krishnamurthi, R., Indrakumari, R., Suresh, P., & Balusamy, B. (2020). Wearable Devices and IoT. *Intelligent Systems Reference Library*, *165*, 245–273. DOI: 10.1007/978-3-030-23983-1_10

Pourbemany, J., Zhu, Y., & Bettati, R. (2023). A survey of wearable devices pairing based on biometric signals. *IEEE Access : Practical Innovations, Open Solutions*, *11*, 26070–26085. DOI: 10.1109/ACCESS.2023.3254499

Puri, J., & Gochhait, S. (2023). Data security in healthcare: Enhancing the safety of data with cybersecurity. In *Proceedings of the International Conference on Computing and Emerging Sciences (ICCES)* (pp. 1779–1783).

Qin, X., & Wang, Z. (2019). Nasnet: A neuron attention stage-by-stage net for single image deraining. arXiv preprint arXiv:1912.03151.

Rachakonda, L., Mohanty, S. P., Kougianos, E., & Sundaravadivel, P. (2021). SaYoPillow: Blockchain-integrated privacy-assured IoMT framework for stress management considering sleeping habits. *IEEE Transactions on Consumer Electronics*, *67*(1), 20–29. DOI: 10.1109/TCE.2021.3054862

Radanliev, P. (2025). Privacy, ethics, transparency, and accountability in AI systems for wearable devices. *Frontiers in Digital Health*, *7*, 1431246. PMID: 40599875

Rafiq, M.. (2025). A deep learning framework for healthy lifestyle monitoring and outdoor localization. *IEEE Access : Practical Innovations, Open Solutions*, *13*, 118695–118705. DOI: 10.1109/ACCESS.2025.3573439

Rahman, F., Titouna, C., & Nait-Abdesselam, F. (2024). Fundamentals of Blockchain and Smart Contracts. *Blockchain and Smart-Contract Technologies for Innovative Applications*, 3–37. https://doi.org/DOI: 10.1007/978-3-031-50028-2_1

Rahman, M. Z. U., Surekha, S., Satamraju, K. P., Mirza, S. S., & Lay-Ekuakille, A. (2021). A collateral sensor data sharing framework for decentralized healthcare systems. *IEEE Sensors Journal*, *21*(24), 27848–27857. DOI: 10.1109/JSEN.2021.3123456

Rajathi, V., Chinnasamy, A., & Selvakumari, P. (2024). DUTC Net: A novel deep ulcer tissue classification network with stage prediction and treatment plan recommendation. *Biomedical Signal Processing and Control*, *90*, 105855. Advance online publication. DOI: 10.1016/j.bspc.2024.105855

Raju, N., & Quazi, F. (2024). Blockchain applications in electronic health records (EHRs) [Preprint]. *SSRN*. https://doi.org/DOI: 10.2139/ssrn.5026829

Ramasubramanian, B., Sundarrajan, S., Rao, R. P., Reddy, M. V., Chellappan, V., & Ramakrishna, S. (2022). Novel low-carbon energy solutions for powering emerging wearables, smart textiles, and medical devices. *Energy & Environmental Science*, *15*(12), 4928–4981.

Rani, D., Kumar, R., & Chauhan, N. (2024). A secure framework for IoT-based healthcare using blockchain and IPFS. *Security and Privacy*, *7*(2), e348. Advance online publication. DOI: 10.1002/spy2.348

Rasmussen, K. B., Castelluccia, C., Heydt-Benjamin, T. S., & Capkun, S. (2009). Proximity-based access control for implantable medical devices. In *Proceedings of the 16th ACM Conference on Computer and Communications Security* (pp. 410–419). ACM. https://doi.org/DOI: 10.1145/1653662.1653712

Rathore, H., Mohamed, A., Al-Ali, A., Du, X., & Guizani, M. (2017, June 26–30). A review of security challenges, attacks and resolutions for wireless medical devices. In *2017 13th International Wireless Communications and Mobile Computing Conference (IWCMC)* (pp. 1495–1501). IEEE. https://doi.org/DOI: 10.1109/IWCMC.2017.7986505

Rathore, H., Fu, C., Mohamed, A., Al-Ali, A., Du, X., Guizani, M., & Yu, Z. (2020). Multi-layer security scheme for implantable medical devices. *Neural Computing & Applications*, *32*, 4347–4360.

Rathore, N., Kumari, A., Patel, M., Chudasama, A., Bhalani, D., Tanwar, S., & Alabdulatif, A. (2025). Synergy of AI and blockchain to secure electronic healthcare records. *Security and Privacy*, *8*(1), e463. Advance online publication. DOI: 10.1002/spy2.463

Rathore, S., Park, J. H., & Chang, H. (2021). Deep learning and blockchain-empowered security framework for intelligent 5G-enabled IoT. *IEEE Access : Practical Innovations, Open Solutions*, *9*, 90075–90091. DOI: 10.1109/ACCESS.2021.3091540

Ray, P. P., Chowhan, B., Kumar, N., & Almogren, A. (2021). BIoTHR: Electronic health record servicing scheme in IoT-blockchain ecosystem. *IEEE Internet of Things Journal*, *8*(13), 10857–10872. DOI: 10.1109/JIOT.2021.3058794

Reegu, F. A., Abas, H., Gulzar, Y., Xin, Q., Alwan, A. A., Jabbari, A., Sonkamble, R. G., & Dziyauddin, R. A. (2023). Blockchain-Based Framework for Interoperable Electronic Health Records for an Improved Healthcare System. *Sustainability (Switzerland)*, *15*(8). Advance online publication. DOI: 10.3390/su15086337

Regalado, P. H., & Han, T. (2025). MediVerse: A secure and scalable IoT-MR framework for real-time health and performance monitoring. *IEEE Access : Practical Innovations, Open Solutions*, *13*, 97511–97528. DOI: 10.1109/ACCESS.2025.3570731

Rehman, A. U., Lu, S., Bin Heyat, M. B., Iqbal, M. S., Parveen, S., Bin Hayat, M. A., & Sawan, M. (2025). Internet of Things in Healthcare Research: Trends, Innovations, Security Considerations, Challenges and Future Strategy. *International Journal of Intelligent Systems*, *2025*(1), 8546245. https://doi.org/10.xxxx/ijis.8546245

Rostami, M., Burleson, W., Koushanfar, F., & Juels, A. (2013). Balancing security and utility in medical devices? In *Proceedings of the 50th Annual Design Automation Conference* (pp. 1–6). ACM.

Rostami, M., Juels, A., & Koushanfar, F. (2013). Heart-to-heart (H2H): Authentication for implanted medical devices. In *Proceedings of the 2013 ACM SIGSAC Conference on Computer & Communications Security* (pp. 1099–1112). ACM. https://doi.org/DOI: 10.1145/2508859.2516658

Roy, C. K., & Sadiwala, R. (2024). Smart environment for IoT based disease diagnosis healthcare framework. *Journal of Integrated Science and Technology*, *12*(2), 731–731.

Saad, H. S., Zaki, J. F. W., & Abdelsalam, M. M. (2024). Employing of ma- chine learning and wearable devices in healthcare system: Tasks and challenges. *Neural Computing & Applications*, *36*, 17829–17849. https: //api.semanticscholar.org/CorpusID:271752210

Saad, H. S., Zaki, J. F., & Abdelsalam, M. M. (2024). Employing of machine learning and wearable devices in healthcare system: Tasks and challenges. *Neural Computing & Applications*, *36*(29), 17829–17849.

Sabry, F., Eltaras, T., Labda, W., Alzoubi, K., & Malluhi, Q. (2022). Machine Learning for Healthcare Wearable Devices: The Big Picture. *Journal of Healthcare Engineering*, *2022*(1), 4653923. DOI: 10.1155/2022/4653923 PMID: 35480146

Said, A., Yahyaoui, A., & Abdellatif, T. (2023). HIPAA and GDPR compliance in IoT healthcare systems. In *Proceedings of the International Conference on Advances in Information Technology*. https://doi.org/DOI: 10.1007/978-3-031-55729-3_16

Salunkhe, V., Tangudu, A., Mokkapati, C., Goel, P., & Aggarwal, A. (2024). Advanced encryption techniques in healthcare IoT: Securing patient data in connected medical devices. *Modern Dynamics: Mathematical Progressions*, *1*(2), 224–247. DOI: 10.36676/mdmp.v1.i2.22

Samimi, H., & Dajani, H. R. (2023). A PPG-based calibration-free cuffless blood pressure estimation method using cardiovascular dynamics. *Sensors (Basel)*, *23*(8), 4145. DOI: 10.3390/s23084145 PMID: 37112490

Sandhiya, D. S., Karthikeyan, M. V., & Shanmuga Priya, M. (2022). Secured health monitoring system using AES. *East Asian Journal of Multidisciplinary Research*, *1*(6). Advance online publication. DOI: 10.55927/eajmr.v1i6.577

Sasikumar, A., Ravi, L., Devarajan, M., Selvalakshmi, A., Almaktoom, A. T., Almazyad, A. S., & Mohamed, A. W. (2024). Blockchain-assisted hierarchical attribute-based encryption scheme for secure information sharing in industrial Internet of Things. *IEEE Access : Practical Innovations, Open Solutions*, *12*, 12586–12601. DOI: 10.1109/ACCESS.2024.3356789

Sasikumar, A., Ravi, L., Devarajan, M., Vairavasundaram, S., Selvalakshmi, A., Kotecha, K., & Abraham, A. (2023). A decentralized resource allocation in edge computing for secure IoT environments. *IEEE Access : Practical Innovations, Open Solutions, 11*, 117177–117189. DOI: 10.1109/ACCESS.2023.3324732

Senevirathna, N., & Kleihorst, R. (2024). 13 reasons why: Rationale and preliminary statistical approach for classifying electromagnetic disturbances in healthcare environments. In *IEEE Joint International Symposium on EMC Italy/APEMC* (pp. 100–103). IEEE.

Seyyedabbasi, A., & Kiani, F. (2023). Sand Cat swarm optimization: A nature-inspired algorithm to solve global optimization problems. *Engineering with Computers, 39*(4), 2627–2651.

Shahzadi, R., Anwar, S. M., Qamar, F., Ali, M., & Rodrigues, J. J. P. C. (2019). Chaos based enhanced RC5 algorithm for security and integrity of clinical images in remote health monitoring. *IEEE Access : Practical Innovations, Open Solutions, 7*, 52858–52870. DOI: 10.1109/ACCESS.2019.2909554

Shajari, S., Kuruvinashetti, K., Komeili, A., & Sundararaj, U. (2023). The emergence of AI-based wearable sensors for digital health technology: A review. *Sensors (Basel), 23*(23), 9498. PMID: 38067871

Shang, X. (2024). The current status and future trends of wearable devices. *Applied and Computational Engineering*. https://api.semanticscholar. org/CorpusID:275091019

Sharma, A. (2025). Securing the Future of Healthcare: Ensuring Privacy and Security in Wearable and Implantable Medical Devices. In *Security, Privacy, and Trust in WBANs and E-Healthcare* (pp. 105-125). CRC Press.

Sharma, R., & Yadav, P. (2024). *Privacy-preserving techniques in AI-based healthcare: A comprehensive review. 2024 IEEE 11th Uttar Pradesh Section International Conference on Electrical, Electronics and Computer Engineering (UPCON),* 1–6. https://doi.org/DOI: 10.1109/UPCON62832.2024.10983387

Sharma, A., Sharma, A., & Malhotra, R. (2023). IoT-based monitoring system for diagnosing adverse drug reactions and enhancing drug compliance in TB patients. *Computer Assisted Methods in Engineering and Science, 30*(2), 187–201.

Sharma, R., & Kshetri, N. (2020). Digital healthcare: Historical development, applications, and future research directions. *International Journal of Information Management, 53,* 102105. Advance online publication. DOI: 10.1016/j.ijinfomgt.2020.102105

Shibi, B., & Ravikumar, S. (2025). Hybrid capsule_CNN for depression detection based sentiment classification using review data. *Biomedical Signal Processing and Control*, *109*, 108013.

Shi, Z., Du, X., Wang, D., Paek, S. C., Kitcharoen, P., Li, J., & Marohabutr, T. (2025). Social capital and health consciousness based on regional differences in China: A cross-sectional study. *Frontiers in Public Health*, *13*, 1598121. Advance online publication. DOI: 10.3389/fpubh.2025.1598121

Shonubi, J. A., & Adelere, M. A. (2024). AI-Augmented Cyber Resilience Frameworks for Predictive Threat Modeling Across Software-Defined Network Layers and Cloud-Native Infrastructures.

shujie Qu & Gao, X. (2020). Analysis of ethical issues involved in wearable equipment for health care. *2020 International Conference on Public Health and Data Science (ICPHDS)*, 406–410. https:// api. semanticscholar. org/CorpusID:232072501

Shuvo, M. M. H., Titirsha, T., Amin, N., & Islam, S. K. (2022). Energy harvesting in implantable and wearable medical devices for enduring precision healthcare. *Energies*, *15*(20), 7495.

Si-Ahmed, A.. (2023). Survey of machine learning-based intrusion detection methods for Internet of Medical Things. *Applied Soft Computing*, *140*, 110227. DOI: 10.1016/j.asoc.2023.110227

Siam, M. K., Saha, B., Hasan, M. M., Hossain Faruk, M. J., Anjum, N., Tahora, S., & Shahriar, H. (2025). Securing Decentralized Ecosystems: A Comprehensive Systematic Review of Blockchain Vulnerabilities, Attacks, and Countermeasures and Mitigation Strategies. *Future Internet*, *17*(4).

Siddiqi, M. A., & Strydis, C. (2019). Towards realistic battery-DoS protection of implantable medical devices. In *Proceedings of the 16th ACM International Conference on Computing Frontiers*. ACM. https://doi.org/DOI: 10.1145/3310273.3321555

Siddiqi, M., Beurskens, R., Kruizinga, P., Zeeuw, C., & Strydis, C. (2021). Securing implantable medical devices using ultrasound waves. *IEEE Access : Practical Innovations, Open Solutions*, *9*, 80170–80182. DOI: 10.1109/access.2021.3083576

Sifaoui, A., & Eastin, M. S. (2024). "Whispers from the wrist": wearable health monitoring devices and privacy regulations in the US: the loopholes, the challenges, and the opportunities. *Cryptography*, *8*(2), 26.

Sikarwar, S. S. (2025). Computation Intelligence Techniques for Security in IoT Devices. *International Journal on Computational Modelling Applications*, *2*(1), 15–27.

Silva-Trujillo, A. G., González González, M. J., Rocha Pérez, L. P., & García Villalba, L. J. (2023). Cybersecurity analysis of wearable devices: Smartwatches passive attack. *Sensors (Basel), 23*(5438). Advance online publication. DOI: 10.3390/s23125438 PMID: 37420605

Silvestri, S., Islam, S., Papangelou, P., & Sookhak, M. (2023). Cyber threat assessment and management for securing healthcare ecosystems using natural language processing. *International Journal of Information Security, 22*(6), 1883–1899. DOI: 10.1007/s10207-023-00735-6

Singh, A. B., Khandelwal, C., & Dangayach, G. S. (2024). Revolutionizing healthcare materials: Innovations in processing, advancements, and challenges for enhanced medical device integration and performance. *Journal of Micromanufacturing*, 25165984241256234.

Singh, A. K., & Kumar, S. (Eds.). (2024). *Security, Privacy, and Trust in WBANs and E-Healthcare*. CRC Press.

Singla, D., Kumar, S., Gulzar, Y., Mir, M. S., Gupta, D., Jaziri, W., Sassi, N., & Arora, S. (2024). Designing and implementing a resilient immutability mechanism for enhanced supply chain management in e-healthcare systems. *Frontiers in Sustainable Cities, 6*, 1403809. Advance online publication. DOI: 10.3389/frsc.2024.1403809

Skh Saad, S. M., & Raja Mohd Radzi, R. Z. (2020). Comparative Review of the Blockchain Consensus Algorithm Between Proof of Stake (POS) and Delegated Proof of Stake (DPOS). *International Journal of Innovative Computing, 10*(2). Advance online publication. DOI: 10.11113/ijic.v10n2.272

Smogavc Cestar, A., & Harer, J. (2023). Mastering Quality System Audits and Inspections for Medical Devices. In *Medical Devices and In Vitro Diagnostics: Requirements in Europe* (pp. 543–584). Springer International Publishing.

Song, Y., Liu, J., Yan, S., Ma, M., Silver Tarimo, C., Chen, Y., Lai, Y., Guo, X., Wu, J., & Ye, B. (2025). Factors influencing health service utilization among 19,869 China's migrant population: An empirical study based on the Andersen behavioral model. *Frontiers in Public Health, 13*, 1456839. Advance online publication. DOI: 10.3389/fpubh.2025.1456839

Spuskanyuk, A. (2024). Ethical implications of wearable digital health tech- nology: Balancing innovation and patient autonomy. *American Journal of Healthcare Strategy*. https: / / api . semanticscholar . org / CorpusID: 274972514

Sreenivasu, S. V. N., Srinidhi, N. N., Chabra, A., Patil, S., Pujari, R., & Kaur, H. 2023, May. An IoT-Based Smart System to Monitor the ECG Continuously and Alert the Medical Practitioner in Case of Emergencies. In *2023 International Conference on Advances in Computing, Communication and Applied Informatics (ACCAI)* (pp. 1-7). IEEE.

Sreerangapuri, A. (2024). *Post-quantum cryptography for AI-driven cloud security solutions.* International Journal for Multidisciplinary Research., DOI: 10.36948/ijfmr.2024.v06i05.29032

Srivastava, S. K., Maakar, S. K., Singh, H. R., Srivastava, D., & Kantha, P. (2023). Supervision of Worldwide Healthcare through an IoT-Based System. In *Intelligent Internet of Things for Smart Healthcare Systems* (pp. 113–131). CRC Press.

Straits Research. (2024). Wearable healthcare devices market report [Accessed: 2025-07-18].

Sultana, S., Hriday, M. S. H., Haque, R., & Das, M. (2025). (in press). Health monitoring through wearables: A systematic review of innovations in cardiovascular disease detection and prevention. *Strategic Data Management & Innovation.*

Sun, S., Folarin, A. A., Ranjan, Y., Rashid, Z., Conde, P., & Stewart, C.RADAR-CNS Consortium. (2020). Using smartphones and wearable devices to monitor behavioral changes during COVID-19. *Journal of Medical Internet Research, 22*(9), e19992. Advance online publication. DOI: 10.2196/19992 PMID: 32877352

Su, R., Huang, X., Chen, R., & Guo, X. (2024). Spatial and social inequality of hierarchical healthcare accessibility in urban system: A case study in Shanghai, China. *Sustainable Cities and Society, 109*, 105540. Advance online publication. DOI: 10.1016/j.scs.2024.105540

Talati, D. V. (2025). *Quantum AI and the future of super intelligent computing. Journal of Artificial Intelligence General Science.* JAIGS., DOI: 10.60087/jaigs.v8i1.329

Tang, Z., Tang, Z., Liu, Y., Tang, Z., & Liao, Y. (2024). Smart healthcare systems: A new IoT-Fog based disease diagnosis framework for smart healthcare projects. *Ain Shams Engineering Journal*, •••, 102941.

Tan, M., Xu, Y., Gao, Z., Yuan, T., Liu, Q., Yang, R., & Peng, L. (2022). Recent advances in intelligent wearable medical devices integrating biosensing and drug delivery. *Advanced Materials, 34*(27), 2108491. PMID: 35008128

Tanveer, M., Ahmad, M., Nguyen, T. N., & Abd El-Latif, A. A. (2022). Resource-efficient authenticated data sharing mechanism for smart wearable systems. *IEEE Transactions on Network Science and Engineering, 10*(5), 2525–2536. DOI: 10.1109/TNSE.2022.3216837

Tanwar, S., Parekh, K., & Evans, R. (2020). Blockchain-based electronic healthcare record system for healthcare 4.0 applications. *Journal of Information Security and Applications, 50.* Advance online publication. DOI: 10.1016/j.jisa.2019.102407

Tariq, M. U. (2024). Introduction to cyber-physical systems 2.0. Cyber Physical System 2.0: Communication and Computational Technologies, 1.

Tariq, M. U. (2025). Challenges and solutions of Internet of Things security in the age of connectivity. In *Human-Centric Integration of 6G-Enabled Technologies for Modern Society* (pp. 327–344). Academic Press.

Tekchandani, P., Pradhan, I., Das, A. K., Kumar, N., & Park, Y. (2023). Blockchain-Enabled Secure Big Data Analytics for Internet of Things Smart Applications. *IEEE Internet of Things Journal, 10*(7). Advance online publication. DOI: 10.1109/JIOT.2022.3227162

Telaprolu, B. S. (2024). *Privacy-preserving federated learning in healthcare – A secure AI framework.* International Journal of Scientific Research in Computer Science, Engineering and Information Technology., DOI: 10.32628/cseit2410347

Templ, M., & Sariyar, M. (2022). A systematic overview of methods to protect sensitive data provided for various analyses. *International Journal of Information Security, 21*(6), 1233–1246. DOI: 10.1007/s10207-022-00887-5

Teng, X.-F., Zhang, Y.-T., Poon, C. C. Y., & Bonato, P. (2008). Wearable medical systems for p-health. *IEEE Reviews in Biomedical Engineering, 1*, 62–74. DOI: 10.1109/RBME.2008.2008248 PMID: 22274900

Tettey, F., Parupelli, S. K., & Desai, S. (2024). A review of biomedical devices: Classification, regulatory guidelines, human factors, software as a medical device, and cybersecurity. *Biomedical Materials & Devices, 2*(1), 316–341.

Thapa, S., Bello, A., Maurushat, A., & Farid, F. (2023). Security risks and user perception towards adopting wearable internet of medical things. *International Journal of Environmental Research and Public Health, 20*(8), 5519. PMID: 37107800

The Patient Safety Documentation. (2019). *Medical devices—Application of risk management to medical devices.*

Thirunavukkarasu, J., & Chinnasamy, A. (2024). Enhancing the preciseness of prediction in heart disease diagnosis by utilizing machine learning. In 2024 *International Conference on Advances in Computing, Communication and Applied Informatics (ACCAI)* (pp. 1–9). IEEE. https://doi.org/DOI: 10.1109/ACCAI61015.2024.10587654

Tiwari, K., & Kumar, S. (2025). Accelerating healthcare data access: A blockchain and decentralized indexing approach. *Concurrency and Computation*, *37*(15–17), e70172. Advance online publication. DOI: 10.1002/cpe.70172

Truong, N. B., Sun, K., Lee, G. M., & Guo, Y. (2020). GDPR-Compliant Personal Data Management: A Blockchain-Based Solution. *IEEE Transactions on Information Forensics and Security*, *15*. Advance online publication. DOI: 10.1109/TIFS.2019.2948287

U.S. Food and Drug Administration. (2025, January). [U.S. Department of Health and Human Services. Retrieved July 19, 2025]. *Medical Devices (Auckland, N.Z.)*.

Umer, M., Aljrees, T., Karamti, H., Ishaq, A., Alsubai, S., Omar, M., Bashir, A. K., & Ashraf, I. (2023). Heart failure patients monitoring using IoT-based remote monitoring system. *Scientific Reports*, *13*(1), 19213. PMID: 37932424

Upadhyay, V., Vaish, A., & Kokila, J. (2024). The need for Lightweight Consensus algorithms in IoT environment: A review. *ACM International Conference Proceeding Series*, 366–376. https://doi.org/DOI: 10.1145/3675888.3676072

Ushimaru, Y., Katoh, T., Sasaki, M., Hata, T., Hosaka, M., Eguchi, H., & Nakajima, K. (2025). Development of medical devices driven by academia-industry collaboration: An internal audit. *Surgery*, *181*, 109289. PMID: 40054052

Vakhter, V., Soysal, B., Schaumont, P., & Guler, U. (2022). Threat modeling and risk analysis for miniaturized wireless biomedical devices. *IEEE Internet of Things Journal*, *9*(15), 13338–13352.

Venkatachalam, S., Padmavathi, T., Vinodh, N., Thilagavathi, J., Joshi, G., Ramachandran, G., & Rajasekaran, B. (2023). Analysis of ethical is- sues associated with wearable medical devices. *2023 5th International Conference on Smart Systems and Inventive Technology (ICSSIT)*, 17– 22.

Verma, A., Gupta, A. K., Kumar, V., & Rajak, A. (2024, July). Secure remote health monitoring: Overall analysis on timely prognosis of disease in primal phase and impart medical assistance using cloud IoT and data mining techniques. In *AIP Conference Proceedings* (Vol. 3168, No. 1). AIP Publishing.

Verma, G. (2024). Blockchain-based privacy preservation framework for healthcare data in cloud environment. *Journal of Experimental & Theoretical Artificial Intelligence, 36*(1), 147–160. DOI: 10.1080/0952813X.2023.2270649

Verma, P., & Ram, B. (2024). Application of blockchain technology in data security. *IP Indian Journal of Library Science and Information Technology, 9*(1), 51–55. DOI: 10.18231/j.ijlsit.2024.009

Vijay, P., Jayashree, K., Babu, R., & Vijay, K. (2024). Deep Learning-Based Chatbots for Patient Queries. In Handbook of AI-Based Models in Healthcare and Medicine (pp. 420-436). CRC Press.

Vijayan, V., Connolly, J., Condell, J., McKelvey, N., & Gardiner, P. (2021). Review of wearable devices and data collection considerations for connected health. In *Sensors* (Vol. 21, Issue 16). https://doi.org/DOI: 10.3390/s21165589

Vimalachandran, P., Wang, H., Zhang, Y., Heyward, B., & Whittaker, F. (2016). Ensuring data integrity in electronic health records: A quality health care implication. In *2016 International Conference on Orange Technologies* (pp. 20–27). IEEE. https://doi.org/DOI: 10.1109/ICOT.2016.8278970

Vineetha Harish, A. (2025). Automated Vulnerability Scanning and Security Audit Framework for Maritime Systems.

Vyas, A., Abimannan, S., & Hwang, R.-H. (2021). Sensitive healthcare data: Privacy and security issues and proposed solutions. In Kanagachidambaresan, G. R., Maheswar, R., Manikandan, V., & Ramakrishnan, K. (Eds.), *Emerging technologies for healthcare: Internet of Things and deep learning models* (pp. 93–127). Wiley., DOI: 10.1002/9781119792338.ch5

Wang, R., Xiao, B., & Xiang, X. (2024, March). An Improved Humboldt Squid Optimization Algorithm Based on Genetic Mutation. In 2024 IEEE 7th Advanced Information Technology, Electronic and Automation Control Conference (IAEAC) (Vol. 7, pp. 573-581). IEEE.

Wang, S., Wei, L., Wang, F., Wang, L., & Mao, J. (2025). Advanced implantable energy storage for powering medical devices. *eScience*, 100409. https://doi.org/DOI: 10.1016/j.esci.2025.100409

Wang, L., Jiang, K., & Shen, G. (2021). Wearable, implantable, and interventional medical devices based on smart electronic skins. *Advanced Materials Technologies, 6*(6), 2100107.

Wang, Y., Zhang, A., Zhang, P., & Wang, H. (2019). Cloud-assisted EHR sharing with security and privacy preservation via consortium blockchain. *IEEE Access : Practical Innovations, Open Solutions*, *7*, 136704–136719. DOI: 10.1109/ACCESS.2019.2943154

Wazid, M., Das, A. K., Kumar, N., Conti, M., & Vasilakos, A. V. (2018). A novel authentication and key agreement scheme for implantable medical devices deployment. *IEEE Journal of Biomedical and Health Informatics*, *22*(4), 1299–1309. DOI: 10.1109/JBHI.2017.2721545 PMID: 28682267

Wu, L., Du, X., Guizani, M., & Mohamed, A. (2017). Access control schemes for implantable medical devices: A survey. *IEEE Internet of Things Journal*, *4*(5), 1272–1283.

Wu, X., Zhou, W., Fei, M., Du, Y., & Zhou, H. (2024). Banyan tree growth optimization and application. *Cluster Computing*, *27*(1), 411–441.

Xie, Y., Lu, L., Gao, F., He, S. J., Zhao, H. J., Fang, Y., & Dong, Z. (2021). Integration of artificial intelligence, blockchain, and wearable technology for chronic disease management: A new paradigm in smart healthcare. *Current Medical Science*, *41*(6), 1123–1133. DOI: 10.1007/s11596-021-2487-8 PMID: 34950987

Xing, X., Li, H., Chen, Q., Jiang, C., & Dong, W.-F. (2024). Blood pressure monitoring with piezoelectric bed sensor systems. *Biomedical Signal Processing and Control*, *87*, 105479. DOI: 10.1016/j.bspc.2023.105479

Xu, F., Qin, Z., Tan, C. C., Wang, B., & Li, Q. (2011). *IMDGuard: Securing implantable medical devices with the external wearable guardian. In 2011 Proceedings IEEE INFOCOM*. IEEE.

Xu, S. S.-D., Chen, C.-H., & Chang, T.-C. (2019). Design of oneM2M-based fog computing architecture. *IEEE Internet of Things Journal*, *6*(6), 9464–9474. DOI: 10.1109/JIOT.2019.2932248

Yang, Q., Mai, S., Zhao, Y., Wang, Z., Zhang, C., & Wang, Z. (2014). An on-chip security guard based on zero-power authentication for implantable medical devices. In *2014 IEEE 57th International Midwest Symposium on Circuits and Systems* (pp. 531–534). IEEE.

Yang, R., Yu, F. R., Si, P., Yang, Z., & Zhang, Y. (2019). Integrated Blockchain and Edge Computing Systems: A Survey, Some Research Issues and Challenges. In *IEEE Communications Surveys and Tutorials* (Vol. 21, Issue 2). https://doi.org/ DOI: 10.1109/COMST.2019.2894727

Yang, E., Schutte, A. E., & Stergiou, G. (2025). Cuffless blood pressure measurement devices—International perspectives on accuracy and clinical use: A narrative review. *JAMA Cardiology*, *10*(6), 624–631. DOI: 10.1001/jamacardio.2025.0662 PMID: 40266607

Yin, S., Li, G., Luo, Y., & Lin, L. (2021). Cuff-less continuous blood pressure measurement based on multiple types of information fusion. *Biomedical Signal Processing and Control*, *68*, 102549. DOI: 10.1016/j.bspc.2021.102549

Zabihi, S., Rahimian, E., Marefat, F., Asif, A., Mohseni, P., & Mohammadi, A. (2022). BP-Net: Cuff-less and non-invasive blood pressure estimation via a generic deep convolutional architecture. *Biomedical Signal Processing and Control*, *78*, 103850. DOI: 10.1016/j.bspc.2022.103850

Zamani, M., & Sharifian, S. (2024). Distributed edge to cloud ensemble deep learning architecture to diagnose Covid-19 from lung image in IoT based e-Health system. *The Journal of Supercomputing*, •••, 1–29.

Zayats, V., Sergeev, I., & Fedorov, D. (2023). Review of promising methods of supplying power to implantable medical devices. *Biomedical Engineering*, *57*(1), 39–44.

Zbiciak, A., & Markiewicz, T. (2023). A new extraordinary means of appeal in the Polish criminal procedure: The basic principles of a fair trial and a complaint against a cassatory judgment. *Access to Justice in Eastern Europe*, *6*(2), 1–18.

Zhang, B., Chen, C., Lee, I., Lee, K., & Ong, K. L. (2025). A survey on security and privacy issues in wearable health monitoring devices. *Computers & Security*, *155*, 104453. DOI: 10.1016/J.COSE.2025.104453

Zhang, G., Choi, D., & Jung, J. (2024). Development of continuous cuffless blood pressure prediction platform using enhanced 1-D SENet–LSTM. *Expert Systems with Applications*, *242*, 122812. DOI: 10.1016/j.eswa.2023.122812

Zhang, Y., Wang, X., Shi, C., Jiang, X., & Ye, Y. (2021). Hyperbolic graph attention network. *IEEE Transactions on Big Data*, *8*(6), 1690–1701.

Zhao, S., Zhang, T., Ma, S., & Wang, M. (2023). Sea-horse optimizer: A novel nature-inspired meta-heuristic for global optimization problems. *Applied Intelligence*, *53*(10), 11833–11860.

Zheng, G., Fang, G., Orgun, M. A., Shankaran, R., & Dutkiewicz, E. (2014). Securing wireless medical implants using an ECG-based secret data sharing scheme. In *2014 14th International Symposium on Communications and Information Technologies* (pp. 373–377). IEEE.

Zheng, G., Fang, G., Orgun, M. A., & Shankaran, R. (2014). A non-key based security scheme supporting emergency treatment of wireless implants. In *2014 IEEE International Conference on Communications* (pp. 647–652). IEEE.

Zheng, G., Yang, W., Valli, C., Qiao, L., Shankaran, R., Orgun, M. A., & Mukhopadhyay, S. C. (2019). Finger-to-heart (F2H): Authentication for wireless implantable medical devices. *IEEE Journal of Biomedical and Health Informatics, 23*(4), 1546–1557. DOI: 10.1109/JBHI.2018.2864796 PMID: 30106744

Zheng, W., & Arakawa, Y. (2025). A review of wearables-based activities of daily living recognition with LLMs: Overview, progress, and trends. *IEEE Access : Practical Innovations, Open Solutions, 13*, 143813–143830. DOI: 10.1109/ACCESS.2025.3598088

Zheng, Z., Xie, S., Dai, H. N., Chen, W., Chen, X., Weng, J., & Imran, M. (2020). An overview on smart contracts: Challenges, advances and platforms. *Future Generation Computer Systems, 105*. Advance online publication. DOI: 10.1016/j.future.2019.12.019

Zhu, G., Li, J., Meng, Z., Yu, Y., Li, Y., Tang, X., Dong, Y., Sun, G., Zhou, R., & Wang, H.. (2020). Learning from large-scale wearable device data for predicting the epidemic trend of covid-19. *Discrete Dynamics in Nature and Society, 2020*(1), 6152041.

About the Contributors

Pandimurugan Vellaisamy serves as an Associate Professor in the Department of Computer Science and Engineering at Acharya University, Bukhara region, Karakul, Uzbekistan. He has over 16 years of professional experience in academia, including more than five years post-Ph.D. His previous appointments include roles as Assistant Professor at SRM Institute of Science and Technology (SRMIST), VIT Bhopal University, and Hindustan University, Chennai. Dr. Pandimurugan's research expertise spans computer networks, security, health informatics, Internet of Things (IoT), and machine learning. He has made significant academic contributions, with 41 Scopus-indexed publications, including 14 in SCI journals, and has authored book chapters and patents. His research has focused on the application of AI and IoT in healthcare, notably developing algorithms for continuous blood glucose monitoring and medical imaging analysis. He has also published on topics such as disease prediction, medical data security, and smart healthcare systems. In addition to his research, Dr. Pandimurugan has served as Head of Department for CSE with a specialization in Health Informatics, project coordinator, and Ph.D. research supervisor. He is an active reviewer for several international journals and has received the Best Teacher Award from INSC Bangalore in 2020. He is a member of the Association for Computing Machinery (ACM) and has contributed to curriculum development and the establishment of research labs in health informatics. Dr. Pandimurugan's academic leadership, research output, and commitment to advancing health informatics education and practice have established him as a recognized expert in his field

Rajaram V serves as an Associate Professor in the Department of Networking and Communications, School of Computing, at SRM Institute of Science and Technology, Chennai. He has over 15 years of academic experience, including three years in his current position and a decade as Assistant Professor at Sri Venkateswara College of Engineering, as well as prior experience at Vel Tech. Dr. Rajaram's research expertise covers wireless sensor networks, wireless communication, Internet of Things (IoT), and digital principles. He holds a Ph.D. in Information and Communication, an M.E. in Communication Systems, and a B.E. in Electronics and Communication Engineering. Throughout his career, Dr. Rajaram has contributed significantly to both teaching and research, focusing on the advancement of wireless and IoT technologies. He has played an active role in curriculum development and has guided numerous student projects and research initiatives in his areas of specialization. Dr. Rajaram's dedication to education, research, and the development of next-generation communication systems has established him as a respected academic and mentor in his field. His commitment to academic excellence and innovation continues to inspire students and colleagues alike.

A. Chinnasamy is currently an Assistant Professor in the Department of Data Science And Business Systems, with nearly 15 years of academic experience. He holds a B.E., M.E., and Ph.D., and has demonstrated expertise in areas such as vehicular ad hoc networks (VANETs), Internet of Things (IoT), machine learning, and wireless communication. Dr. Chinnasamy has made significant research contributions, with 13 publications indexed in Scopus, 4 in Web of Science, and a total of 22 in Google Scholar. His work has garnered over 100 citations, reflecting his impact in the field. He has authored book chapters, published in reputed journals, and presented at both national and international conferences. His research includes the development of secure routing protocols for VANETs, anomaly detection in sensor-based cyber-physical systems, and IoT-based health assistance systems. He also holds a granted patent on cooperative sensing and control in IoT networks using machine learning algorithms, and has filed another on emotion recognition for fitness applications. In addition to his research, Dr. Chinnasamy is actively involved in academic leadership and service. He is an Anna University recognized Ph.D. supervisor, guiding nine research scholars, and serves as a reviewer for several SCI journals. He has contributed to curriculum development, coordinated departmental activities, and organized workshops and seminars. His professional memberships include the Computer Society of India (CSI), International Association of Engineers (IAENG), Indian Society for Technical Education (ISTE), and IEEE. Dr. Chinnasamy's dedication to teaching, research, and academic service has established him as a respected educator and researcher in computer science and engineering, with a strong commitment to advancing knowledge in wireless networks, IoT, and intelligent systems.

S. Sountharrajan serves as Associate Professor and Chairperson of Computer Science and Engineering at the School of Computing, Amrita Vishwa Vidyapeetham, Chennai Campus. With over 19 years of academic and research experience, he has held key academic and leadership roles at leading institutions, including VIT University Bhopal and Bannari Amman Institute of Technology. Dr. Sountharrajan's research expertise spans artificial intelligence, machine learning, cybersecurity, cloud computing, data science, and the Internet of Things (IoT). He has made substantial scholarly contributions, with over 69 Scopus-indexed publications, 35 international journal articles, 10 book chapters, and a patent in IoT-based smart vehicle systems. His research has addressed a wide range of topics, including AI-driven healthcare analytics, secure cloud infrastructure, wireless sensor networks, and optimization algorithms for big data and medical imaging. In addition to his research, Dr. Sountharrajan has played a pivotal role in academic administration and curriculum development. He has designed and implemented innovative programs in AI, machine learning, cloud computing, health informatics, and cybersecurity. He has established multiple Centers of Excellence and advanced laboratories in cloud computing, robotics, and high-performance computing across various institutions.

Amudhavel Jayavel Senior Lecturer, De Montfort University, Leicester, United Kingdom Expert in Generative Adversarial Networks, Deep Computational Imaging & Image Reconstruction Dr. Amudhavel Jayavel is a seasoned academic and researcher specializing in computational imaging and deep learning, with a focus on Generative Adversarial Networks (GANs). With over a decade of teaching, research, and leadership experience across institutions in India and Europe, he currently serves as a Senior Lecturer at De Montfort University, Leicester, UK. Prior to this, he held key research and academic roles at the University of Tartu (Estonia), VIT Bhopal University, KL University, and Sri Manakula Vinayagar Engineering College. His research interests span generative models, image reconstruction, computer vision, and deep learning frameworks such as TensorFlow, PyTorch, and Keras. His work has led to significant advancements in visual data enhancement, including super-resolution imaging, noise reduction, and the recovery of corrupted visual data. Dr. Amudhavel has published extensively in Web of Science and Scopus-indexed journals and is known for his contributions to computational techniques that address complex imaging challenges. He holds a Ph.D. in Computer Science and Engineering from Pondicherry University, where he was awarded the prestigious INSPIRE Fellowship. He has also earned several academic accolades, including being a gold medalist in M.Tech and achieving All India Rank 15 in the national M.Tech entrance examination. In addition to his research credentials, Dr. Amudhavel has been actively involved in digital outreach, curriculum development, and student mentorship. His certifications in cloud computing and blockchain further complement his technical repertoire.

***

Arun. A completed his B.E from University of Madras in 2003 & M.TECH from SRM Institute of Science and Technology in 2005. He was awarded Doctorate Degree in the year 2020 by Anna University, Chennai in Information & Communication Engineering. He is currently pursuing his Post Doc from National Kaohsiung University of Science and Technology, Taiwan. He has more than 19 years of teaching experience. Currently he is working as Associate Professor, Department of Networking and Communications, SRM Institute of Science and Technology, Chennai. He has published more than 30 papers in renowned International Journals with good Impact Factor. He has 8 patents published and two design patent grants to his credit. He is also guiding four students in their Ph.D work. His area of research includes Image Processing, IOT, Networking, VLSI Design and Embedded Systems.

Smita Agrawal is working as an Associate Professor in Computer Science and Engineering Department since 2009. She has a teaching experience of over 20 years. She received her Master of Computer Applications degree from Gujarat Vidhyapith in 2004. She completed her doctoral studies in the field of Big Data Analytics from CHARUSAT University in 2019. She works in the area of Big Data Analytics, Parallel Processing, Web Development and IoT. She is a Senior Member of IEEE, Member of CSI, ACM, and ISTE. She has published several Scopus/SCIE-indexed research papers in national and international conferences and journals. Dr Smita has conducted ISTE approved short-term training Programme in the field of Web Services using PHP. She is involved in teaching courses at both undergraduate and postgraduate levels. She also serves as a member of the Programme committees and session chair for international conferences and as a reviewer for indexed international journals.

N Nasurudeen Ahamed, Received the Bachelor's Degree in Computer Science and Engineering, The Master Degree in Computer Science and Engineering and Ph.D. Degree in Computer Science and Engineering. He is Currently Serving as an Postdoctoral Fellow, College of Information Technology, United Arab Emirates University,UAE. He has 12+ Years' of Teaching Experience. His Research Interests Include Blockchain, Cyber Security, Supply Chain Management, Industry 4.0, Deep Learning.

Munir Ahmad is a seasoned professional in the realm of Spatial Data Infrastructure (SDI), Geo-Information Productions, Information Systems, and Information Governance, boasting over 25 years of dedicated experience in the field. With a PhD in Computer Science, Dr. Ahmad's expertise spans Spatial Data Production, Management, Processing, Analysis, Visualization, and Quality Control. Throughout his career, Dr. Ahmad has been deeply involved in the development and deployment of SDI systems specially in the context of Pakistan, leveraging his proficiency in Spatial Database Design, Web, Mobile & Desktop GIS, and Geo Web Services Architecture. His contributions to Volunteered Geographic Information (VGI) and Open Source Geoportal & Metadata Portal have significantly enriched the geospatial community. As a trainer and researcher, Dr. Ahmad has authored over 50 publications, advancing the industry's knowledge base and fostering innovation in Geo-Tech, Data Governance, and Information Infrastructure, and Emerging Technologies. His commitment to Research and Development (R&D) is evident in his role as a dedicated educator and mentor in the field.

Anorgul Ashirova is working as an Associate Professor at the Department of General Professional Sciences, Mamun University, Khiva, Uzbekistan

S. Ida Evangeline, presently working as an Assistant Professor in the Department of Electrical and Electronics Engineering at the Government College of Engineering, Tirunelveli, Tamilnadu, India. She obtained her Bachelor’s in Electrical and Electronics Engineering from Manonmaniam Sundaranar University in 2003, and Master's in Power Systems Engineering from Anna University, Chennai, Tamilnadu, India in 2005. She completed her PhD degree in 2023 at Anna University, Chennai, Tamilnadu, India. She has published six research papers in international journals. Her current research interests include optimal power flow, renewable energy, soft computing, machine learning, and deep learning.

J Sreemathy is presently an Assistant professor in the Department of Computer Science & Engineering, Sri Eshwar College of Engineering, Coimbatore, Tamil Nadu, India. She has more than 12 years of teaching experience. She received the B.E. degree from Anna University, Chennai and M.E from Karpagam University, Coimbatore. She is pursuing her PhD in Anna University, Chennai. She has published more than 15 papers in refereed international journals and conferences. Her research interests include Data Analytics, Big Data. She is an active member in various professional society.

Mayur Jariwala is a seasoned Project Manager with over 15 years of diversified experience across product design, manufacturing, financial services. With a proven track record of leading cross-functional teams to complete complex projects on or ahead of schedule and within budget, he excels in all phases of project management. His expertise extends to both Waterfall and Agile methodologies, change management, quality assurance, and system integration. Currently pursuing a PhD in Information Technology at the University of the Cumberlands, he holds masters degrees in Project Management and Business Administration and is certified as a Project Management Professional (PMP)®, Lean Six Sigma Green

Belt, and SAFe® 5 Scrum Master. He is also an accomplished reviewer for several prestigious journals. As an author, he has contributed significantly to the fields of cybersecurity and AI with publications such as "The Cyber Security Roadmap: A Comprehensive Guide to Cyber Threats, Cyber Laws, and Cyber Security Training for a Safer Digital World," and numerous research articles on topics ranging from blockchain's potential in space missions to AI in project management frameworks. These contributions underscore his commitment to advancing the fields of project management, AI, and cybersecurity.

Yathaarth Jariwala is a Research Scholar in the Engineering Physics program at the University of Colorado Boulder, USA. His academic focus lies at the intersection of physics, computational modeling, and artificial intelligence, with a strong emphasis on applying machine learning techniques to robotics, sensor design, and control systems. As a Research Scholar, he has led interdisciplinary projects in robotics and automation, integrating advanced AI algorithms into mechanical and electrical subsystems for real-time optimization and precision control. Yathaarth's interests extend to data-driven decision systems, predictive analytics, and sustainable technology design.

Jawahar Jonathan K is an Assistant Professor in the Department of Computer Science and Engineering at Acharya Institute of Technology, Bangalore, India. Previously, he served as a Senior Faculty member at Anudip, Bangalore, and as an IT Trainer at UDS, Chennai, Tamil Nadu. He earned a B.E. in Computer Science and Engineering from Hindusthan College of Engineering and Technology, Coimbatore, and an M.E. in Computer Science and Engineering from K.C.G. College of Technology, Chennai, India. With over seven years of experience spanning academia and industry, his expertise lies in computer networks and network security.

Hemalatha Karnan pursued B.Tech. Bioengineering in SASTRA University during 2002 2006. She received her ME Applied Electronics degree from Anna University, BIT campus, Tiruchirappalli in the year 2012 and Ph.D. from the Department of Instrumentation & Control Engineering in National Institute of Technology, Tiruchirappalli. Her research areas are Bio- signal processing and machine learning techniques for clinical data analysis. She has also interests in image processing and its usage in point-of-care device design. She has over 15 years of research experience. She has presented her research findings in 15 different International and 3 National Conferences. Her publications are on learning model development and optimization with publishers like CRC press, Wiley and etc. She has filed a patent on her recent research work on the design of wearable system for geriatric care.

Thangavel Murugan is a Senior IEEE member serving as an Assistant Professor in the Department of Information Systems and Security, College of Information Technology, and as a Faculty Fellow in the Center for Excellence in Teaching and Learning, United Arab Emirates University, Abu Dhabi, United Arab Emirates. He received a Doctorate from the Madras Institute of Technology (MIT) Campus, Anna University – Chennai. He received Post Graduate degree as M.E. Computer Science and Engineering from J.J. College of Engineering and Technology, Trichy under Anna University – Chennai (University First Rank Holder & Gold Medalist) and Bachelor's degree as B.E. Computer Science and Engineering from M.A.M College of Engineering, Trichy under Anna University – Chennai (College First Rank Holder & Gold Medalist). He currently holds over 12 years of Teaching and Research experience from various academic institutions. He has published 15+ articles in International Journals, 7+ edited books, 3+ authored books, 20+ book chapters in International Publishers, 5+ patents, 45+ in the proceedings of International Conferences, and 3 in the proceedings of national conferences /seminars. He has been actively participating as a reviewer in international journals and conferences. He has attended over 100 workshops, FDPs, and conferences at various higher learning institutions, including IIT and Anna University. He has organized over 50 workshops, FDPs, contests, and industry-based courses in the past few years of his experience. He has been a technical speaker in various Workshops/FDPs/Conferences. His research specialization is Information Security, Cloud Computing, Ethical Hacking, Cyberforensics, Blockchain, AI Applications, and Educational Technology.

Prasath N has obtained his Doctoral Degree from Anna University, Chennai in 2017 and Master of Technology from SASTRA University in 2009 and Undergraduate degree under Anna University Chennai in 2006. He is having 17+ years of experience in teaching and Industry. He has published 8 patents and published more than 40+ research papers in refereed conferences and in journals. He is a member in many professional societies. His research interests include MANET, Sensor Networks, IoT and Cloud, Cyber Physical System.

Parita Oza is a faculty member in the Department of Computer Science and Engineering at Nirma University, Ahmedabad. She completed her Ph.D. focusing on breast cancer diagnosis using deep learning. Her work contributed to the development of the first Indian mammography dataset. Dr. Oza has published several papers in reputed journals and conferences, with research interests in medical image analysis and AI in healthcare.

Soniya R is a assistant professor in the Engineering Department, specializing in Computer Science & Engineering, at the University of Visvesvaraya technological

University, she served as an lecture at BGS pu college, Bengaluru and also served as lecture in Sri Chaitanya pu college, Bengaluru also served as lecture in scholars pu college, Bengaluru and having 5 years of experience in teaching.

Selvaraj Balachandran is an accomplished mathematician and researcher specializing in graph theory and topological indices. He is currently serving as an Assistant Professor of Mathematics in the Department of Mathematics at SASTRA University, Thanjavur, India, where he has been on the faculty since 2006. He earned his Ph.D. in Mathematics from SASTRA University in 2014 under the supervision of Dr. S.K. Ayyaswamy, with his doctoral thesis focusing on A Study on Energy and Indices of Graphs. Earlier, he completed his M.Phil. in Mathematics from Bharathidasan University (2002), his M.Sc. in Mathematics from A.V.C. College, Bharathidasan University (2000), and his B.Sc. in Mathematics from the same institution in 1997. From 2017 to 2020, Dr. Balachandran worked as a Postdoctoral Researcher at the University of the Free State, Bloemfontein, South Africa, under the mentorship of Prof. Tomas Vetrik. His research continues to center on topological indices of graphs and graph theory, with numerous contributions to extremal problems and chemical graph theory. He has been actively involved in the global mathematical community as a reviewer for several international journals, including Ars Combinatoria, Applied Mathematics and Computation, Discrete Applied Mathematics, Graphs and Combinatorics, Journal of Combinatorial Optimization, and others. A prolific researcher, Dr. Balachandran has authored and co-authored numerous publications in high-impact journals, addressing topics such as Zagreb indices, Randic indices, Sombor indices, harmonic indices, and other mathematical measures associated with graph theory. His works often focus on extremal problems, chemical graph theory, and structural properties of trees, unicyclic, and bicyclic graphs. Through his extensive research, teaching, and professional activities, Dr. Selvaraj Balachandran has established himself as a dedicated scholar in mathematics, particularly in the field of graph theory, contributing significantly to both theoretical advancements and applications.

Hariharan S is a highly committed and enthusiastic graduate with a strong ambition to contribute significantly to the field of wearable healthcare technologies. His core areas of interest include IoMT system design, biosignal processing, medical image analysis, and Artificial Intelligence-driven healthcare solutions. Throughout his academic and research journey, he has gained substantial experience working with prestigious institutions, including the Dr. Shyama Prasad Mukherjee International Institute of Information Technology. He has published his research findings in reputed international and national journals, conference proceedings, and has also contributed to a book chapter, reflecting his strong academic and technical impact. He has filed a patent for his innovative work titled "Intelligent EDGE-Enabled Fall Tracking System for Geriatrics."

S. Srividhya is an Assistant Professor in the Department of Data Science and Business Systems at SRM Institute of Science and Technology, Kattankulathur, Chennai. She holds a Ph.D. in Computer Science and Engineering from SRM Institute of Science and Technology, completed in 2022. She also earned an M.Tech in Advanced Computing from Sastra University in 2014 and a B.Tech in Information Technology from Anna University in 2012. She has 10 years of experience and her research interests are diverse, encompassing Wireless Sensor Networks, Database Management Systems, Data Structures, Data Analytics, IoT Protocols, Fuzzy Set, and Clustering in Wireless Sensor Networks. She has a notable academic profile with 19 articles and 84 citations indexed by Scopus and in International Conferences.

S.P.Maniraj is working as Assistant Professor in the Department of Data Science and Business Systems at SRM Institute of Science and Technology, Kattankulathur campus. He holds a Ph. D degree in the field of Medical Image Processing from Sathyabama Institute of Science and Technology since 2022. He has 14 years of teaching experience with good programming skills. He got certified in various courses from NPTEL, Coursera, Udemy and Cisco. He also got a NPTEL Discipline and Motivated Learner Award. He has published more than 25 articles in National and International Journals, Conferences and Symposiums.

Biswajit Saha has more than 23 years of academic experience which includes teaching at both under graduate and post graduate level of Computer Science and Engineering. He has authored numerous journal and conference publications and contributed book chapters with highly reputed publishing houses. His broader interests include machine learning, health informatics, AI in education, and outcome-based pedagogy.

Index

A

B

C

D

E

F

H

R

S

www.ingramcontent.com/pod-product-compliance
Lightning Source LLC
LaVergne TN
LVHW080912300926
849162LV00003B/652